10th Edition

Understanding
Human Behavior

A Guide for Health Care Professionals

Alyson Honeycutt, M.A., N.C.C.

Australia • Brazil • Canada • Mexico • Singapore • United Kingdom • United States

Understanding Human Behavior: A Guide for Health Care Professionals, **Tenth Edition**

Alyson Honeycutt

SVP, Product: Cheryl Costantini

VP, Product and Marketing: Thais Alencar

Portfolio Product Director: Jason Fremder

Associate Portfolio Product Director:
Laura Stewart

Product Manager: Andrea Henderson

Product Assistant: Jannell Whitted

Learning Designer: Deb Myette-Flis

Senior Content Manager: Kenneth McGrath

Digital Delivery Quality Partner: Lisa Christopher

Director, Product Marketing: Neena Bali

Product Marketing Manager: Joann Gillingham

IP Analyst: Erin McCullough

Production Service: Lumina Datamatics Ltd.

Designer: Felicia Bennett

Cover Image Credits: cover and interior;
1633124830 imtmphoto/Shutterstock.com;
422341813 Pressmaster/Shutterstock.com;
1537293188 fizkes/Shutterstock.com;
2150323261 PeopleImages.com -
Yuri A/Shutterstock.com;
2085176281 LightField Studios/Shutterstock.com

For product information and technology assistance, contact us at **Cengage Learning Customer & Sales Support, 1-800-354-9706**

For permission to use material from this text or product, submit all requests online at **www.cengage.com/permissions**. Further permissions questions can be e-mailed to **permissionrequest@cengage.com**

Library of Congress Control Number: 2023932104
ISBN: 978-0-357-61860-8

Cengage Learning
200 Pier 4 Boulevard
Boston, MA 02210
USA

Cengage is a leading provider of customized learning solutions. Our employees reside in nearly 40 different countries and serve digital learners in 165 countries around the world. Find your local representative at **www.cengage.com.**

To learn more about Cengage platforms and services, register or access your online learning solution, or purchase materials for your course, visit **www.cengage.com.**

Notice to the Reader

Publisher does not warrant or guarantee any of the products described herein or perform any independent analysis in connection with any of the product information contained herein. Publisher does not assume, and expressly disclaims, any obligation to obtain and include information other than that provided to it by the manufacturer. The reader is expressly warned to consider and adopt all safety precautions that might be indicated by the activities described herein and to avoid all potential hazards. By following the instructions contained herein, the reader willingly assumes all risks in connection with such instructions. The publisher makes no representations or warranties of any kind, including but not limited to, the warranties of fitness for particular purpose or merchantability, nor are any such representations implied with respect to the material set forth herein, and the publisher takes no responsibility with respect to such material. The publisher shall not be liable for any special, consequential, or exemplary damages resulting, in whole or part, from the readers' use of, or reliance upon, this material.

Printed at CLDPC, USA, 03-23

Contents

Contents

Preface

Introduction

Understanding Human Behavior: A Guide for Health Care Professionals is designed to assist students in health care education programs to learn basic principles of human behavior. These principles provide a basis for increased self-understanding and improved interpersonal relationships. With technological advances in diagnostic and therapeutic procedures, it is easy for a health care professional to focus on procedures and routines. Patients, however, want personalized care that conveys respect for the patient as a person.

Patients' expectations are more likely to be met when health care professionals aim for effective interaction with each patient. By consciously attending to each interaction with patients, the health care professional will experience greater job satisfaction.

Organization

Understanding Human Behavior: A Guide for Health Care Professionals, Tenth Edition, is organized to proceed from relatively simple information to more complex concepts, from the known to the unknown, and from application to self to application in a variety of interpersonal situations. For that reason, Chapters 1 through 18 are designed for *sequential study.*

Chapters 19-21 do not follow the sequential pattern. Chapter 19 describes historical content and current developments in health care; Chapter 20 explores the nature of healing and suggests guidelines for evaluating the legitimacy of various therapies. Each of these chapters can be studied independently at any point in the course. Chapter 21 introduces the importance of managing stress and can potentially be assigned early in the program, so students can start practicing stress management. Undertaking the role of a student, introduction to the clinical setting, and care of the sick all include stressful experiences. Preparing to become a health care professional includes learning the importance of self-care, and stress management is an essential component of self-care.

Section I (chapters 1-3) provides an orientation to the role of health care professional, the importance of accepting each patient as a worthwhile human being, the challenge of striving for self-understanding, and guidelines for personal and professional growth. Section II (chapters 4-8) presents information about various influences on human behavior: the role of heredity, basic physical and psychological needs, developmental factors, role of the social environment, emotions and their power to influence behavior, and adjustment as a composite of all these factors. Section III (chapters 9-12) presents more complex concepts related to human behavior: stressful events that occur in the lives of most people, domestic violence and bullying, and the mental and emotional effects of traumatic experiences. Many victims of a traumatic event subsequently require health care. For both personal and professional reasons, health care professionals need to be aware of the mental/emotional and physical effects of these traumatic experiences, as well as the potential for long-term adverse effects on the victim. The remainder of Section III covers other factors related to one's adjustment: common defense mechanisms, inner conflict, and frustration.

Section IV (chapters 13-15) explores the components of effective communication. Practice exercises are designed to help students become better communicators by improving their skills in sending, receiving, and observing verbal and nonverbal exchanges. These exercises can involve all students and be accommodated readily within a class period. Section V (chapters 16-18) provides an overview of practices in relation to death and dying and legislation related to the rights of patients to participate in health care decisions, especially those related to end-of-life care. The grief process is discussed in detail, with guidelines for assisting the bereaved.

Section VI (chapters 19-22) is designed to encourage students to accept the changes that inevitably will occur in the dynamic health care system. Chapter 19 provides a historical overview that reflects the roots of current practices, including holistic health care. Chapter 20 describes the emergence of the holistic emphasis and spotlights several complementary healing modalities that have gained widespread acceptance with the public. The reader is encouraged to maintain an open mind in conjunction with a healthy skepticism in evaluating various treatment modalities. Chapter 21 addresses stress management.

Changes to the Tenth Edition

Understanding Human Behavior, Tenth Edition, includes the following updates and additions:

- In Section I: Becoming a Health Care Professional, Chapter 3 includes an expanded discussion of growth mindset.

- In Section II, Understanding Human Behavior, Chapter 5 describes the connection between nutrition and resistance to illness, and Chapter 6 contains an exploration of the need for balance between independence and interdependence. Chapter 8 provides an expanded discussion of positive emotions, including gratitude and joy, and addresses the influence of culture on the expression of emotion. Chapter 8 includes a discussion of how social media can impact adjustment, and Chapter 9 addresses the influence of national and world events, including the COVID-19 pandemic, on adjustment.

- In Section III: Behavior and Problems in Living, Chapter 10 describes the traumatic impact of the COVID-19 pandemic. Chapter 11 includes updated information about substance use in the US, and Chapter 12 now includes a discussion of discrimination can be a source of frustration.

- In Section IV: Effective Human Relations and Communication, Chapter 13 now includes a discussion of how financial concerns and cultural background impact behavior of patients and their families. Chapter 14 provides practical strategies for setting personal matters aside while at work. Chapter 16 discusses cultural differences in how individuals express grief.

- In Section V: Death and Loss, Chapter 18 discusses how financial concerns impact family decisions about end-of-life care.

- Section VI: Trends in Health Care, Chapter 20 is streamlined, providing guidelines for evaluating the validity of alternative and complementary treatments. Chapter 21 explores the connection between stress and health.

Instructor & Student Resources

Additional instructor and student resources for this product are available online. Instructor assets include an Instructor's Manual, Educator's Guide, PowerPoint® slides, Solution and Answer Guide, and a test bank powered by Cognero®. Student assets include PowerPoint® slides. Sign up or sign in at **www.cengage.com** to search for and access this product and its online resources.

MindTap

MindTap is a fully online, interactive learning experience built upon authoritative Cengage Learning content. By combining readings, multimedia, activities, and assessments into a sin- gular learning path, MindTap elevates learning by providing real-world application to bet- ter engage students. Instructors customize the learning path by selecting Cengage Learning resources and adding their own content via apps that integrate into the MindTap framework seamlessly with many learning management systems.

To learn more, visit www.cengage.com/training/mindtap.

Using *Understanding Human Behavior*

The effectiveness of *Understanding Human Behavior* depends on the instructor's choice of activities: class time to clarify various concepts and specific activities to encourage student participation, especially the sharing of experiences, discussion of problem situations, and selection of effective behavior for real and hypothetical situations. The instructor's own cre- ative use of the text material is the key to students' achievement.

No one ever completely masters human relations skills. Those who sincerely want to relate effectively to others must become lifelong students of human behavior. They must con- sciously practice human relations skills in order to improve their sensitivity to the possible meaning of observed behavior and select appropriate responses. The immediate challenge is to gain as much as possible from this course, as a foundation for the lifelong challenge of developing a high level of skill in human relations.

About the Author

Alyson Honeycutt, M.A., N.C.C., is a National Certified Counselor, holds a License in School Counseling from the North Carolina Department of Public Instruction, and has advanced degrees from North Carolina State University at Raleigh and Appalachian State University. She has taught parenting and literacy classes, has been an instructor in English at the col- lege level, has taught students with emotional and behavioral disabilities, has served as a district-level behavior support coordinator in the public schools, and has worked as a health and wellness coach and yoga instructor.

Reviewers of the Tenth Edition

Brett Brandon, RMA, AA, BS, MPAS
Allied Health Instructor
Sarasota, FL

Elizabeth MacQuillan, PhD, RDN, CHSE
Program Director and Assistant Professor
Grand Rapids, MI

Beverly Marquez, M.S., RHIA
Director
Sedalia, MO

Kat Slusser, PhD, RN
Falculty, Program Coordinator
Santa Rosa, CA

Joshua Snyder, MBA, EMT-P
Clinical Coordinator
McKinney, TX

Becoming a Health Care Professional

This section introduces some of the challenges, responsibilities, and satisfactions of being a health care professional. People from all walks of life require health care. As a health care professional, you will be challenged to serve each person effectively. Section I is designed to help you become aware of the realities of a health career and to help you learn strategies to succeed as both a student and a health care professional.

Challenges and Responsibilities of Health Care Professionals

Objectives

After completing this chapter, you should be able to:

- Describe the challenges and satisfactions of working in health care.
- Explain the importance of client-centered care for health care professionals.
- Explain how your study habits as a student relate to your future work habits as a health care professional.
- Explain the meaning of **empowerment** and apply the concept of empowerment to real-life situations.

Key Terms

Client-centered care
Empowerment

Self-confidence
Self-reliance

Standards of
performance

Congratulations! You have decided to become a health care professional. During your educational program, you will have the satisfaction of learning new information and developing new skills. As a health care professional, you will be able to make a significant contribution to your community. This chapter introduces some of the challenges, responsibilities, and satisfactions of being a health care professional.

Challenges and Satisfactions in Health Care

Your career choice indicates that you like people and have a strong desire to help others. Although you could possibly make more money in some other field, a career that provides opportunities to help others may be very rewarding. You will also be part of one of the largest and fastest growing industries in the world. As you gain skills and experience, you will have opportunities to work in many different locations and different types of facilities. Qualified health care professionals are expected to be in high demand in the future.

Challenges

Health care providers have always faced challenges, including long work hours, staff shortages, and potential job burnout. In recent years, events such as changes in the health insurance system and the COVID-19 pandemic have increased these challenges. Many health care facilities experience high turnover, and health care professionals often cite stress, burnout, and long hours as factors in their decision to leave their jobs. Yet many health care professionals also report finding great satisfaction in their work. The habits and attitudes you practice now as a student will impact your effectiveness and your satisfaction in your work later.

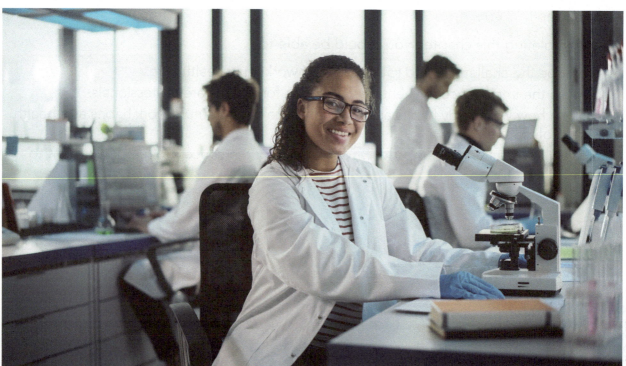

© Gorodenkoff/Shutterstock.com

FIGURE 1-1 Qualified health care professionals are expected to be in high demand in the future.

Approval versus Inner Satisfaction

We all admire those who can do something extremely well; each of us would like to be admired by others. We enjoy receiving approval from others, yet this good feeling is only temporary. Athletes may enjoy hearing the cheers of the crowd, but the deepest satisfaction comes from knowing that they performed with great skill. True satisfaction is an inner feeling of pride in doing something well, regardless of whether the performance is applauded by others.

As a health care professional, you will find your greatest satisfaction in trying to give each patient appropriate care. By meeting each patient's needs to the best of your ability, you will complete the day with an inner feeling of pride. The opposite approach—to view your work as a series of assignments to be completed so that you can get off work or go on break—results in finishing the day by saying, "Whew, I'm glad that's over!" Stop now and consider this very important question: How will you approach your work? As a challenge that provides satisfaction and a sense of accomplishment? Or as work you must do to get a paycheck?

Setting Goals for Inner Satisfaction

Performing your work well can provide **self-confidence** and a deep sense of satisfaction that is not dependent on praise from others. By working to improve your performance each day, you will increase your level of skill. Excellence lies in that little bit of extra effort given to achieve a superior performance. *In the health field, that little bit of extra effort may make the difference between safe and unsafe practice.*

The habits you form as a student carry over into your performance as a health care professional. Now is the time to develop habits that will lead to skillful performance, self-confidence, and pride in your work.

Setting Standards of Performance

Only you can set the standards that will guide your performance over the coming years. At times, you may be tempted to take a shortcut. Sometimes a piece of equipment will be contaminated and obtaining sterile materials to complete the procedure will require extra effort and time. Only you will know whether or not sterile technique was violated and the contaminated equipment was used—unless, of course, the patient develops an infection as a result. Your own standards should include accuracy in measurements, observations, and reporting. Your **standards of performance** determine whether you experience the inner satisfaction that comes from knowing the job was well done.

One key skill that will serve you well as a student and as a professional is the ability to focus your full attention on the task at hand. Modern life is full of distractions, and most of us are accustomed to multitasking. Many students complete assignments while having a conversation, watching a video, or texting a friend. Consider this now: Would an effective health care provider be distracted while checking a patient's vital signs or administering medication? If you make it a habit to set study goals and give each task your full attention, you will be better equipped to perform your job duties effectively in the future.

For Discussion and Reflection

Do you often multitask, for example, by completing assignments while checking social media or texting friends? In the future, what types of tasks might need your full attention, without distractions?

When making that little bit of extra effort to do tasks well has become a habit, it becomes an essential part of your performance. Thus, excellence as a health care professional will depend upon setting high standards of performance for yourself now.

Excellence and Patient Safety

In the health field, all professionals should strive for excellence. *Anything less than excellence can endanger the patient.* The nurse should give the correct medicine to each patient. The medical assistant should use correct technique in all situations that require asepsis. The laboratory assistant should report test results correctly; the dental assistant should sterilize instruments correctly; the ambulance attendant should move the accident victim correctly. *Careless or incorrect performance can have disastrous effects for the patient.*

Providing Client-Centered Care

As a health care professional, you will work with many different people, each of whom is a unique individual—a physical, emotional, mental, and spiritual being. Each has a history of experiences, a life within the context of a specific family and community, beliefs and values, and a unique genetic makeup. To provide the best possible care, you will need to show concern about the patient as a person rather than as someone for whom a specified procedure must be carried out ("the knee replacement").

As a Student

Your commitment to providing quality, **client-centered care** begins now, while you are a student. Your first responsibility as a student is to take full advantage of every opportunity to learn. Try to see the purpose in each assignment; look at it as an *opportunity to learn,* rather than as a chore to complete. With this attitude toward learning, you will not be tempted to skip class without good reason.

Your second responsibility is to decide what standards will guide your performance as a student. Imagine that your school has set a certain grade, such as 70, as passing in your program. Now imagine yourself saying, "I'll study this material until I know it well enough to make 75." In many courses of study, a grade of 75 is acceptable; a deficiency in the student's knowledge of subject matter is unlikely to cause harm to someone else.

In an allied health course, however, the implications of "just passing" are much more serious. Any gaps in your knowledge and performance of skills can affect every patient served. Do you want your future services to patients to be of "just passing" quality? Or do you wish to give the very best service you can give? If your educational program is preparing you to provide health services, can you be content to learn only 70 percent of what your teachers expect you to learn? Can you be content to develop your skills just enough to get a passing grade in a laboratory course?

For Discussion and Reflection

1. Explain the importance of setting high standards for yourself as a student and as a health care professional.

2. Tell about a time you felt proud of something you worked hard to accomplish. What made your accomplishment so satisfying?

Of course, you won't earn perfect scores on every assignment or test, nor should you expect to. Grades can be viewed as feedback from your instructor about what material you have mastered and what you need to review. Make it a habit to look back over your graded tests and assignments to see which topics you need to revisit. If you are uncertain, ask your instructor to discuss the test or assignment with you, not in an effort to raise your grade, but in order to increase your understanding and skills. The mark of a good student is not someone who receives a high score every time, but rather someone who uses each assignment, especially difficult ones, as an opportunity to learn more.

Practicing Habits That Lead to Success

In setting standards for achievement, plan to *do your best,* rather than trying to be the best student in the class. How can you do your best? Develop a study routine and establish the habits that work best for you. To get started, consider the following guidelines:

- Tell family and friends that you have set aside a certain time of day as your study period. Do not allow them to violate your schedule by interrupting you unless there is an emergency.

- At the beginning of each study period, write out a list of specific things you need to complete; then rank the items in order of importance. Complete task #1 (most important) first, and then move on to task #2. If one of the tasks is something you dislike but must get done, let it be task #1 so that you get it out of the way.

- If your list of study assignments is too long to complete today, set up tomorrow's list so today's remaining assignments come first; then put the items on that list out of your mind until tomorrow and give your full attention to today's list.

- Set up a calendar or special notebook for assignments, due dates for projects or reports, and test dates. Note on your calendar the dates/times you will work on specific assignments or study for a test. By planning, you can avoid last-minute rushes to meet a deadline.

> **For Discussion and Reflection**
>
> What study techniques have been most effective for you in the past? What challenges do you foresee in creating a study routine?

Practicing Empowerment

Adults should control most aspects of their lives. During adolescence, learning to make decisions is an important developmental task. If you entered adulthood with a tendency to let your parents, spouse, friends, or anyone else make decisions for you, it is time to recognize that you are giving away your power—the power to be a **self-reliant**, responsible adult.

When you are planning to eat out with a friend, who decides which restaurant? Do you usually say, "Oh, I don't care—you choose"? Does your significant other give you a choice? If you do not participate in small decisions that affect you, how can you expect others to include you in big decisions?

How does empowerment affect you? Suppose you have informed the family that your study hour will begin at 9:00 each evening. During the second day of this plan, your teenager calls you to the phone at 9:15; the caller is a relative, who talks about their problems for a full half hour. Two days later, your 10-year-old opens the door at 9:30 and says, "I need a note for my teacher about the field trip next Monday." Each time you permit these violations of your study hour, you are giving away your power. You gave your two children the power to interrupt your study hour. You gave your relative the power to use 30 minutes of your study time for their own purposes. You probably responded to these requests because you are accustomed to meeting the needs of others, even if doing so interferes with your own needs.

When you take an active role in making decisions, you are *taking responsibility for your life.* If you have not been in the habit of making your own decisions, you can start claiming your power by requiring others to respect your needs. For example, after informing all members of your family that a certain time is your study time, do not permit any violations to occur. Remind those who interrupt you that you are not available during study hour. If you are consistent, the interruptions will eventually stop.

Then you can use the same approach with another of your needs. You may choose to make the next decision about where to eat or which movie to see, instead of allowing someone else to make that decision. You may wish to inform your partner or friend that you want to be involved in any decisions that affect you. This change will not occur rapidly; be content with small changes initially. By persisting, you will eventually gain more control over your life. Do not be surprised if others resist your decision, especially if you are just beginning to participate in making decisions. Give your family and friends time to accept your change in behavior. Ideally, decision making is a give-and-take situation. Sometimes your decision is accepted, whereas at other times another person's decision prevails.

FIGURE 1-2 **Empowerment contributes to patients' self-esteem and sense of well-being.**

As a health care professional, you should also recognize the importance of empowerment to patients' self-esteem and sense of well-being. Patients who are dependent on others for their personal needs may express anger about their helplessness. Many patients need help in regaining some control over their life situations. By respecting their wishes and involving patients in decisions, *when appropriate,* you contribute to feelings of empowerment.

Choosing to enter this educational program for the health field was an important decision in your life. Now, it is time to make another decision—what kind of health care professional will you be? Excellent? Or "just passing"? Remember, the standards of performance that will characterize you as a health care professional will be influenced by the standards you set for yourself now.

> **For Discussion and Reflection**
>
> Sometimes even a self-reliant person has an experience that gives rise to feelings of helplessness or at least requires asking for help. For each situation below, describe one or more actions that would indicate self-reliance rather than dependence on others.
>   a. You have a flat tire on the way to class.
>   b. You have locked your keys in the car.
>   c. You are going to lunch with two classmates and realize that you left your wallet at home.

Activities

1. Interview someone who works in health care to ask about what challenges they experience in their job and what they find satisfying about their job.

2. Describe the steps you can take as a student to prepare yourself to provide client-centered care in your future work.

3a. Complete each of the following using Worksheet A (see page 11) at the end of this chapter.

    a. List the things you *have to do* each day.

    b. List the things you *have to do* each week, but not every day.

    c. List the things you *have to do* occasionally.

    d. Beside each item in a, b, and c, write the name of someone who could help you complete that task, at least some of the time. For example, could you and a friend rideshare so that you alternate days picking your children up from day care or school?

3b. Use Worksheet B (see page 12) at the end of this chapter to develop a tentative study plan. Note times you have class, work, or other commitments. Decide when you will study each day, and when you will devote time to other tasks or hobbies. Try this plan for two weeks. If your plan seems to be effective, continue to use it. If it is not effective:

    a. List problems that interfered with the effectiveness of the plan.

    b. Modify the plan by changing the schedule, the place where you study, or other details. If other people are part of the problem, try to involve them in developing the "improved plan" to increase the probability of getting their cooperation.

4. Explain what empowerment means and why it is important for adults to control most of the decisions about their own lives. To what extent do you make your own decisions about the following: your finances, your daily schedule, your meals, and your relationships with others? Are there areas of life in which you would like to take a more active decision-making role?

Reference

CHG Healthcare. (2021, April 6). Survey: Healthcare career satisfaction drops, burnout rises amid COVID-19. https://chghealthcare.com/blog/survey-healthcare-career-satisfaction-drops-burnout-rises-amid-covid-19/

Worksheet A

Tasks I Have to Do

Every day:

Once a week:

Occasionally:

Worksheet B

Study Plan

Time	Monday	Tuesday	Wednesday	Thursday	Friday	Saturday	Sunday
6 A.M.							
7							
8							
9							
10							
11							
12 Noon							
1 P.M.							
2							
3							
4							
5							
6							
7							
8							
9							
10							
11							
12 Mn							

The Philosophy of Individual Worth and Equitable Care

Objectives

After completing this chapter, you should be able to:

- Explain the philosophy of individual worth.
- Define and give examples of bias.
- Discuss barriers to equity in health care.
- Explain cultural awareness.
- Describe how cultural competence contributes to improved health care outcomes.

Key Terms

Bias
Cultural awareness

Cultural competence
Equity

Socioeconomic

As a health care professional, you will meet people from many different backgrounds. Patients have varying incomes, educational levels, and occupations. Your coworkers and patients will likely represent many cultural groups and nationalities. In addition to background, each person has unique qualities that make them who they are, including their gender identity, sexual orientation, religious beliefs, value system, interests, abilities, and preferences. As a health care professional, you are responsible for showing respect to coworkers and providing quality care to all patients.

The Meaning of Individual Worth

The philosophy of individual worth is the belief that everyone, regardless of personal circumstances or personal qualities, has worth and is entitled to respect as a human being. For health care professionals, this means that the quality of service does not vary because of the patient's race, nationality, religion, gender identity, sexual orientation, age, economic level, occupation, education, diagnosis, or any other characteristic.

Each patient is an individual. Each should receive health care that takes into consideration both the person's individuality and the specific health problem. The philosophy of individual worth has many implications for patient care. Health care professionals who do not accept the philosophy of individual worth may interact differently with patients from a culture other than their own while remaining unaware of any differences in the care they are providing.

© Rawpixel.com/Shutterstock.com

FIGURE 2-1 Everyone, regardless of personal circumstances or personal qualities, has worth and is entitled to respect as a human being.

What Is Bias?

Bias refers to making assumptions or judgments about a person, group, or situation based on our own beliefs, expectations, or previous experiences. When we encounter people with whom we have something in common, our expectations and assumptions tend to be positive, and we are more likely to give others the benefit of the doubt. When we perceive a person or situation as unfamiliar, we may feel cautious or unsure. If a person or situation reminds us of a negative experience or a strongly held belief we have, we may assume the worst or approach the person with a judgmental attitude.

Feeling some degree of bias in our encounters with others is normal. However, effective health care professionals learn to recognize and question their own biases. Rather than making assumptions or judging a patient or a situation, they practice an attitude of openness, curiosity, and willingness to recognize each person as a unique, valuable individual.

For Discussion and Reflection

Have you ever felt that another person's behavior toward you reflected bias based on your race, ethnicity, gender identity, religion, **socioeconomic** status, lifestyle, or other factors? How did the person's behavior show bias, and how did you respond?

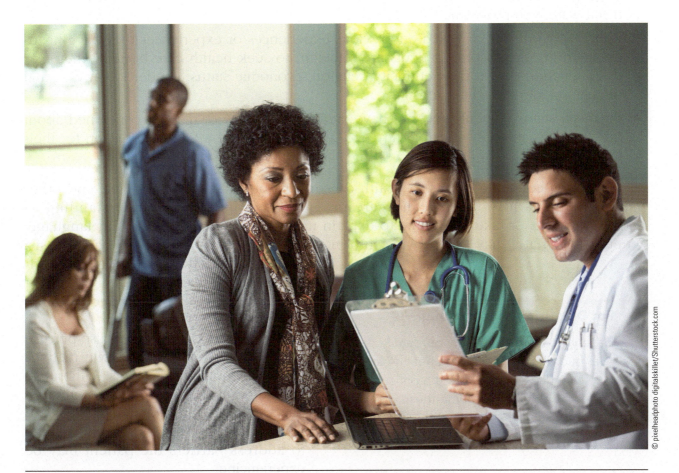

© pixelheadphoto digitalskillet/Shutterstock.com

FIGURE 2-2 For health care professionals, quality of service does not vary because of the patient's race, nationality, religion, gender identity, sexual orientation, age, economic level, occupation, education, diagnosis, or any other characteristic.

Promoting Equity in Health Care

Patients' attitudes toward health care, their ability to access health care, and their previous experiences with health care professionals also vary. Some patients are accustomed to seeking care when needed and are comfortable asking questions and advocating for their own needs. Other patients feel unsure of how to access care and are nervous about speaking to a professional about their needs. In accessing health care, patients may face one or more of the following barriers:

- Location and availability of providers: In some communities, there are too few health care facilities, facilities may be located far from patients' homes, and appointments may fill up quickly.

- Transportation and childcare: Patients may have difficulty traveling to health care facilities or may need assistance caring for children or other family members while they attend an appointment.

- Lack of knowledge or access to technology: Patients may be unsure how to access medical care or what type of provider to call. They may lack access to a computer to complete online intake forms or to view test results through a patient portal.

- Language: Patients may need a translator to schedule appointments and to discuss their health care with providers.

- Fear of discrimination: Based on previous experiences or experiences they have heard about from others, some patients are reluctant to seek health care because they fear discrimination due to race, ethnicity, religion, economic status, gender identity, sexual orientation, or other characteristics.

- Financial status: Patients may not have medical insurance or may be concerned about how to cover the cost of care. They may also fear creating a financial burden for their families.

Promoting equitable access to health care means being sensitive to these and other barriers patients may face. Health care providers can listen with understanding to patient concerns or take extra time to explain medical information in familiar language. When appropriate, they can provide information about community resources to assist with finances, transportation, or childcare. They can be familiar with their employer's procedure for accessing an interpreter.

Health care providers can also practice self-awareness about their own feelings and reactions toward patients. Rather than judging or making assumptions about a patient's behavior, providers can seek to understand the patient's perspective and to address barriers the patient may be experiencing.

For Discussion and Reflection

Have you or a member of your family ever had difficulty accessing health care? If so, what barriers created the difficulty? Were you able to overcome these barriers? If so, what helped? If not, what resources were needed?

FIGURE 2-3 Promoting equitable access to health care means being sensitive to barriers patients may face.

Practicing Cultural Awareness

Cultural awareness refers to understanding that everyone's habits and behaviors are shaped by their culture, accepting differences and similarities among cultures, and appreciating the diverse characteristics of different cultures. Some cultural differences are easy to observe, such as clothing styles, language, and food. Other behaviors, beliefs, and practices that vary by culture include the following:

- Hygiene and personal care practices
- Family structures and roles
- Parenting and discipline styles
- Religious or spiritual practices
- Gender roles and expectations
- Attitudes toward dating and sexual relationships
- Attitudes toward education and work

For Discussion and Reflection

Describe a culture or group you consider yourself to be part of. How has culture has shaped your behaviors or beliefs in two or more of the areas listed above?

Cultural awareness also means recognizing that *culture* is not limited to groups from a specific region or ethnic group but can include any group of people who identify themselves as sharing similar beliefs, values, or practices. For health care professionals, practicing cultural awareness means remaining open, curious, sensitive, and respectful of the culture of each patient.

Cultural Competence and Health Care Outcomes

Developing cultural awareness is an important first step. Health care organizations and health care professionals have a responsibility to practice cultural competence as well. For organizations, **cultural competence** includes creating policies, procedures, or programs that actively seek to create **equity** in hiring and patient care. For example, organizations may actively reach out to underserved populations to identify and remove barriers to accessing health care. Many organizations provide employee training in diversity and inclusion.

For you as a health care professional, practicing cultural competence means listening to patients' values, needs, and expectations. While maintaining professional best practices, you can tailor care to best fit the needs of each patient. You can be familiar with resources in your organization and community that assist patients in overcoming barriers to care such as those listed earlier in this chapter. Most importantly, you can practice understanding and respect, even in situations that you find challenging.

Studying a Situation

It is not easy to serve all patients equally well. Sometimes there is a strong desire to escape—to carry out an assigned task and leave the patient as quickly as possible. If you find yourself trying to avoid a patient, consider the situation carefully: Why do you find this patient difficult to serve? Have you tried to understand this patient's personal and health needs? Have you tried to see the situation as the patient sees it? If you make a habit of studying such situations, applying your knowledge about human behavior, you will grow in your ability to form effective relationships with your patients.

Improving Health Care Outcomes

Developing positive relationships with patients leads to improved health care outcomes. Patients who feel respected and heard are more likely to keep appointments, follow treatment plans, and call to ask questions about their health care. They are more likely to seek care when a health problem arises rather than waiting until the problem has become severe. Assistance with translation, scheduling appointments, transportation, childcare, and other logistics can determine whether patients are able to receive the care they need.

Practicing a Philosophy of Individual Worth

It is easy to state the philosophy of individual worth; it is quite difficult, however, to practice it day after day when there is a busy schedule and a wide variety of patients to take care of—unless you form certain ways of thinking about your patients. The following suggestions provide a starting point for developing and applying a philosophy of individual worth to your relationships with patients:

- Accept each patient as an individual with a unique personality.
- Recognize that each person tries to meet their needs with patterns of behavior that have developed over a lifetime; these patterns cannot be changed easily.
- Make a conscious effort to understand each patient's behavior.
- Accept that many of your patients will not behave as you want them to behave.
- Do not expect a sick person to adapt to you. As a health care professional, you should adapt to the patient.
- Consider each patient with a cultural background different from yours as an opportunity for you to learn.
- Make it a habit to treat all patients with respect, regardless of their backgrounds.

Activities

1. In your own words, explain the philosophy of individual worth. What attitudes, words, and actions can you take to practice this philosophy?

2. Notice how social media, television, movies, and politicians speak about different groups of people. Can you find examples that reflect a philosophy of individual worth? Which examples illustrate bias?

3. Review the list of barriers to care listed in this chapter. Research online resources in your community that can assist patients in overcoming these barriers. Based on your research, what additional resources does your community need?

4. Think about someone you know whose background is different from your own. Describe how this person's life (past and present) is similar to or different from your life.

5. Consider how you can apply cultural competence to these patient situations:

    a. A 15-year-old patient is pregnant and is afraid to tell their family.

    b. A patient states that they do not want to take a prescribed medication because they read online that weight gain is a common side effect.

    c. A patient who has had a heart attack states that it is difficult to follow the doctor's dietary recommendations because their partner does the cooking, and the family enjoys eating traditional meals together.

    d. A patient who has been diagnosed with colon cancer declines treatment because they do not wish to place a financial burden on their family.

    e. A patient tells you that some aspects of the treatment plan outlined by their doctor conflict with their religious beliefs.

References and Suggested Readings

Greene-Moton, Ella, & Minkler, Meredith. (2019). Cultural competence or cultural humility? Moving beyond the debate. *Health Promotion Practice, 21*(1), 142–145. doi:10.1177/1524839919884912.

Henderson, Saras, Horne, Maria, Hills, Ruth, & Kendall, Elizabeth. (2018). Cultural competence in healthcare in the community: A concept analysis. *Health & Social Care in the Community, 26*(4), 590–603. doi.org/10.1111/hsc.12556.

Radix, Asa, & Maingi, Shail. (2018). LGBT cultural competence and interventions to help oncology nurses and other health care providers. *Seminars in Oncology Nursing, 34*(1), 80–89. doi.org/10.1016/j.soncn.2017.12.005.

Sharifi, Majmeh, Adib-Hajbaghery, Mohsen, & Najafi, Maryam. (2019, November). Cultural competence in nursing: A concept analysis. *International Journal of Nursing Studies, 99*(103386). doi.org/10.1016/j.ijnurstu.2019.103386.

Shepherd, Stephane M., Willis-Esqueda, Cynthia, Newton, Danielle, Sivasubramaniam, Diane, & Paradies, Yin. (2019). The challenge of cultural competence in the workplace: Perspectives of healthcare providers. *BMC Health Services Research, 19,* 135. doi.org/10.1186/s12913-019-3959-7.

Self-Awareness

Objectives

After completing this chapter, you should be able to:

- Distinguish between *learning information*, *applying skills*, and *modifying your behavior*.
- Explain the benefits of a growth mindset.
- Explain why health care professionals must clearly understand their role.
- Identify your life roles and appropriate behaviors for each role.
- Discuss time management strategies.

Key Terms

Ethics
Fixed Mindset
Growth Mindset

Procrastinate
Proficient
Role

Self-Awareness

You are studying to become a health care professional. When you graduate, you will likely work at an agency that provides health services to the community. How best can you, the student of today, prepare to become you, the health care professional of tomorrow?

Understanding Learning

As a student, you must gain knowledge, learn to apply it appropriately to a wide variety of situations, and develop skills in performing certain procedures. Your teachers have created learning experiences to guide your progress toward a future **role** in health care. To benefit from these experiences, you will need the desire to learn, the willingness to make the necessary effort, and the determination to gain as much as possible from each learning experience.

Learning Information

Based on past experiences, many students view learning as a series of terms to memorize and tests to pass. If you can answer the questions on a test, but do not apply that information in appropriate clinical situations, have you *really* learned? Do you approach assignments as though you are storing information that can be played back on demand? Memorizing information is just a first step toward becoming **proficient**, or developing the professional skills you will use daily in your work as a health care professional.

Applying Skills

Do you constantly ask yourself how a new idea can be used? Does new information guide you in selecting appropriate behavior for situations where that information is relevant? If you can answer "yes" to these questions, then you are truly learning. You are using mental processes such as thinking, reasoning, selecting, decision making, and evaluating for conscious control of your behavior.

Modifying Your Behavior

Learning new skills begins with studying and continues with practicing and applying new skills. With practice, your new skills become routine parts of your behavior. Each time you begin a new topic of study in class, ask yourself the following questions:

- What do I already know about this topic?
- What do I want to find out about this topic?
- How will I apply this information now? In my future career?

When you connect new information to ideas you have previously learned, the new information becomes more meaningful and easier to remember.

For Discussion and Reflection

Think of a skill that you can perform well now but once had to learn, such as riding a bicycle, playing a sport, driving a car, or cooking. What was your first attempt like? How did you become *proficient* at this skill?

FIGURE 3-1 Honestly assessing your strengths and weaknesses is a first step in developing your potential.

Taking a New Look at Yourself

A first step in developing your potential is to practice **self-awareness**. Notice your habits and behavior patterns. Identify your feelings and thoughts in various situations. Be honest with yourself about your strengths and weaknesses.

The first question to ask yourself is "Am I willing to make changes in myself?" When someone criticizes you, do you nurse your hurt feelings or express anger toward your critic? Do you reject the criticism or make excuses for your behavior? Or do you see criticism as a possible indication that you need to change some aspect of your behavior? Willingness to change is necessary so that you can learn and grow as a person.

Strengths and Weaknesses

Your next question might be "What are my strengths and my weaknesses?" To develop your potential, you must know your weak points, for these will need your attention and greatest effort. For example, do you put off tasks until the last minute? This habit can lead to many undesirable results: being late to class, not being prepared for a test, not practicing a skill until you have achieved a high level of proficiency. By correcting a tendency to **procrastinate**, you can spare yourself the emotional strain of doing things at the last minute. You may even escape the irritation others express when your last-minute efforts inconvenience them.

For Discussion and Reflection

Regarding your habits and personal traits, which of the following statements best reflects your attitude? What are the pros and cons of each of these attitudes?
  a. "This is just the way I am; other people need to accept that."
  b. "I try to learn from each experience and become a better person over time."

An honest appraisal of your personal traits, including your work habits, is the key to planning ways of developing your potential. If you change behaviors that interfere with good performance, you will improve your ability to perform well in a variety of situations.

Adapting to New Conditions

A third question to ask yourself is "How well do I adapt to change?" Do you still follow ineffective habits formed early in your school years? If so, these habits are probably not working very well in your current educational program. No longer can you depend on the teacher. No longer can you expect the teacher to go over the same material until you have passively absorbed it. *You* must assume primary responsibility for learning.

In the future, you may be in a new situation and find yourself saying or thinking, "But I learned to do it a certain way, not the way they do it here." For most tasks, there is more than one acceptable procedure; adapting to the new setting requires that you perform according to the procedures of the new setting. *Basic principles, however, do not vary.* For example, aseptic technique requires certain steps and certain precautions, regardless of the setting or the precise sequence of steps for the total procedure.

Using Experience to Learn

A fourth question is "Do I learn from my experiences?" Let's take a look at how two people reacted to an embarrassing experience. When Maria and Darian gave oral reports, they both showed signs of nervousness and performed poorly. For each of them, this was a very embarrassing experience.

Maria reviewed the situation, admitted to putting little effort into the assignment, and made plans to be well prepared for the next oral report. Maria decided to have the information better organized, to study the material thoroughly, to prepare good notes, and to rehearse the presentation until it was smooth. Maria also spoke with the instructor after class about ways to improve the presentation.

Darian, on the other hand, used the same approach to prepare the next oral report, which proved to be another poor performance. In addition to being no better prepared for the second report than for the first, Darian was developing a fear of oral reports that would have a negative effect on future efforts to speak in front of others.

Maria used an uncomfortable experience constructively, making careful plans to prevent a recurrence of this particular embarrassment. With additional practice, Maria will give oral reports with confidence. Darian, on the other hand, allowed the experience to create self-doubt and fear of oral reports. Which of these students will grow as a person?

Developing a Growth Mindset

Stanford researcher Carol Dweck popularized the term **growth mindset**. Dweck found that students who believed that their abilities and intelligence were fixed, or unchanging, traits were less successful than students who believed that they could develop and increase their abilities through effort and practice. Statements such as "I'm just not good at math" indicate a **fixed mindset** and can make it more difficult to learn new skills.

Students with a growth mindset, on the other hand, tend to have the following attitudes and beliefs about learning:

- While not everyone will become a "genius," anyone can learn and improve their skills.

- By reviewing what has or has not worked previously, we can determine whether a new strategy or approach is needed.

- An unsuccessful attempt should not be viewed as a failure, but as feedback about how to improve future efforts.

Dweck (2015) cautions that while effort is an important part of the growth mindset, effort alone may not lead to improvement. Rather, Dweck says, "Students need to try new strategies and seek input from others when they're stuck" (pp. 20, 24).

Consider these differences in how individuals with a fixed mindset tend to approach learning and life situations, compared to how individuals with a growth mindset approach these same situations. Someone with a fixed mindset may avoid challenges and new experiences, while someone with a growth mindset may seek out challenges. After making a mistake, someone with a fixed mindset may hide the mistake or blame others, while someone with a growth mindset will ask, "What can I learn from this situation? How can I do better next time?" Someone with a fixed mindset may avoid asking others for help, not wanting to look weak, or may say, "Can you do this for me? I don't know how." Someone with a growth mindset is more likely to ask for help by saying, "Can you show me how to do this so I can learn?"

No one has a fixed mindset or a growth mindset all the time, in all areas of life. Most people have a fixed mindset in some areas of life and a growth mindset in other areas. For example, Darian (from the public speaking example earlier in this chapter) may have a fixed mindset about giving oral presentations but a growth mindset about learning to play a sport. What about you? How would you describe your mindset toward learning? Toward certain subjects such as math, reading, or science? By noticing how you think about your abilities in these areas, you can intentionally choose a growth mindset that will support your progress in your health care preparation courses.

For Discussion and Reflection

Do you have a particular subject area or skill that you tell yourself "I'm just not good at?" On the other hand, do you have skills that you have worked hard to develop through effort and practice? How do the concepts of a fixed mindset and a growth mindset apply to either of these skills?

Your Role As a Health Care Professional

Role Perception

An additional question to ask yourself is "What is my role?" The present program of study will help you understand your future role as a health care professional. For every role there are appropriate and inappropriate ways of behaving. Whether a particular behavior is appropriate depends not only on the specific *type* of health care professional you are preparing to become, but also on the *level* of that role in relation to other health team members.

Certain behaviors that are appropriate for a specific health care role may not be appropriate for personnel in a different role. For example, the behaviors appropriate for laboratory personnel are distinct from those appropriate for nursing personnel. Also, within individual departments there are differences in roles based on level: Within nursing there are nursing assistants, licensed practical nurses, registered nurses, head nurses, and supervisors, all of whom have specific roles; similarly, within the hospital laboratory, there are numerous roles such as pathologist, medical technologist, clinical laboratory assistant, and others. The same is true of other hospital departments such as physical therapy, radiology, food service, and so on, as well as for medical offices. In the dental field, dentists, dental hygienists, dental assistants, and dental laboratory technologists are all concerned with oral health. Their roles vary according to the specific functions and educational preparation of each.

Knowing one's role is essential to effective functioning. Most roles within the health field require accepting instructions from someone at the next higher level. If you do not like "taking orders," then you may not be happy as a health care professional. If you feel anger or distrust toward persons in authority, you are likely to resent the **ethics** of the health field; the policies of your health agency; and relationships with those on the health team who have responsibility for giving instructions, making assignments, and evaluating performance. On the other hand, if you can accept a defined role, function within that role to the fullest extent of your educational preparation, and accept the limitations of the role, then you are likely to find much satisfaction as a health care professional.

Your Life Roles

How many roles do you play? Probably several. You are a student now and hope to have a role as a health care professional in the future; you may be an employee, a spouse or partner, parent, or sibling. Within each role, you have a set of behaviors and responsibilities to fulfill.

Role as an Influence on Relationships

There are similarities in the child-parent relationship and the teacher-student relationship during the school years. In a health occupations education program, the teacher-student relationship is between two adults, even though one adult is a student. What difficulties in role perception might occur if the student is a mature, 50-year-old person, and the teacher is a 25-year-old health professional? Or if a doctor is 35 and the medical office assistant is 55, with 20 years of experience?

Making a Distinction between Roles

The roles you play at home, in community activities, as a health occupations student, and as a neighbor are all different. To some extent, each role requires different behavior patterns. Do not confuse the health care professional role with other roles in your personal life. Some friends may try to get "free medical advice," but the role of friend and the role of health care professional are different. Medical practice acts, which are state laws, make it illegal for nonphysicians to diagnose and prescribe. Therefore, this type of role confusion is dangerous.

The Value of Studying Human Behavior

Note that the sequence of growth is from understanding self to understanding others. Therefore, *the ability to understand others is limited until you have begun to understand yourself.*

Human behavior is very complex. In any situation, the behavior of a person is influenced by many different factors. The remainder of this course will introduce some of these influences. Understanding of oneself and others must be based on knowledge about human behavior in general.

Managing Your Time

An important aspect of understanding yourself is to recognize how you use your time. Have you ever asked yourself at the end of the day, "Where did the time go?" Have you ever wondered why some people seem to get everything done, whereas others are perpetually late or behind on their assignments? Learning to manage your time can make you more effective as a student and a professional.

To help you identify how you spend your time, try for a day or two to write down hourly what you are doing. You will gain a realistic estimate of how long household tasks or childcare take as well as how much time you spend on nonessential activities, such as television, social media, or games. Once you know how you are spending your time, you can decide what changes you would like to make in your daily routine.

The following strategies may help you use your time more effectively:

- Write down tasks or goals you hope to accomplish each day.
- Prioritize your goals so that you tackle the most important or most urgent first.
- As much as possible, focus on completing one task at a time.

© Daniel M Ernst/Shutterstock.com

FIGURE 3-2 Learning to manage your time will reduce stress and help you meet deadlines.

- Throughout the day, stop periodically and ask yourself, "Am I working to meet my goals? Am I doing what I am supposed to be doing?"
- Review your list of goals each evening, mark off those that were completed, and plan the list for the next day.
- Start tasks well ahead of time to avoid the stress of having to rush.
- Break large tasks into small chunks and tackle one chunk at a time.

Personal Growth

Consider the following strategies you can use to understand yourself and set goals for personal growth and achievement as a student and health care professional:

- Recognize that learning occurs only if you make the effort to learn, if you are willing to change, and if you recognize opportunities for learning.
- Study yourself in relation to specific traits, such as willingness to change, ability to be honest with yourself, and readiness to correct weaknesses and change habits.
- Identify your strengths and make full use of them to achieve your goals.
- Identify your weaknesses—the traits or habits you need to change to be more effective in each of your roles.
- Study your various roles in terms of desirable behavior. Identify differences, such as habits used at home that are not appropriate at school, interpersonal relations between a parent and child that are not appropriate between the health care professional and a pediatric patient, or relations between friends that are not appropriate between a hospital employee and a patient.
- Study your ability to make distinctions between different life roles and change your behaviors accordingly.
- Study your tendency to use old habits in new situations. Do you allow habits to determine your behavior in any situation? Do you need to improve in adapting your behavior to each situation?
- Mentally review past experiences to understand how your own behavior contributed to the outcome. Consider the important question "Would the outcome of that experience be improved if I had behaved differently?" This practice can serve as a "rehearsal" for future similar experiences.

By considering the questions above on a regular basis, you will identify ways you can grow in your personal life and in your role as a health care professional.

Activities

1. Describe learning strategies you have used in the past, both in class and in nonschool activities such as sports or learning a new hobby. Which strategies are likely to be effective in your health care preparation program? Which strategies are not likely to be effective?

2. Identify one area of your life in which you have a fixed mindset and one area in which you have a growth mindset. What differences do you notice about how you approach each of these areas?

3. Identify one behavior in your personal life that is not an acceptable behavior with patients or coworkers.

4. Which of the following roles do you play in your current life situation? Add other roles to the list as needed.

   Student in a health-related educational program

   Spouse or partner

   Parent of a child

   Family member

   Employee

   a. Beside each role that applies to you, estimate how much time per day you devote to that role.

   b. Mark the role that you value most with an asterisk (*).

   c. If other demands (e.g., job, school) limit the amount of time you devote to the role you value the most, describe how you can improve your approach to that role so that *quality* can compensate for lack of *quantity*. For example, "When in the role of _____, I will give it my full attention and not allow concerns about my other roles to distract me."

5. Consider a situation in which you ran out of time to complete a task. Discuss how time management strategies might help you handle a similar situation more effectively in the future.

References and Suggested Readings

Dweck, Carol. (2015, September 23). Carol Dweck revisits the "growth mindset." *Education Week, 35*(5), 20, 24.

Elliot-Moskwa, E. (2022). *The growth mindset workbook: CBT skills to help you build resilience, increase confidence, and thrive through life's challenges.* Oakland, CA: New Harbinger.

Robbins, M. (2021). *The high 5 habit: Take control of your life with one simple habit.* Carlsbad, CA: Hay House.

Understanding Human Behavior

The interpersonal skills of health care professionals are very important to the patient. The health care professional who can build rapport with patients increases confidence in the health team, promotes faith in the treatment plan, and is more likely to gain the patient's full cooperation. If a health care professional is unable to develop rapport, then the opposite may occur. The patient may have negative feelings toward members of the health team, may distrust them, and may not comply with the health care plan. The skillful health care professional can recognize behavior that indicates negative feelings and attitudes and respond to them. Section II explains some of the many factors that influence human behavior.

Influences on Behavior

Objectives

After completing this chapter, you should be able to:

- Identify the basic purpose of human behavior.
- Discuss how people are alike and different.
- Describe genetic influences on behavior.
- Summarize the developmental process.
- Describe how the physical and social environments influence development and behavior.
- Discuss the importance of taking responsibility for one's behavior.

Key Terms

Behavioral genetics	Genes	Heredity
Chromosomes	Genetics	Human Genome Project
Congenital	Genotype	Phenotype
DNA	Hereditary	Rapport

The Basis of Human Behavior

At the most basic level, any behavior can be seen as a person's attempt to either *obtain* or *avoid* something. From birth, we instinctively seek food, warmth, and comfort. We attempt to avoid cold, pain, and loud noises. As we grow, we develop an increasingly complex repertoire of behaviors to obtain what we need or want. We also develop behaviors that help us avoid experiences we find unpleasant. But what causes different people to behave in different ways, even though they are attempting to meet similar needs?

Human behavior is influenced by many factors. Heredity, environment, and culture all play a role in shaping our behavior. Researchers continue to explore the ways in which each of these factors contributes to behavior and to our mental processes.

How People are Alike and Different

Behavior is influenced by factors that all people have in common, as well as by individual differences.

All of us are alike in many ways:

- We have basic physical needs for food, water, shelter, sleep, oxygen, and physical safety.
- We also share basic psychological needs, such as the needs for acceptance, belonging, love, self-esteem, and opportunities to develop our talents and abilities.

Most behavior can be understood as an individual's effort to meet one or more of these needs. However, individual and cultural differences cause us to meet these needs in diverse ways. Three major forces interact to create a specific individual:

- Heredity
- Developmental process
- Physical and social environments

Genetic Influences on Behavior

Each person is a unique individual. At the time of conception, **hereditary** traits are inherited from the biological parents to form a unique combination of traits. Since thousands of traits are involved, the possible combinations are limitless. That is why we say that no two people have exactly the same **heredity**, except in the case of identical twins. You are likely learning about heredity in other courses. Therefore, our concern here is to emphasize that *each person, from the time of conception, possesses a unique combination of traits that will affect that individual throughout life.*

The Physiology of Heredity

At the time of conception, 46 **chromosomes** are organized into 23 matched pairs (23 from each parent). There are two sex-linked chromosomes: X for biological females and Y for biological males. The combination of chromosomes from the two biological parents provides the individual's **genotype**, a unique set of inherited traits. The **phenotype** is the result of all genes that, in combination, provide traits that determine the individual's physical appearance.

Genes are segments of DNA that occupy specific locations on each chromosome. Each gene is composed of molecules of a protein called deoxyribonucleic (de-oxy-ri-bo-nu-cle-ic) acid, or **DNA**. DNA is made up of four basic chemicals—adenine, thymine, guanine, and cytosine—arranged as strands that wrap around each other to form a spiral known as the double helix. DNA is present in every cell of the body in the form of genes. These chemicals are arranged on the gene in a particular sequence, and it is this sequence that establishes the trait or traits carried by that gene, just as the arrangement of letters makes up a specific word. The "words" are larger protein molecules, and each has a specific function—control of a specific cellular activity. The discovery of DNA and subsequent discovery of molecular sequences on strands of DNA were exciting scientific breakthroughs. This led to the rapid development of human **genetics** as a scientific field of inquiry and the discovery of much new information on heredity.

The Genetic Basis for Individuality

A particular characteristic of an individual may be due to:

- One specific gene
- The sequential arrangement of molecules on each gene
- A particular pair of genes
- A group of genes interacting with each other
- The influence of environmental factors on a gene or genes

Some traits are expressed, meaning that the individual will manifest that trait. Other traits are unexpressed but predispose that individual to manifest the trait under certain conditions. A person may have the gene for a specific hereditary disease but will develop the disease only under certain conditions. A person who has the gene for a disease but does not develop symptoms is known as a *carrier*; that gene can be passed on to their children, who may manifest the disease.

Like chromosomes, genes are paired so that a given trait is determined by the contribution of either or both parents. A dominant trait will be expressed, even if inherited from only one parent; a recessive trait will manifest only if matched with a recessive gene from each parent. Some traits are sex-linked, meaning they are inherited through the X chromosome of the biological female or are linked to the Y chromosome of the biological male. For example, red/green color blindness is expressed only in biological males but is inherited from biological females because the gene for color blindness is carried on the biological female's X chromosome.

Health Implications

Genetics, the study of heredity, has expanded rapidly and is making significant contributions to medicine. Research to locate the genetic basis of diseases is ongoing, with new findings announced frequently.

A genetic disorder is one that results from an individual's genetic makeup. It may be apparent at birth, may appear as a developmental disorder, or may appear later in life as a disease or health problem. A single-gene disorder is due to the absence or alteration of one gene specific to that trait. Tests are available for many single-gene disorders, such as cystic fibrosis, hemophilia, and red/green color blindness. A multifactorial disorder is one involving variations in several genes. Obviously, identifying several defective genes is more complex than identifying a single gene. There are also chromosomal disorders; for example, persons with Down syndrome have three, rather than two, copies of chromosome 21.

Gene therapy has emerged as a specialty in medicine; therapy consists of modifying a defective gene to treat or prevent a specific disease. Genetic testing is used to identify certain single-gene disorders, confirm a diagnosis, identify carriers, and identify persons who are at risk for developing a disease but are currently free of symptoms.

From the moment of conception, then, an individual has a unique combination of hereditary traits—a blueprint that will guide growth, development, and numerous processes throughout that individual's life. Some genes are so specific that their traits cannot be modified by environmental influences or therapy. Other genes require pairing (one from each parent) for a trait or disorder to develop. Some genes are sex-linked—specific to the X or Y chromosome. Some genes provide a trait that will manifest only if environmental conditions foster its development.

Genetic Testing

In 1990, the U.S. Congress funded the **Human Genome Project**, a 13-year project to map the sequencing of all the genes on all the chromosomes. The project was completed in 2003. This map, or pattern, of the chromosomal and gene arrangement is called the human genome, the basis for human genetics. Identification of the genetic basis for certain disorders has resulted in the development of genetic testing that surpasses the development of improved therapies. Scientific advances in genetics have raised questions about privacy rights and the right of each patient to participate in health-related decisions.

DNA tests are proving valuable in areas other than health-related genetics. An individual's DNA can be used to determine paternity, to identify a body, to prove or disprove family relationships, and to investigate crimes; DNA samples have been used as proof to establish the guilt or innocence of an accused person.

Genetic testing is expensive. It also involves certain risks that should be made known to anyone who is considering genetic testing. Insurance companies and employers (or potential employers) can demand the results of genetic testing. There are examples of people who were denied insurance or lost their jobs when genetic tests indicated the presence of a gene for some specific disease (e.g., breast cancer, Huntington's disease). Although a negative test can relieve one's anxieties, a positive test has profound psychological effects on the individual and their loved ones.

For Discussion and Reflection

What have you heard about genetic testing in the media? For example, has DNA testing played a key role in solving a crime? Determining the paternity of a child? What do you see as the pros and cons of genetic testing in these situations?

If your parent died at age 49 of Huntington's disease, you may or may not develop this incurable disease. Genetic testing could remove this terrible cloud over your life if you do not have the specific gene. On the other hand, if you do have the gene, you will be faced with the certainty of developing the disease, probably between ages 30 and 50. Would you choose to live with uncertainty? Or would you want to know, even if a positive test might cost you your job, insurance coverage, and relationships with those who cannot face the prospect of caring for you through a long illness? A positive approach to knowing that you have the gene would be to acknowledge your own mortality, accept that you will not have a long life, use your remaining years of health to live life to the fullest, and make end-of-life decisions while you are still in good physical and mental health.

Behavioral Genetics

Genetics research has also given rise to the field of **behavioral genetics**, which seeks to understand human behavior in terms of hereditary or biological influences. Researchers note that some behaviors tend to run in families. Studies of twins and adoptees have been used for some time to explore the effects of heredity on behavior. Research suggests that some behaviors are more closely linked to heredity; some are more closely linked to environmental influences, and some are linked to a combination of heredity and environment. For example, researchers have found evidence that aggressive behavior is linked to genetic factors, past or present substance use, and socioeconomic status (van Dongen et al., 2021).

The Developmental Process

Heredity establishes the basic physical/mental/emotional makeup and all the personality traits of each person. But many other influences determine how these ingredients will be molded as individuals grow and develop from babies into adults. One important difference is the built-in developmental rate, a hereditary factor. You have likely known children who appeared "big for their age" or "mature for their age" as well as children who are smaller or less mature than their same-age peers. Thus, physical development proceeds at one rate for one child and at another rate for their sibling. The study of a child must always consider the apparent rate of development.

Prenatal Influences

The developmental process is subject to tremendous environmental influence, especially during the prenatal period. Ideally, the birthing parent's body provides the embryo with a physical environment that is favorable to healthful development. This prenatal environment is affected by the birthing parent's general health, nutritional status, pathogenic organisms such as those that cause syphilis or measles, and the presence in the blood of any substance that is toxic to the embryo.

Research indicates that the birthing parent's daily habits have tremendous influence on the embryo:

- Smoking during pregnancy increases the risk of complications of pregnancy, premature birth, low birth weight, stillbirth, and infant mortality.

For Discussion and Reflection

Consider yourself as a child, as compared to your siblings or friends. Were you small or large for your age, or were you of average size? In school did you learn quickly, or was it a struggle to keep up? Were you ever told that you were mature (or immature) for your age?

© B-D-S Piotr Marcinski/Shutterstock.com

FIGURE 4-1 Nutrition is critical to healthy prenatal development.

- Consumption of alcoholic beverages by a pregnant parent places the infant at risk of various **congenital** defects, including fetal alcohol syndrome (FAS).

- The role of nutrition during the prenatal period is critical to healthy prenatal development. For example, spina bifida is caused by a deficiency of folic acid. If a birthing parent supplements their diet with folic acid *after* becoming pregnant, it is already too late to prevent this neural tube defect.

Anyone who may become pregnant should be concerned about nutrition, especially adequate intake of vitamins and minerals. Individuals who have decided to start a family should practice good nutrition and a healthy lifestyle.

The experiences and emotions of a pregnant individual have profound prenatal effects. Fear, anger, and grief—normal reactions to stressful and traumatic experiences—can affect the developing fetus. If the birthing parent is in an abusive relationship, the abuse may accelerate during pregnancy; the birthing parent's emotional reactions to such abuse affect the fetus, even in the absence of physical trauma. On the other hand, positive experiences have a positive effect. Some pregnant individuals listen to classical music daily; some read and talk to their unborn child. Studies of young children reveal that a child's personality and developmental rate are related to such prenatal influences.

How Physical and Social Environments Shape Behavior

The environment is another major influence on the development and the expression of certain hereditary potential. Much has been written about the relative importance of heredity and environment. With increasing knowledge about heredity and with growing awareness of the power of the physical and social environments to affect the developmental process, it is now apparent that many forces interact to determine the traits of an individual. Heredity provides the basic ingredients and the blueprint, but environmental factors and events that affect the developmental process determine what aspects of the blueprint will be expressed.

Physical Environment

Environment, in its broadest sense, means many things. The physical environment includes home conditions, climate, community conditions, means for meeting physical needs, and resources for developing one's potential. Children who live in a large city have a physical environment that differs greatly from that of children who live in a rural community. Many factors vary based on children's physical environments:

- Exposure to pollution
- Access to cultural resources such as museums and concerts
- Ability to spend time outside
- Participation in team sports, clubs, or community organizations
- Opportunities to learn skills such as gardening, tending livestock, or building repair
- Ability to spend time with other children outside one's own family

All aspects of the physical environment affect personality. Some personality traits tend to develop in one kind of environment, whereas a different environment fosters the development of other traits.

Those who care for a child create the child's immediate physical environment. It may be as safe as thoughtful adults can make it, or it may contain many hazards. Unless adults make a conscious effort to control risks in the home and childcare facility, the child may experience serious injuries from falls, burns, or poisoning. Although some such injuries are correctible, some are fatal, and others leave lifelong scars. In addition to environmental hazards, some personal habits of adults also affect the child. Exposure to secondhand smoke increases the risk of sudden infant death syndrome (SIDS) in infants, and the chance of developing asthma is higher in babies and young children who are frequently exposed to secondhand smoke.

Social Environment

The social environment involves people. A baby's experiences provide important first learnings about the world and people. The baby may learn that the world is a friendly place—that they can depend on others to correct such discomforts as hunger, cold, and a wet diaper. Or the baby may learn the world is a hostile place—that they cannot rely on others to relieve hunger and cold. These infant experiences lay the foundation for future relations with other people: distrust or trust, expectations of comfort and nurturing from others, or accepting discomfort without expecting help from others.

For Discussion and Reflection

How would you describe the physical environment in which you grew up? What activities or resources did you have access to because of your environment? What resources were not available to you?

FIGURE 4-2 The physical and social environments has a significant effect on a child's development.

Role models are powerful influences on children. Every adult in a child's world has the potential to serve as a role model, whether they are within the home (immediate or extended family), the neighborhood, a place of worship, or school. Role models influence children in many ways—value system, parenting style, career choice. The role model's influence may be positive or negative. It may last a lifetime, or it may be temporary. A child may have only one role model or may adopt different role models at various life stages. An adult may even be unaware that they are serving as a role model for a specific child.

Culture and Socioeconomic Level

Children are strongly influenced by the culture in which they grow up. Culture refers to the ideas, beliefs, values, and customs shared by a group of people. These shared ideas may be based on religion, ethnicity or nationality, geographic region, or other factors. Put simply, children learn from the adults around them what is important and how they are expected to act in certain situations.

Socioeconomic level also influences children's early learning. According to the National Center for Children in Poverty (NCCP), 38 percent of children in the United States live in low-income families (NCCP, 2021). These children may be at increased risk for learning and behavioral problems. In some cases, it is more difficult for them to access educational resources in the community due to lack of funds, transportation, or caregivers' work schedules.

Influences During Childhood

The basic heredity of a child, plus environmental influences, exerts a powerful influence on development. Throughout the early years, a child continues to learn about people and the world. If relationships with caregivers are positive and nurturing, the child develops a sense of security and finds the world a place for exploring and satisfying curiosity. If the child experiences a chaotic environment and harsh relationships with caregivers, the child learns to distrust other people and tends to fear new experiences or strange places.

Home The home environment is of great importance in the young child's development. Physical and mental health as well as emotional and individual growth depend largely on a child's home and family:

- How well does the family provide for the child's physical needs?
- What health practices are followed?
- Is the home atmosphere democratic or authoritarian?
- Do the parents overprotect the child, or do they allow the child to develop self-reliance gradually?
- Is there a parent who feels anxious and repeatedly warns the child about getting hurt?

The child's home may include a parent who is abusive. Child abuse is widespread, and many parents who are abusive experienced being abused as children. The abuse may be physical, mental, or emotional. Mental and emotional abuse may be inflicted verbally (with put-downs or statements that arouse guilt) or by specific actions (isolation, darkness). Physical abuse may be in the form of beatings or sexual activities. The person acting abusively may even threaten to harm the child if this "secret" is revealed to anyone. The child who has experienced abuse may be impacted in many ways. In addition to physical trauma, the child must deal with fear, anger, and guilt. Unless they get help, children who have experienced abuse are at a higher risk of becoming parents who are abusive.

What is the neighborhood environment? Is it safe or full of hazards for children? Are there opportunities for a wide variety of experiences? Are there relatives and neighbors who care about the child, or is the social climate of the neighborhood hostile? Are the parents from another culture? If so, do they require the child to behave in ways appropriate for the parents' culture, but inappropriate in the present community?

The School Years When the child enters school, the physical and social environments are greatly extended. If development has proceeded according to schedule, the child is ready for this expansion of experience. If the physical or social environment of early life inhibited some aspect of development, then the child may not be ready to benefit fully from school. Early school experiences may be so frustrating that they inhibit development. Elementary school students show marked differences in development and in behavior patterns; these differences reflect both hereditary and environmental influences:

- Some children readily adapt to being with a group of their own age; others are reluctant to join the group.
- Some see the teacher as absolute authority, to be obeyed without question; others show rebellion toward authority.
- Some students work independently; others seek the teacher's assistance for every task.
- Some are bubbling with ideas and participate fully in every activity; others sit quietly and participate only when told to do so.

These differences are not accidental. They are the result of both heredity and early influences on patterns of behavior.

Assuming Responsibility for Behavior

Early learning continues to influence our behavior throughout life, often without our realizing. On the other hand, we can learn to recognize certain early influences on behavior and, when needed, modify our behavior pattern. *As children we do not choose our heredity, our home environment, or our developmental influences. However, as we mature into adults, we can become self-directing:*

- Adults can recognize undesirable behavior patterns and choose to change.
- Adults can work to understand the basis for particular behaviors and, with such understanding, resist or eliminate the effects of early influences.
- An adult can leave an unhealthy situation and seek a more favorable environment.

These options are not available to children, who are trapped in specific living situations. As adults, we can choose not to remain trapped in past patterns but to change our behaviors, habits, and living conditions.

Modifying Early Learnings

Prejudice is one example of early learning that can influence behavior throughout life unless we choose to examine behavior patterns and their apparent origins. Prejudice is usually learned early in life from the people around us. In its most common form, prejudice consists of negative feelings toward people from a different race or subculture. If parents and their friends speak in unkind terms about members of another group, children may learn to show hostility or disrespect toward members of that group. As adults, however, we can change these early learnings. We can reexamine our attitudes, considering new knowledge and personal experience. Often, we find that our prejudice does not hold up against rational examination. *As adults, we can modify early learnings and take control of our own behavior, attitudes, and beliefs.*

An example of unexamined prejudice is the behavior of people who belong to one of the "hate groups." The leaders of such groups depend on "us versus them" thinking to arouse strong feelings and mobilize people to behave as the leaders wish them to behave. Televised reports of demonstrations show people who are controlled by their emotions, rather than by clear thinking. Those emotions probably have their roots in early learning that has not been reexamined during adulthood. People who blindly accept the policies of a group, a political party, or even of a government, are allowing others to do their thinking, determine their beliefs, and control their behavior. *Throughout adult life, we benefit from continuously evaluating and modifying our beliefs and value systems.*

Interests

Interests also influence behavior. They determine where we direct our attention. They influence the decisions we make, the activities we pursue, the occupations we choose, and the types of recreation we select for our leisure time. People who have many interests are well prepared for

FIGURE 4-3 Having a variety of interests will help you relate to different people.

forming effective relationships with a variety of people. Those whose only activities are work, television, and social media do not have much to offer others in the way of interesting companionship. Developing a variety of interests is one way to become a more interesting person, find greater satisfaction in living, and form satisfying relationships.

For Discussion and Reflection

What are your interests? What activities do you enjoy? Do these interests and activities provide topics of conversation or other ways to interact with others?

Value Systems

A value system is the degree of importance we attach (largely unconsciously) to various beliefs, ideas, or material things. Each person's values have a strong influence on behavior. Our daily choices provide evidence of our values:

- Did you give up watching a movie to do an assignment for today? Then you placed a higher value on being a student than you did on recreation, at least in this instance.
- Did you return the extra dollar you received as change at the grocery store? Then you placed a higher value on honesty than on "getting the best of the other person."
- Did you cheat on that last test to improve your grade? Then you placed a higher value on a grade than on honesty or true learning.

The value system includes many things: character traits such as honesty and truthfulness, personal achievement, the symbols of achievement, love and friendship, material possessions, religion, recreation, work, and family living. Each person's values begin to form early in life, influenced by the rewards or punishments that followed specific types of behavior. Throughout life, the value system exerts a powerful influence on behavior, particularly when there is a choice to be made. Your enrollment in this educational program indicates that you value education enough to attend classes and do your assignments.

Standards of Behavior

Standards of behavior consist of our own personal rules and regulations, our own "dos" and "don'ts," that are part of our self-concept. There is a close relationship between our value system and our standards of behavior. Both are learned early in life and continually modified according to life experiences.

Deciding to change our standards of behavior should be an intentional decision, not an impulsive one. Teenagers are often subjected to pressure from their friends to abandon home teachings and adopt the group's code of behavior. This can be a difficult decision for a young person, since peer acceptance is very important during adolescence.

There is a difference between current standards and those of the past. Standards of behavior are a frequent source of misunderstanding between parents and adolescents. There are also wide differences in standards of behavior from one subculture to another. Standards of behavior, including sexual behavior, vary between socioeconomic levels, cultural groups, and generations.

For Discussion and Reflection

When you were a child, what behaviors or activities did your caregivers reward? What behaviors resulted in punishment? What values were communicated by these rewards and punishments?

Taking time to consciously examine your own beliefs and standards of behavior will help you make your own choices as an adult rather than simply deferring to "the way you were brought up" or "what everyone else is doing." You may decide to maintain some or all of the standards of behavior you were taught as a child, or you may not. Either way, you benefit from making a conscious choice.

Sleep and Nutrition

Our behavior is also influenced by whether we get enough sleep and appropriate nutrition. The need for sleep is discussed in greater detail in Chapter 5. In short, insufficient sleep weakens the immune system, affects mood, and inhibits our ability to think clearly. You have likely noticed that you (or your family members) tend to be more short-tempered or accident-prone when you have not had enough sleep. Similarly, eating nutritious food without artificial colors or preservatives has been found to have a positive behavioral effect, particularly in children.

As you can see, the human personality is the result of many ingredients. It is continuously molded by the environment and by life experiences. It is always subject to further change as a result of future life situations.

When we were children, our early learnings were determined by circumstances beyond our control. As adults, we have a choice:

- We can continue to live without consciously directing our lives, or we can take control.
- We can nurture certain aspects of our personalities and dial down other aspects.
- We can learn to make informed decisions.
- We can learn to recognize ineffective behaviors that may prevent us from reaching our goals.

By becoming aware of our behavior, we can become intentional and self-directing instead of living by patterns of thought and behavior established during childhood. Even more important, as adults we can think through various issues, decide what our values are, set our own standards of behavior, and accept or reject the values and standards proposed to us by others.

The Health Care Professional and the Patient

As a health care professional, you will find great satisfaction in your work if you make a conscious and continuous effort to study behavior—both your own and that of other people. You will meet people from many different backgrounds. With some, it will be easy to establish a pleasant relationship, one in which the patient believes that *you understand* and that *you are sincerely concerned*. Such a relationship is said to have **rapport**.

With some patients, you will find it more difficult to communicate. Perhaps the patient's behavior makes you uncomfortable. Perhaps you just do not find the patient "interesting" as a person. If this climate exists between you and the patient, rapport will not be established.

Any patient who has been labeled "difficult" needs special attention from the health team. The behaviors that cause the patient to be labeled "difficult" may be signs that the patient's needs are not being met. On the other hand, the pleasant, agreeable patient may be covering up true feelings and may have just as much need for understanding and concern. In other words, as a health care professional, you will need to apply interpersonal skills to *establish rapport with each patient* as an individual. Some patients will be more of a challenge than others, but all need your understanding and sincere interest if you are to make a positive contribution to their health care.

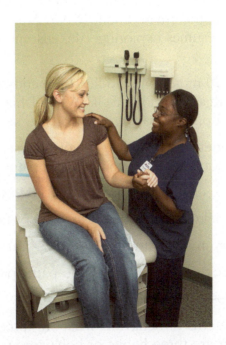

FIGURE 4-4 As a health care professional, you will need to apply interpersonal skills to *establish rapport with each patient as an individual.*

Activities

1. List five behaviors or activities that you engage in several times per week. For each behavior, identify which physical or psychological needs or wants this behavior fulfils. Does each behavior help you obtain something you need or want, avoid something you don't need or want, or both?

2. List five of your interests. State how each interest will be helpful to you as a health care professional.

   a. Review the list of interests you made. Estimate the amount of time you have spent on each interest during the past seven days. Place a star by those interests to which you have devoted as much as five hours.

   b. For two of the interests on your list, write ways each of them could provide opportunities to connect with other people.

   c. Discuss your list of interests with one or more classmates, noting where your interests are similar and where they differ.

3. If one of your parents died at age 42 of a disorder that is known to be genetic, would you choose to undergo genetic testing to determine if you have the gene for that disorder (yes or no)?

   a. Write a brief explanation for your answer.

   b. If the test result is positive, what is the likely effect of that information on your life?

4. Consider the following scenarios and describe what each child is learning.

   a. Alex is a 15-month-old who is developing walking, running, and climbing skills while actively exploring the environment. When Alex falls, the parents say, "Uh-oh," and Alex gets up and resumes exploring. Alex also now reacts to a fall by saying, "Uh-oh."

   b. The parent of Dhia, a 20-month-old toddler, frequently calls out, "Don't run. Don't climb on that. You'll fall and hurt yourself." When Dhia does fall and starts to cry, the parent picks the child up, often saying angrily, "You know you shouldn't do that!"

5. Based on your own experiences and those of your classmates, discuss how each of the following influences has contributed to your current patterns of behavior.

   a. Size and location of the city or cities in which you grew up

   b. Cultural or religious background of your parent(s) or guardian(s)

   c. The type of elementary, middle, and high schools you attended

   d. Sports, arts, or other community activities you participated in

   e. Friends or other groups with whom you spent time

6. Consider your current patterns of behavior. What are three habits or behaviors that you consider beneficial? What are three habits or behaviors you would like to change? For each behavior you would like to change, list one specific action you could take to begin changing that behavior.

References and Suggested Readings

Isen, J., Tuvblad, C., Younan, D., et al. (2022). Developmental trajectories of delinquent and aggressive behavior: Evidence for differential heritability. *Child Psychiatry Hum Dev, 53,* 199–211 https://doi.org/10.1007/s10578-020-01119-w.

National Center for Children in Poverty (NCCP). (2021). Facts about low income children: Children under 18 years, 2020. https://www.nccp.org/publication/basic-facts-about-low-income-children-children-under-18-years-2019/.

National Human Genome Research Institute. (2020). The human genome project. https://www.genome.gov/human-genome-project.

van Dongen, J., Hagenbeek, F. A., Suderman, M., et al. (2021). DNA methylation signatures of aggression and closely related constructs: A meta-analysis of epigenome-wide studies across the lifespan. *Mol Psychiatry, 26,* 2148–216. https://doi.org/10.1038/s41380-020-00987-x.

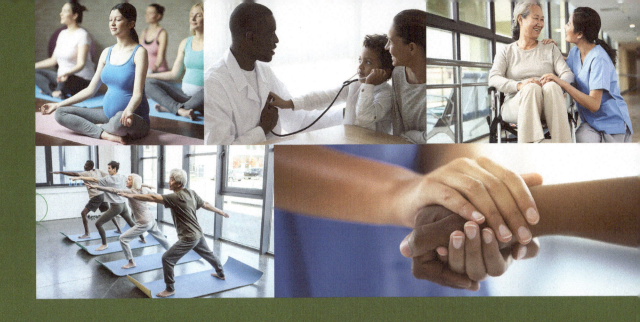

Physical Needs

Objectives

After completing this chapter, you should be able to:

- List the levels of human needs as proposed by Maslow.
- Explain why Maslow stated these needs as a hierarchy.
- List physical needs that are essential to survival.
- Describe safety needs.
- Explain behavior as an attempt to satisfy our needs.

Key Terms

Compensation
Consequences
Dehydration

Hierarchy
Necrosis

REM sleep
Suffocation

All humans share certain basic needs that we are driven to satisfy. However, we are all different in the ways we attempt to satisfy these needs. What satisfies one person may not satisfy another. Most patterns of behavior can be understood as a person's effort to fulfill one or more needs.

Psychologists and sociologists engaged in the study of human behavior have described these needs in various ways. The most useful approach for our purpose is the model provided by psychologist Abraham Maslow. This model is known as Maslow's Hierarchy of Needs.

Maslow's Hierarchy of Needs

Maslow's **hierarchy** identifies the following needs. Maslow theorized that each level of need must be satisfied before an individual can focus on satisfying of the next level of need:

1. Physiological or survival needs
2. Safety needs
3. Love, affection, and belongingness needs
4. Esteem needs
5. Need for self-actualization

This chapter discusses the physical needs, which include levels 1 and 2. Levels 3, 4, and 5 are discussed in Chapter 6.

Importance of the Hierarchy of Needs

Like other animals, humans are biologically programmed to survive. By instinct, we seek food, water, warmth, and safety. Until these needs are met, they will consume most or all of our time, energy, and attention, and we will find it difficult to focus on anything else. For example, children who lack food or who live in unsafe home environments often have difficulty concentrating on their assignments at school. Adults may worry about "putting food on the table" and "keeping a roof over the family's heads." In everyday conversation, we often refer to a preoccupation with maintaining these basic needs as "being in survival mode." Until individuals are able to consistently meet their physiological and safety needs and to feel secure that these needs will continue to be met, they will have difficulty pursuing the social and psychological needs described in levels 3, 4, and 5.

Physical Needs

Some physical needs are essential to life; others contribute to comfort and satisfaction. The physical needs that are essential to life are oxygen, water, food, protection, and sleep. These needs are not only essential to the life of the total organism, but also to the survival of individual cells. For example, a body part that does not receive a continuous supply of oxygen and nourishment will die. If this body part is a vital organ, then the individual will also die. If, however, the body part is a finger, the affected finger can be surgically removed and the individual will survive, minus the finger. Death of tissues in a limited area is called **necrosis**. It is usually due to lack of an adequate blood supply that deprives the cells of oxygen and nourishment. As you work in the health field, you may see patients with necrosis of some body part or area.

© Piateresca/Shutterstock.com

FIGURE 5-1 Maslow's hierarchy of needs: Maslow theorized that each level of need must be satisfied before an individual can focus on the next level of need.

Importance of Oxygen

The physical need for oxygen pertains to every cell in the body. Submersion of the face in water for more than a few minutes can result in death due to drowning. Although some people have been resuscitated after about 20 minutes under water, in such cases there is serious risk of permanent brain damage because the brain needs a continuous supply of oxygen. If deprivation of oxygen is due to the face being covered, as in a cave-in, the death is called a **suffocation**. Accidental drowning or suffocation may be the result of carelessness, failure to use appropriate precautions (e.g., not wearing a life jacket when going out in a boat), or inappropriate sleeping arrangements (in the case of a baby). The American Academy of Pediatrics recommends that babies be placed on their backs to sleep on a firm surface (in a crib or bassinet) without blankets or stuffed toys that could interfere with breathing.

Importance of Water

The body must have adequate water for various functions. More water is needed if you work or exercise vigorously or spend time outside during hot weather. Water provides liquid and is the carrier for various nutrients that cannot be digested and absorbed without a liquid medium. Eight to ten cups (64 to 80 ounces) of water is often recommended, but research shows that individual needs for water vary based on body size, physical activity, and other factors. One indicator of proper hydration is the color of the urine. Pale yellow or colorless urine indicates proper hydration, while dark yellow or orange urine may indicate dehydration. Note that some medications and nutritional supplements can change the color of the urine as well.

When the body does not receive adequate water each day, chronic **dehydration** develops, and certain body functions are affected. When the body loses water, as through diarrhea, persistent vomiting, or high fever, dehydration develops. Severe dehydration leads to an imbalance in body chemistry, a life-threatening condition. In hospitals, intravenous fluids are used for patients who cannot drink enough fluids to prevent dehydration. Persons who are stranded where there is no water available, as in a desert, can survive only a few days. For this reason, survival training includes learning how to extract water from plants and use liquids from other sources to maintain life until rescue help arrives.

Importance of Food

Because of its ability to store food in various tissues and organs, the body can survive without food for longer periods of time than it can survive without oxygen or water. Prolonged lack of food results in stored nutrients being used for basic metabolic processes and for the energy needed for physical activities. Even thinking requires energy! Muscle movement requires a lot of energy. If lack of food continues, tissues shrink and body wasting occurs. When body reserves have been exhausted, death occurs due to starvation.

Regular intake of food, then, is essential for providing the body with the nutrients needed to carry out metabolic processes, build and repair tissues, and produce energy for various activities. The nutrients needed include proteins, fats, carbohydrates, vitamins, minerals, amino acids, and essential fatty acids. Optimal health requires that *all* of these nutrients be included in one's daily diet, since even a slight deficiency of certain nutrients results in less efficient body functions.

Even more significant, a slight deficiency in certain nutrients, especially vitamins, minerals, and amino acids, can lead to symptoms. For example, a prolonged clotting time or a tendency to bruise easily may indicate a serious health problem or may simply indicate that the individual needs additional vitamin C or vitamin K. There is currently a trend in health care to acknowledge the relationship of certain nutrients to specific body functions. Health care professionals should become informed about nutrients in order to protect their own health and that of their families. Sometimes it may be appropriate to suggest dietary changes to a friend or patient or to recommend a consultation with a nutritionist.

The importance of nutrition gained additional urgency during the COVID-19 pandemic, which began in 2020. While data specific to COVID-19 continue to be gathered, researchers have pointed out that nutritional status is clearly linked to immunity, influencing a person's susceptibility to infection, severity of illness, and ease of recovery. For example, adequate intakes of zinc, selenium, and vitamin D have been associated with resistance to viral infections. At the same time, the nutritional status of many individuals declined during the lockdowns of 2020 due to decreased access to fresh foods, increased consumption of unhealthy foods, and reduced physical activity (Antwi, 2021).

Importance of Protection

In its broadest sense, protection includes the safety and security of having a home that protects one from the elements, using safety precautions to avoid accidents, having a lifestyle that includes healthful eating and drinking clean water, avoiding exposure to extremes of heat and cold, and avoiding substances that can harm the body.

Commonsense measures, such as avoiding times and places where one might be attacked and practicing safe driving, can decrease the likelihood of a serious accident or traumatic experience. Small children, especially, need protection against a variety of hazards in the community and in the home. It is a responsibility of adults to "child-proof" the home, so that children do not have access to household cleaners, medicines, and other harmful substances. Adults have a responsibility to provide safe and healthful lifestyles for themselves and their children.

For 2020, the Centers for Disease Control and Prevention (CDC) reported that accidents and unintentional injuries were the fourth-highest cause of death in the United States, causing over 200,000 deaths that year. Not all accidents can be avoided. However, maintaining safety in homes, schools, and workplaces can prevent many injuries.

Importance of Sleep

Sleep is essential to life and health, but people are more inclined to deprive themselves of sleep than of water, food, and air. The body's demand for sleep can be resisted, or even ignored, more easily than hunger, thirst, and the need for air. Of the various aspects of lifestyle that are *essential* to health, recent research indicates that sleep ranks third, behind diet and exercise.

Although individual needs for sleep vary, the average person needs one hour of sleep for every two hours of wakefulness. Sleep needs are biologically determined; a person who needs 10 hours of sleep is not "lazy" and will be healthier if that need is respected. On the other hand, persons who claim to need only a few hours of sleep per night place their health at risk. According to the CDC, lack of sleep can contribute to accidents, decrease efficiency, and increase the risk of depression and various chronic health conditions.

> **For Discussion and Reflection**
>
> Think about your usual sleep pattern. How many hours do you sleep on weeknights? On Saturday nights? On Sunday nights? If you are sleeping less than seven to eight hours each night, list reasons that you stay up too late to get a full night's sleep or get up before you have had seven to eight hours of sleep.

The CDC recommends the following amounts of sleep:

- 9–12 hours per night for school-age children
- 8–10 hours per night for teens
- 7 or more hours per night for adults

A third of adults in the United States reported sleeping less than the recommended amount (CDC, 2020). Chronic sleep deprivation can affect a person's emotions, behavior, and performance at school or work.

The Sleep Cycle

Sleep consists of two phases that alternate throughout the sleep period: **REM sleep** and non-REM sleep. The latter phase is a period when most body processes slow down, the muscles are relaxed, and the eyes are relatively still. This phase includes four stages of progressively deeper sleep. Following a complete cycle of the four stages, the REM (rapid eye movement) phase begins. In this phase, there is an increase in mental activity, dreaming occurs concurrently with bursts of rapid eye movement, breathing is irregular, and pulse and blood pressure rise and fall. In normal young adults, the first non-REM phase lasts about 90 minutes and is followed by about 15 minutes of REM sleep. The frequency and duration of REM sleep periods increase during the final hours of sleep, especially between the sixth and eighth hours.

The dreaming that occurs during REM sleep is thought to be a major factor in stress management. The entire sleep period is a time when the brain cleanses itself of the day's accumulated sensory input and prepares for the next day's mental activity; it is also the time when the brain replenishes its stock of neurotransmitters. Although people vary in the amount of sleep they need to awaken rested and refreshed, less than eight hours of sleep deprives the body of some periods of REM sleep. Research conducted in sleep laboratories has revealed that deprivation of REM sleep has the same effects as sleep deprivation.

Effects of Sleep Deprivation

After the loss of one night of sleep, a person has poor concentration and coordination; usually irritability is increased. Anyone who is deprived of sleep for several days will experience hallucinations and exhibit psychotic behavior.

Sleep deprivation is an increasing problem in American society. The temptations of television and social media are causing large numbers of people to get as little as two or three hours of sleep per night.

Some health care professionals work double shifts, and those who regularly work the night shift may experience 24- to 30-hour periods without sleep before or after their days off. These people should make a special effort to ensure adequate sleep and rest, for both personal health and avoidance of errors due to fatigue and lack of sleep.

Satisfaction of Physical Needs

Physical needs have an important characteristic that sets them apart from psychological needs—*they can be satisfied in only one way.* An abundant supply of oxygen cannot make up for a lack of food. Abundant food stored within body tissues cannot provide survival for the worker who has just been buried in a cave-in and has no supply of oxygen. The need for sleep can be satisfied only by sleeping; though eating may enable one to delay going to sleep, food cannot satisfy the body's need for sleep. *Each essential physical need can be met only by a specific substance or condition.* Neither substitution nor **compensation** is possible. In contrast, people often use compensation or substitution to address social and emotional needs when they are not able to meet the actual need directly. Social and emotional needs will be explored in the upcoming chapters.

Comfort and Safety Needs

There are also physical needs that we very much want to meet but that are not essential to life. These needs are related to comfort and a sense of well-being. Labor-saving devices, soundly built homes, running water, comfortable clothing, and automatic heat seem like essential needs to those who are accustomed to them. Though some of these comforts are not essential for survival, they do meet safety needs and contribute to health and well-being.

The satisfaction of sexual needs falls into two categories: emotional needs and physical needs. Intimacy can contribute to a sense of belonging—an especially important need of adolescents. Sexual activity was formerly considered an adult activity, but currently many young people—adolescents and children—are sexually active. This is an issue for families and individuals to address in terms of beliefs and standards of behavior. The issue of *responsibility,* however, extends beyond the family to the larger community because of health issues and the risk of pregnancies that produce children who are unwanted or whose parents cannot or will not provide for them.

Anyone who is sexually active, regardless of age, should practice safe sex. For young people who are not prepared to assume the adult responsibilities of parenting (which includes financial support), prevention of pregnancy requires the use of protection. For everyone who is sexually active but is not in a stable, one-partner relationship, responsibility means protecting oneself against sexually transmitted diseases. Safe sex, then, has two very important purposes: (1) avoidance of an unwanted pregnancy and (2) prevention of a sexually transmitted disease.

Physical Needs and Behavior

Each person has specific ways they try to meet needs. The baby cries when hungry but is dependent on others to provide nourishment. Throughout childhood each of us learned which behaviors were successful or unsuccessful in meeting our needs within the home and in the subculture. *The child tends to repeat any behavior that results in satisfaction of a need and to abandon behaviors that do not get results.* Behavior patterns are established on the basis of **consequences**—what happens following a specific behavior.

If you find yourself or someone else repeating a particular pattern of behavior, try to identify the consequence (outcome) that reinforces the behavior. A typical example is a young child whining for candy at the store. If the parent first says "no" but later buys the candy to stop the child's whining, the parent has reinforced the behavior of whining. The child has learned that whining gets them what they want.

Cultural Influences

A person living in a city may purchase food at the grocery store but is dependent upon a complex system of marketing and distribution to keep a supply available. A person living in a rural area may purchase only staples and depend on a garden and livestock to provide most of the family's food. A family living in a large city with an income below the federal poverty level may depend upon public services for food. Patterns of behavior used to meet these needs are learned in childhood and influenced by the customs and practices of the family, neighborhood, and community. Patterns of behavior are also influenced by individual factors, such as the desire to obtain the comforts of life and the value placed on conforming to group standards.

For Discussion and Reflection

1. If you have children, have you ever "given in" to negative behavior as described? If you do not have children, think of ways you have seen adults complain or threaten to get what they want from others.
2. When someone receives what they want as a result of a negative behavior, how likely are they to continue using negative behaviors in the future?

A

B

FIGURE 5-2 Our life situation influences behavior patterns for meeting basic needs.

Understanding Behavior in Terms of Physical Needs

There are certain physical needs that people must meet in order to survive. There are other needs that make people more comfortable or free them from routine tasks so they may do other things that are more satisfying. In having these needs, people are alike. In the specific ways they meet these needs, people are different. Each person behaves in ways that have been learned by imitating members of one's subculture and from personal experiences. Each person tends to repeat the behavior that has been successful in satisfying a particular need. This repetition becomes established as a behavior pattern.

Most people meet their needs in ways that are acceptable within the laws, customs, and religious beliefs of their group. Some people choose or are forced by circumstances to violate the laws or customs of the group in order to satisfy their needs. These people may be meeting their needs in the only way they know. Here, too, the health care professional's philosophy of individual worth can be applied to understanding, rather than judging, a patient.

Activities

1. List the five human needs proposed by Maslow, giving an example of a need for each level.

2. Explain in your own words why physiological and safety needs must be met before individuals can focus on the needs at Maslow's levels 3, 4, and 5.

3. If you have ever experienced any of the following, describe how it affected you physically, mentally, and emotionally.

    a. Difficulty in getting air for several minutes

    b. No water (or any other beverage) for eight hours

    c. No way to obtain food for two days

    d. Exposure to severe weather, without any way to get to shelter for several hours

    e. Deprivation of sleep for 36 hours

4. Think of a situation in your community where someone died due to an accident or injury. Using all the information available to your class, discuss the circumstances and identify actions individuals or the community could take to protect others from similar dangers in the future.

5. Consider your own cultural background, including your family of origin and the community in which you grew up. How did your family and others in the community go about meeting their needs for food, shelter, and safety? If you have lived in different communities, what differences have you observed in the ways people meet these basic needs?

References and Suggested Readings

American Academy of Pediatrics. (2022). *Tips for keeping infants safe during sleep from the American Academy of Pediatrics.* https://www.aap.org/en/news-room/news-releases/aap/2020/tips-for-keeping-infants-safe-during-sleep-from-the-american-academy-of-pediatrics/.

Antwi, J., Appiah, B., Oluwakuse, B., & Abu, B. A. Z. (2021, December). The nutrition-COVID-19 interplay: A review. *Current Nutritional Reports, 10*(4), 364–374. doi: 10.1007/s13668-021-00380-2. Erratum in *Current Nutritional Reports* (2021, December 14).

Centers for Disease Control and Prevention (CDC). (2017). How much sleep do I need? https://www.cdc.gov/sleep/about_sleep/how_much_sleep.html.

Centers for Disease Control and Prevention (CDC). (2020). Sleep and sleep disorders. https://www.cdc.gov/sleep/index.html.

Centers for Disease Control and Prevention (CDC). (2022). Leading causes of death. https://www.cdc.gov/nchs/fastats/leading-causes-of-death.htm.

Merck & Co. (2022). Symptoms and signs of nutritional deficiency. *Merck Manual, Professional Version.* https://www.merckmanuals.com/professional/multimedia/table/symptoms-and-signs-of-nutritional-deficiency.

U.S. Department of Agriculture. (2020). 2020–2025 dietary guidelines for Americans. https://www.dietaryguidelines.gov/sites/default/files/2020-12/Dietary_Guidelines_for_Americans_2020-2025.pdf.

Social and Emotional Needs

Objectives

After completing this chapter, you should be able to:

- Explain social needs.
- Define self-concept, self-esteem, and self-awareness.
- Discuss how success and failure, goal setting, problem solving, and establishing good habits contribute to self-actualization.
- Describe how environment and culture shape the ways we seek to fulfil social and emotional needs.
- Discuss ways to practice social/emotional competence as a health care professional.

Key Terms

Aptitudes

Autonomy

Compensation

Conformity

Empathy

Martyr complex

Self-awareness

Self-concept

Sympathy

Remember Maslow's Hierarchy of Needs? In Chapter 5, we discussed physical needs, which include levels 1 and 2 of the hierarchy. This chapter discusses level 3, love and belongingness; level 4, esteem needs; and level 5, self-actualization. These social and emotional needs are just as important to comfort and happiness as physical needs, though they are less obvious. As we discussed in Chapter 5, most human behavior is an attempt to meet a need. However, people use a variety of behaviors to meet their social and emotional needs, based on their own unique blend of heredity, cultural and environmental influences, previous experiences, and personal preferences.

Social Needs

For the most part, physical needs can be met either alone or in the company of others. However, sharing with others is more satisfying than meeting these needs alone. You enjoy your dinner more if you have pleasant company than if you eat alone or with someone you dislike. When physical needs and social needs are met simultaneously, you are more likely to experience enjoyment and a sense of well-being.

Types of Social/Emotional Needs

The third level of Maslow's Hierarchy of Needs is love and belongingness. This level includes social/emotional needs, which can be met through interactions with other people. There are many kinds of social/emotional needs: psychological, emotional, intellectual, spiritual, and recreational. These terms overlap because each term refers to groups of needs that are closely related.

Some social needs can be partially met alone, but relationships with other people are necessary for full satisfaction. For example, the person who enjoys studying a subject can partially meet intellectual needs alone. Greater satisfaction might be experienced, however, if there are opportunities to discuss the subject with others who share the same interest. *Satisfying relationships with other people lead to full satisfaction of the social/emotional needs.*

Some social/emotional needs are related to the self; other needs are related to contact with other people. Each of us needs to feel important as a person, to have a sense of achievement, and to feel worthy. We also need to feel that we are important to others, that other people approve of us, and that we are accepted as a member of the group.

A

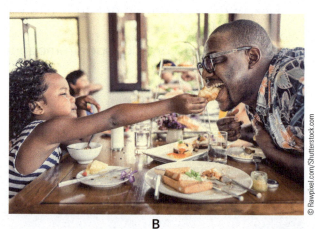

B

FIGURE 6-1 Basic physical needs can be met alone, while social needs are met by interacting with others.

Compensation

You have learned that each of the physical needs can be met only in a specific way. With the social/emotional needs, a type of substitution known as **compensation** is possible. It is important to remember, however, that *compensation does not satisfy a basic need*; it is a device that provides temporary relief from the discomfort felt when a basic social/emotional need is not being met.

Do you know a person who habitually talks loudly, tends to brag, is a showoff, or dresses in flashy clothes? Is this person popular? Is this person accepted by the group? Probably not, for these are attention-seeking behaviors. For some people it is better to be noticed, even disapprovingly, than to be ignored. Behavior that gets attention can relieve the inner discomfort of being ignored. Attention-seeking behavior is an example of compensation. This behavior temporarily relieves inner discomfort and gains attention from the group. Obtaining approval meets a basic need; getting attention compensates for not gaining approval. People who compensate are usually unaware that they are getting temporary relief from inner discomfort instead of the full satisfaction that comes only from meeting basic social/emotional needs.

The Importance of Acceptance

Social/emotional needs can be met fully only through satisfying relationships with other people. Satisfaction of social/emotional needs requires both self-approval and approval and acceptance by others. The person who has achieved self-approval finds it easier to gain approval and acceptance by others. On the other hand, acceptance by others makes us feel more comfortable with ourselves. So these two needs are closely tied together; the person who can grow in self-approval can become increasingly acceptable to others and vice versa.

Each of us needs to believe that others accept us as a worthwhile person. To satisfy this need, we must see and hear expressions of approval from time to time, in order to remain convinced of this acceptance. We also need to believe that others understand our viewpoint, our feelings, and our problems. Obviously, satisfying the need for acceptance requires receiving indications of approval and caring from other people.

Friendships develop and are maintained on the basis of whether or not two people meet each other's needs. Ideally, a relationship between two people involves a balance of give-and-take. This ideal can be met only if the behavior of each person helps the other to satisfy basic social/emotional needs. In some relationships, the balance of give-and-take appears to be one-sided. One person exerts much effort to please the other and seems to get little in return. If the relationship continues over a long period without a change in this balance, both parties are satisfying certain needs. Self-sacrificing behavior is sometimes referred to as the **martyr complex**, meaning that the individual actually derives satisfaction from being taken advantage of by another person.

To a great extent, we can understand our behavior and that of others in terms of basic needs—behaviors that satisfy a basic need, and behaviors that compensate for not being able to satisfy a basic need. Usually, a person puts up with certain circumstances or with

For Discussion and Reflection

Have you or someone you know experienced a relationship (either as a friend or as a romantic partner) in which one person seemed to repeatedly take advantage of the other? If this pattern continued over time, what needs do you think each person in the relationship was meeting?

the behavior of others because some need is being met. Perhaps compensation is taking place. Perhaps the need is unhealthy, as illustrated by martyr behavior. If no need is being met, the individual will usually engage in behavior that either changes the situation or provides escape.

The Importance of Approval from Others

Have you ever expected to be praised for something you did, but instead you were criticized? How did it make you feel? How did you behave? How did you feel about the person who was critical instead of approving? This person, in failing to give approval, deprived you of a basic need. Each of us has had such experiences. The one who failed to give us our earned approval may have been a parent, friend, classmate, teacher, or boss. The hurt associated with such experiences is proportional to the importance we attach to the other person.

Now consider the other side of the coin. Have you ever had a friend show you something new, yet you failed to express approval? Has a friend ever won an honor, but for some reason you could not bring yourself to offer congratulations? If so, you were depriving this person of approval. Why did you withhold your approval?

Hunger for Approval

Being deprived of approval early in life can create a hunger for approval that never seems satisfied. Do you know someone who "looks for compliments"? How do you feel about this person? Seeking compliments usually indicates a strong need for expressions of approval. The next time you observe such behavior, will you recognize the need for approval? Assuming it is deserved, will you express your approval freely and sincerely? If so, you will be helping that person meet an important need. You will be contributing to that person's inner comfort, but the cost to you is only the effort it takes to state your sincere approval.

The Need to Believe That Others Care

Another social/emotional need that requires appropriate responses from other people is the need to believe that other people care. The extent to which we believe that someone cares about us influences how we feel about that person. Expressions of caring promote strong ties between people.

Sympathy   As a health care professional, you will be hearing the terms **sympathy** and **empathy**. Perhaps you think of sympathy as "feeling sorry for someone." Actually, few people want or expect pity from others, and some would react to expressions of pity with anger. But most people, when sick or experiencing some type of difficulty, need to believe that their loved ones and friends care, share their feelings, and regret that they are having a bad experience. Sympathy, then, implies sharing and feeling with another, while retaining one's own point of view.

Empathy   Empathy is similar to *some* of the meanings of sympathy, but it is not the same. Empathy means identifying with another person in such a way that we see another person's situation from their point of view, rather than from our own perspective.

As a health care professional you will be exposed to many situations in which an effort to feel empathy for the patient and the family—*to see the situation as they see it*—will help you understand their behavior. Most patients do not want others to feel sorry for them. They *do* want others to care about them, to understand what they are experiencing, and to care about their feelings and beliefs.

The Need for Appreciation

Each of us needs to believe that someone appreciates us. We especially need to feel appreciated by those who are important to us. Appreciation may mean "being grateful," by saying "thank you," or "having respect," as shown by the statement "She has great appreciation for modern art."

Expressing appreciation might indicate either of these meanings and might even imply approval or caring as well. For example, a child's first attempt to help with a household task will be unsuccessful by adult standards, yet the child may be proud of the effort. The adult reaction will affect future efforts. For a positive effect, the parent could show gratitude for the attempt to be helpful, could show respect for the child's effort, or could show caring and pleasure related to the child's intent to help. All of these should be shown sincerely, even though the result of the child's performance may not meet adult standards.

Expressions of approval, appreciation, and caring provide a sense of satisfaction. The absence of any such expressions can have as negative an effect as open criticism or disapproval. If a task has been attempted but not performed well, sincere *approval* cannot be given; yet it is quite likely that an expression of *appreciation* would be appropriate. If suggestions for improvement are needed, these suggestions are less likely to appear as criticism if they are preceded by an expression of appreciation, caring, and understanding. Thus, there are some situations where approval should be expressed, but indications of appreciation or caring are not necessary. At other times, approval is not needed or has not been earned, but appreciation could be shown. Sometimes neither approval nor appreciation can be expressed, yet an expression of caring would be appropriate.

Our social/emotional needs are interrelated. The person who is aware of the importance of social/emotional needs will recognize opportunities to contribute to the satisfaction of another's needs. The person who is unaware may blunder through life, experiencing frequent frustrating, awkward, or unsatisfying interactions with others.

Self Esteem, Self-Concept, and Self-Awareness

Each of us has an image of "self." We think of ourselves as a certain kind of person, possessing specific characteristics. **Self-concept** may be thought of as all the things a person thinks are true about the self. It is a mental image of "me." Self-esteem refers to our *feelings about self at a given moment* and is often based on recent experiences. Self-awareness refers to the ability to identify our own thoughts, feelings, and beliefs and to identify how these influence our own behavior.

Behavior as an Indicator of Self-Concept

The person with a realistic self-concept thinks of the self in terms that are consistent with their behavior. Usually, behavior is an accurate indicator of a person's self-concept. The person who has a realistic self-concept can be honest about the real self. Such a person's behavior accurately reflects the person's own beliefs, values, and standards.

The person whose self-concept is unrealistic is not ready to set goals for personal growth until the self-concept has been revised. "What is" must be acknowledged before considering "what can be." An unrealistic self-concept may be either idealized or self-derogatory.

For example, Amina has great difficulty with high school subjects, but thinks of herself as a person who can do anything she attempts. Her ambition is to be a scientist. Amina's *idealized self-concept* may trap her into setting goals that she cannot achieve. In contrast, Enrique is an excellent student but lacks self-confidence. He has an older sibling who is a good student and an outstanding athlete. Because Enrique has always compared himself unfavorably with his sibling, he thinks of himself as a second-rate person, yet he has tremendous potential and can probably succeed in any field of study he undertakes. Enrique has a derogatory *self-concept*, meaning that he is overly critical of himself and does not fully recognize his abilities and talents. Unless Enrique revises his self-perception, he may settle for goals less challenging than those he could achieve.

Building a Realistic Self-Concept

A realistic self-concept requires conscious and thoughtful consideration of "what is." By honestly appraising your strengths and weaknesses, identifying your interests, and clarifying your values, you will get in touch with the "real you." This is the starting point for planning ways to develop your potential and gaining greater satisfaction from living.

Formation of the Self-Concept

The self-concept begins to form at a very early age and is well established by about age 6. The self-concept is greatly affected by all life experiences, but it is most susceptible to the influence of other people *during the early formative years and during adolescence.* The young child's relationships with other people establish the early pattern. Is the child considered a person with rights and feelings? Many adults demand expressions of courtesy from a child yet fail to use courteous behavior toward the child.

A positive self-concept develops if the young child has positive experiences and positive verbal interactions with the important adults of their social environment:

"You are sweet."

"I love you."

"You are so strong."

"You are special."

"It's fun being with you."

"I like for you to ask questions."

Busy adults may forget to tell children that they are loved and are important. Children need to hear such positive statements to think of themselves as loved and are important to other people. Children also need positive nonverbal messages: hugs and kisses, a squeeze of the hand, a pat on the shoulder, and other appropriate forms of touch. The most important message is conveyed through time spent with the child, time in which the child is the primary focus of a parent's attention. Parents should plan for quality time with the child each day—reading, playing, walking, and talking.

The form of discipline used with a child also has an extensive influence on the child's self-concept. If children are repeatedly told that they are "bad," they begin to think of themselves as being "bad." Why try to be "good" if you have learned to think yourself as "bad" and you believe that everyone expects you to be "bad"?

During adolescence, the peer group exerts a powerful influence on self-concept. Teens experience pressure to conform to the group's standards and values. Adolescents may label those who do not conform. Even if peers do not actively pressure them to conform, teens may feel an internal sense of pressure to be like others they see in the community or on social media. A teenager must have a strong self-concept to resist those pressures, to stand up for personal beliefs and values, and at the same time gain acceptance from the peer group.

In these and many other ways, the people around a young child mold the developing child's self-concept. In the following sections, we will explore three aspects of personality development: independence (being a strong, capable person), dependence (being a person who relies excessively on others), and interdependence (being someone who interacts and works together effectively with others). The tendency to remain dependent on others, versus the ability to be self-reliant while still working cooperatively with others, influences a person's self-concept.

Learning Independence

One of the most important aspects of development during childhood and adolescence is a gradual increase in independence, with less and less dependence on others. The need for self-reliance is an inborn force. Many infant behaviors reflect the need for this type of development: efforts at self-feeding, attempts to help with dressing and undressing, and attempts to "do it myself!" A child's angry reaction when an adult interferes in something the child is trying to do reflects this need for independence.

Autonomy, Dependence, and Interdependence The struggle between self-reliance and dependence on others continues throughout life. Each of us has a need for **autonomy**, the ability to function independently without outside control. No one ever achieves complete autonomy. We are social beings, and in many ways our welfare depends upon our being able to function as a member of the group. The mature person has learned to live harmoniously with their fellow humans, functioning autonomously in many ways and accepting that dependence on others for some things is a matter of necessity.

Autonomy must be achieved over time, by gradually learning to be self-reliant in the simple tasks of daily living (e.g., dressing and eating) and then progressing to self-reliance in more complex situations. It is impossible to be dependent on others throughout childhood and adolescence and then suddenly, at age 18 or 21, become a self-directing, autonomous adult. Effective parenting provides for the gradual development of independence throughout childhood by encouraging the child to do simple tasks. It also requires being available when help is requested, or frustration becomes more than the child can handle.

This struggle for a compromise between autonomy and dependence reaches its peak during adolescence. The young person struggling for autonomy rebels against dependence on others. The parents may resent the young person's insisting on greater independence than they believe the child can handle. Young people who do not successfully resolve this conflict may carry the struggle for autonomy into adulthood, usually as rebellion toward any form of authority, such as the teacher or the "boss." You may find it interesting to study examples of rebellious behavior in terms of the struggle for autonomy.

In addition to developing autonomy throughout childhood and adolescence, individuals begin to develop skills for working together effectively with others. The psychological need for independence is complemented by the realization that we are also interdependent, needing the help and cooperation of others to survive and thrive. For a young child, learning interdependence takes the form of learning to share toys, take turns, and follow the rules when playing a game. For many children and adolescents, team sports and group activities such as scouting or band provide opportunities to develop interdependence. As adults, we benefit from working cooperatively with others at our jobs and in our communities.

For both children and adults, the appropriate balance between independence and interdependence varies greatly based on family, community, and cultural values. For some, an extremely high value is placed on "being yourself" and choosing your own interests, beliefs, career, and more. For other families and cultures, following the expectations of the family and community is emphasized above personal satisfaction and fulfilment. As an individual, it is up to you to decide which values to live by: your own, those of your community, or a combination of the two. As a health care professional, you should be aware that some clients may value their autonomy highly, while some may value the expectations of family and community above their own personal wants and needs.

For Discussion and Reflection

If you are a parent, how have you encouraged your child to develop independence by doing tasks for themselves? If you are not a parent, recall a task your own parents encouraged you to do independently.

Self-Esteem

Self-esteem is closely related to self-concept but is not the same. Although self-concept is established during the early years and is relatively permanent, self-esteem is quite changeable and is affected by life experiences. A person's self-esteem may be high in the morning; then some negative experience may plunge that person's self-esteem to a very low point. For most people, a period of low self-esteem is short-lived. If a negative experience, such as being unemployed, extends over a period of weeks, then self-esteem may remain low throughout that period. Effectively dealing with a life problem usually restores self-esteem to a high level. Good life experiences tend to maintain self-esteem at a high level, whereas negative experiences can lower a person's self-esteem.

For Discussion and Reflection

Have you had a teacher, coach, relative, or friend who inspired you or helped you recognize your own strengths? What did this person do or say that contributed to your self-concept?

You should now become more aware of the role others play in determining how you feel about yourself at a particular time. Your interactions with some people almost always make you feel good. Some people say and do things that make you feel good about yourself. Other people tend to have the opposite effect: They make put-down statements, are often critical, play the one-upmanship game, or otherwise have a diminishing effect on your sense of self.

FIGURE 6-2 Interactions with other people can have a negative or positive effect on self-esteem.

If there are many such people in your daily life, you are probably struggling to maintain a positive level of self-esteem. In order to correct the situation, you have certain choices:

1. Avoid such people.
2. Be assertive about not accepting negative statements.
3. Learn ways to respond to communications that have a negative effect on you.

Obviously, the first choice is not available to you if members of your family or your coworkers have a negative effect on you. In that case, you can begin to learn how to deal with such people through various activities, such as reading about effective relationships and participating in assertiveness training and communication skills.

In summary, positive relationships can help one to develop a strong self-concept and maintain high self-esteem most of the time. Negative relationships can have a destructive effect on self-concept and may result in a chronic state of low self-esteem.

Self-Actualization

The fifth level of Maslow's hierarchy of needs is *self-actualization*, fulfilling your potential and becoming the best you can be. Having a satisfying life depends largely on how you define success for yourself, how you approach challenges and obstacles, and how you handle the disappointments and losses that are inevitable parts of everyone's life.

Effects of Success and Failure

Have you ever had a task so difficult that you did not believe you could complete it? Perhaps it was a reading assignment that just did not make sense when you read it. Perhaps it was a written assignment, and you did not know how to proceed.

What was your approach to this task that appeared so hopeless? Did you try your best and find that you could do it, after all? How did you feel about your accomplishment? You should have felt good, for you overcame obstacles and successfully completed a difficult task. Each successful experience should be consciously recognized as a success. Each success should help you believe in *yourself as a person who can overcome obstacles.*

On the other hand, you may have found a particular task just as hard as you expected and were unable to complete it. No doubt you still have some negative feelings about this experience. Perhaps you were angry at yourself for not finishing it. Perhaps you were angry with the person who assigned the task to you. In either case, your self-confidence was threatened. You were discouraged and probably approached the next difficult task with greater self-doubt.

Meaning of Failure Expectation Discouragement and a sense of failure can be quite damaging to self-confidence, especially if they are experienced frequently. But this is only part of the problem. When failure occurs too frequently, there is a tendency to develop "failure expectation." Each failure adds to self-doubt; self-doubt creates failure expectation; failure expectation interferes with performance. Thus, there is an increased probability that the next task will result in another failure. If this cycle becomes well established, the individual may need professional help to break the pattern and believe in the possibility of future successful performances.

Success Expectation For most people, however, the problem is lack of self-confidence rather than an established failure expectation. Self-confidence might be thought of as "success expectation." The key to building self-confidence is recognizing that life includes both successful experiences and disappointing experiences. Self-confidence also comes through practicing a growth mindset, the belief that with work and practice, you can learn and improve your skills. Viewed from a growth mindset, an obstacle or failure, while frustrating, is an opportunity to learn, to improve your skills, or to try a new approach.

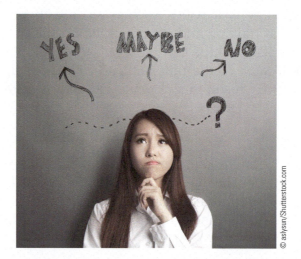

FIGURE 6-3 An obstacle is an opportunity to learn, to improve your skills, or to try a new approach.

It is possible to use such experiences as opportunities to identify factors that may have contributed to an undesirable outcome:

- Did I begin the task without proper preparation?
- Did I attempt to do the task too rapidly? Did I give enough attention to details (or technique)?
- Did I allow too little time for the task?
- Did I use efficient work habits? If not, what work habits might have been more effective?
- Did I use the appropriate method for this task? If not, what method would have been better?
- Did I give up too soon?
- Did I have control over the outcome, or was the outcome controlled by someone else?

Successful experiences in life make it easier to accept the occasional failures that all of us have. If you can maintain a reasonable balance between successes and failures and experience satisfaction after each success, then your self-esteem will likely be high most of the time, and any periods of low self-esteem will be brief.

Defining Success Do you think of "success" as making a lot of money, gaining power, having an expensive car, or perhaps becoming a social media influencer? Only a few people get to the top, and some of those who do get to the top in their field find that their "success" does not provide happiness.

Influence of Success Each of us has many opportunities for success if we recognize daily accomplishments and grant ourselves the right to feel good about them. Each time a job is done well, you should feel inner satisfaction. If others notice and express approval, this should add to your enjoyment. But even when you do not gain approval from others, you should feel good when you know, deep inside, that you did a job well.

If you recognize and acknowledge daily successes, each one will build your self-confidence and prepare you for succeeding in the next task you undertake. Each success diminishes the probability that self-doubt will interfere with success in future undertakings.

> **For Discussion and Reflection**
>
> How do you define success? Describe a past experience in which you felt successful. Now consider your definition of future success. What would a successful career or life look like to you?

Developing Problem-Solving Skills

You can also deal with problems more effectively by using a systematic method. The following steps to choosing successful behavior can be applied to a variety of situations:

1. Identify the problem. Think it through. Discuss it with someone who might help you understand it or see the problem in a new light. Write out a statement of the problem.
2. Collect information and/or ideas that might help you understand the problem better.

3. Consider all available information, then look at your statement of the problem. Reconsider what the problem is and rewrite the statement, if necessary.

4. Write down every imaginable solution. In a second column beside each possible solution, write out the possible consequences of trying that solution.

5. Select the solution that seems most likely to lead to the desired outcome and carry out the actions required.

6. Evaluate the outcome. If the result was not satisfactory, try another solution that appears likely to succeed.

> **Note**
>
> At this point, your perception of the problem may have changed completely. You may eventually see the problem as being entirely different from what you initially thought.

It requires practice to become skillful in using a problem-solving approach, but if you apply it to daily problems, you will soon become skillful in thinking through these steps. In other words, thinking through a problem may become a work habit. Skill in problem solving enables a person to choose a specific behavior for a desired result.

Setting Goals

Your true interests and **aptitudes** influence the success you are likely to experience and the satisfaction you are likely to gain from certain types of activities. Each of us tends to do best those things that we enjoy doing. Also, we learn more easily and perform best those activities for which we have an aptitude. A realistic appraisal of "what is" provides the foundation for setting goals, or "what may be."

Goals that are in accordance with your true interests and aptitudes are more likely to be achieved than goals set for you by someone else. If your goals offer a challenge, then reaching them will provide much satisfaction—the feeling of having overcome obstacles and of being a person who can achieve goals. This is self-approval. When goals are too high for your aptitudes or readiness, then you may experience disappointment, failure, and self-doubt. Goals that are too low are easily reached, do not challenge you to develop your potential, and provide only limited satisfaction.

It is desirable to have both short-range and long-range goals. Short-range goals are the stepping stones that lead to long-range goals. If Carissa wants to study medicine and is qualified to do so, her high school curriculum and college courses will be a series of short-range goals leading to the long-range goal of becoming a physician. If there are financial problems, Carissa may use a health occupations course as a short-term goal, obtaining job skills that enable her to work part time while attending college. Thus, Carissa may eventually reach her long-range goal through a series of intermediate goals. Intermediate goals provide inner satisfaction and a sense of achievement that can help one persist in striving for the long-range goal.

Modifying Habits

In order to build self-confidence, you must be realistic. You have many, many personal traits. Some are so highly developed that they characterize you as a person; in trying to describe you, someone would mention those traits. Other traits are not so prominent, but can be developed if you give your attention to them. Some traits are favorable; others are unfavorable. Try to identify the traits that will help you as a person and as a health care professional and strive to develop those traits to a high degree. Also, identify those traits that hold you back and work to minimize or eliminate them from your behavior patterns.

It takes persistence to replace an undesirable habit with a more desirable one. The following steps can help:

1. Identify the habit you want to change.
2. Identify the function, or purpose, that the habit serves. Does it help you relax? Reward yourself? Avoid an undesirable task?
3. Select a replacement behavior that serves the same function as the bad habit without the negative effects.
4. Develop a plan or routine for when you will use the replacement behavior.
5. Start small, but be consistent. For example, if beginning an exercise routine, start with just five or ten minutes, but do it every day.
6. As your new behavior becomes a habit, add to it if appropriate. For example, gradually lengthen your exercise session.

For Discussion and Reflection

Have you ever worked to change a bad habit? Were you successful? If so, what strategies helped you change your habit?

Environmental and Cultural Influences on Social/Emotional Needs

Just as people fulfil the physical and safety needs described in Chapter 5 in a variety of ways, people also fulfil social and emotional needs is ways that are consistent with their preferences, beliefs, and values. For most people, family, community, and culture play a significant role in shaping the way social and emotional needs are met. Some of the factors that are shaped by our environment and culture include:

- Our attitude toward time
- Our understanding of family, including our responsibilities toward family
- Religious and spiritual beliefs
- Definition of success
- The importance of individual fulfillment versus meeting social expectations

If you are aware that cultural differences influence people's behavior in these and other areas, you can more easily resolve potential misunderstandings. For example, in some cultures, if you are invited to someone's home at 7 P.M., you are expected to arrive promptly or to call if you are running late. In other cultures, arriving an hour or more after the stated time would be completely acceptable.

In some cultures and families, children are encouraged to discover their own interests and choose their own college major and career field. In other cultures and families, young people are expected to conform to their family's expectations about college studies, career fields, or even whom to marry. Success may be defined as "finding what makes you happy," or it may be defined as having a highly respected and well-paying job, regardless of personal happiness.

Likewise, some cultures place high value on individualism, or "being your own person," while other cultures value a person primarily in terms of their contribution to the group—the family, the community, or the company that employs them. As you interact with individuals from diverse backgrounds and cultures, you can benefit from being curious and willing to learn about their beliefs, values, and experiences, especially when those are different from your own. At the same time, keep in mind that even among people from the same or a similar cultural background, personal beliefs, values, and preferences can vary greatly.

Conformity

Conformity means acting in accordance with the behaviors, beliefs, and values of a specific group. Conformity expectations of group members may extend to lifestyle choices, including manner of dress, food, sexual behavior, and relationships with the group's authority figures. In groups that emphasize conformity, individuality is not valued and may be perceived as rebellion against the group's beliefs. The person who "dares to be different" may be excluded from the group; if allowed to remain within the group, that person may be viewed with suspicion and watched closely for evidence of unacceptable behavior.

Being overly concerned about conformity places one at risk of allowing others to make decisions that mature people make for themselves. A person who readily accepts the opinions of others, without becoming informed and giving thought to the situation, depends upon conformity as a means of gaining acceptance.

Importance of Acceptance during Adolescence

Have you ever arrived at a party and found you were dressed differently from most of those present? Perhaps you dressed casually and the others "dressed up." If you were among friends, you were probably not overly uncomfortable. But if you were trying to gain acceptance by the members of this group, discovering that you dressed inappropriately may have made you very uncomfortable.

During adolescence the need for acceptance by the peer group is very strong, and conformity is almost necessary to gain acceptance. Parents are often distressed to find that their teenager is more concerned about the opinions of friends than about their parents' beliefs. Some people never outgrow depending on conformity to win the acceptance of the group to which they wish to belong.

Rawpixel.com/Shutterstock.com

FIGURE 6-4 During adolescence the need for acceptance by the peer group is very strong.

Social/Emotional Competence for Health Care Professionals

For health care professionals, being aware of the social/emotional needs of others can mean the difference between effective and ineffective relations with patients and their families. People under the physical and psychological stress of illness are more likely to cope with their illness successfully if caregivers help them meet social and emotional needs, as well as physical needs.

As a health care professional, you can be more effective if you study human behavior. Perhaps you are now more aware of the complexity of human behavior. One person seeks approval by strict conformity to a group's standards of behavior, another by getting good grades, another by acquiring symbols of success, another by doing favors for people, and still another by being the life of the party. Some people find effective patterns of behavior that lead to self-approval and acceptance by others. Some people compensate with behavior that temporarily relieves their inner discomfort but fails to satisfy basic social/emotional needs.

All behavior is caused; it does not just happen. However, it is seldom possible to pinpoint one particular cause of a specific action. The causes of behavior are numerous and complex. Some of these causes lie in the situation in which the behavior occurs; other causes are within the individual, as a result of past experiences and their continuing influence on behavior. Many behaviors are goal-oriented; that is, they represent an individual's efforts to achieve some goal, such as satisfying the need for acceptance. We can increase our understanding and tolerance for the behavior of others by being more aware of possible contributing causes, some apparent and others hidden. It is also helpful to study behavior in terms of its effectiveness—the degree to which it satisfies some basic need.

You know that basic needs, both physical and social/emotional, continue during illness. However, the need for relieving distress and releasing emotions such as fear may temporarily push the need for approval or acceptance into the background. On the other hand, some patients try to cover up their own emotional distress by being pleasant and cooperative to win acceptance from health care professionals.

Developing social/emotional competence will enable you to meet your own social and emotional needs more effectively as well as improve your effectiveness as a health care professional. Social/emotional competence involves several skills (CASEL 2020).

- **Self-awareness**: Identifying and acknowledging our own emotions, thoughts, beliefs, and values

- Self-management: Handling emotions and stress effectively; setting and working toward goals

- Responsible decision making: Making decisions which consider ethical standards, safety, benefits, and consequences of an action on yourself and others

- Social awareness: The ability to understand and empathize with others from diverse backgrounds

- Relationship skills: The ability to maintain effective personal and professional relationships with diverse people

Practicing these skills will be an ongoing process throughout your life and throughout your career. Improving your social/emotional skills increases your ability to deal with difficulties; to find satisfaction in daily life; and to interact effectively with coworkers, supervisors, and clients in the workplace.

Activities

1. Consider your own life, past and present. What groups of people have you tuned to for love or a sense of belonging? What role have family, friends, classmates, teachers, sports teams, musical groups, religious activities, or other groups played in providing a sense of belonging and connection?

2. Explain the difference between self-concept, self-esteem, and self-awareness.

3. After reviewing the section about self-actualization in this chapter, describe the factors you believe to be most important in fulfilling your potential or becoming the best you can be.

4. Describe how your own family, community, or cultural background has influenced your attitude toward each of the following: time, responsibility toward family, definition of success, your right to "be yourself," and your duty to others in your community.

5. For each of the following social/emotional competencies, rate yourself on a scale of 1 to 10 (1 = not strong; 10 = very strong). Which competencies are your strongest? Which areas could use improvement?
   - Self-awareness
   - Self-management
   - Responsible decision making
   - Social awareness
   - Relationship skills

References and Suggested Readings

Collaborative for Academic, Social, and Emotional Learning (CASEL). (2020). *CASEL's SEL framework.* https://casel.org/casel-sel-framework-11-2020/

Eaude, Tony. (2019). The role of culture and traditions in how young children's identities are constructed. *International Journal of Children's Spirituality, 24*(1), 5–19. doi:10.1080/1364436X.2019.1619534

Chapter

7

Emotions and Behavior

Objectives

After completing this chapter, you should be able to:

- Describe the meaning, importance, and physiological effects of emotions.
- Define stress, distress, and stressor.
- Give examples of positive and negative emotions.
- Explain how emotional patterns are formed.
- Identify ways to use emotions constructively.

Key Terms

Adrenaline	Mental chatter	Stress
Altruism	Noradrenaline	Stressors
Compassion	Physiological	Suppression
Cynicism	Repressed	
Hostility	Resentment	

Meaning, Importance, and Physiological Effects of Emotions

Emotions are the inner feelings that all of us have. They are responses to life situations, varying in type and intensity according to the experience of the moment. Many different terms are used to describe emotions. Some of these terms describe the *type* of feeling; other terms imply the *intensity* of the feeling.

Emotions are neither good nor bad. We all experience these inner feelings according to what is happening to us and how we perceive the experience. To think of any emotion as good or bad, in a moral sense, is as pointless as considering hunger to be morally good or bad. Both positive and negative emotions are natural reactions to life experiences. However, as adults, we are responsible for expressing and managing our emotions in a healthy way.

Importance of Emotions

Emotions have physical and mental effects. Indirectly, emotions determine the amount of satisfaction we get from life, the degree of success we have in solving life problems, the satisfaction we find in relations with other people, and, ultimately, our *physical* and *mental* well-being throughout life.

The relationship between negative emotions and physical health is now well established by research. Anger, when experienced frequently, tends to evolve into **resentment** (chronic, low-level anger), **hostility** (an angry attitude toward a specific person or group), or **cynicism** (an attitude of contempt or distrust of others). Thus, anger can influence the personality.

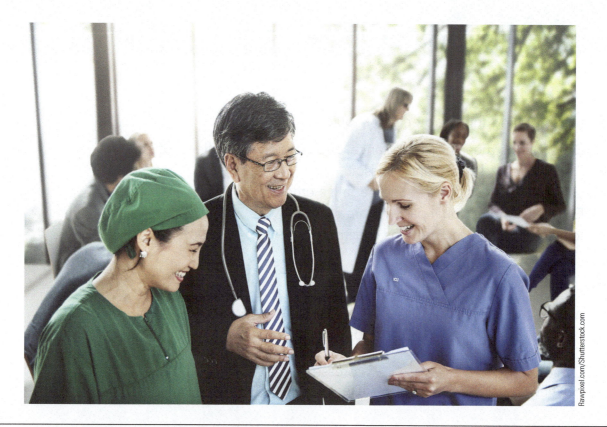

FIGURE 7-1 Appropriate expression of emotions in any job situation influences relations with coworkers, supervisors, and patients/clients.

Since our emotions have powerful mental and physical effects, it is important that we learn to use emotions effectively, rather than allowing emotions to control our behavior. The person who has learned to express feelings in socially acceptable ways is competent in dealing with life situations—both good and bad. A person who has not learned to use emotions constructively is likely to lose control when feelings become strong. The sudden eruption of powerful feelings may result in impulsive behavior that is ineffective in dealing with a situation. Appropriate expression of emotions in any job situation influences relations with coworkers, supervisors, and patients/clients.

Physiological Effects of Emotions

Emotions influence physical functioning, with particular effect on the autonomic nervous system, which influences the functioning of internal organs. Through this indirect influence, the emotional state can stimulate certain organs and inhibit the activity of others. If the emotion is strong, the effect is of short duration. If it is a long-term emotion, as in chronic anxiety, internal processes are kept in a state of "semi-emergency alert." Over a period of time, this long-term **physiological** situation can lead to actual physical changes.

Studies of body reactions to situations that arouse fear or anger show that the adrenal glands discharge large amounts of **adrenaline**, and the sympathetic nervous system produces **noradrenaline**. These two hormones speed up the circulation of blood, accelerate blood clotting, dilate the blood vessels that serve the skeletal muscles, and increase the respiratory rate. The purpose of these changes is to prepare the body for unusual activity—that is, a "fight or flight" state—to deal with the emergency situation. While the body's resources are being mobilized to strengthen the musculoskeletal system, other areas of the body have a diminished supply of blood. These physiological changes are adaptive, meaning that they enable the individual to deal physically with a threatening situation.

Stress

Dr. Hans Selye studied the physiological effects of unusual life situations for over 30 years. Dr. Selye noted that there is a *generalized* body reaction in addition to the alarm ("fight or flight") reaction. He labeled the latter response **stress** and the generalized reaction *general adaptation syndrome*, the sum total of physiological changes that occur in a state of stress. The stress response is essential to survival; it occurs in response to either a positive or a negative emotional state. Thus, a happy event such as marriage or the birth of a baby, as well as an unhappy experience, can trigger the generalized stress reaction.

Extreme emotional states are generally of short duration; they can be measured in terms of minutes or hours. The "fight or flight" arousal generally subsides as soon as the emergency has passed, although the aftereffects, such as sweaty palms and trembling, may continue for several hours, until the levels of adrenaline and noradrenaline in the bloodstream have returned to normal. On the other hand, stress (the generalized response) does not subside quickly; when this aroused state exists for a long period, the body is in a state of distress. The physiological arousal interferes with normal body functions. Stress over a period of years can lead to depletion of the adrenal glands. The term *stress* refers to the adaptive response itself. The outside influences that create a state of arousal are **stressors**.

FIGURE 7-2 The capacity for feeling love has a powerful effect on physical and mental health.

Dr. Selye's research led to the discovery that the stress reaction includes increased body resistance to outside agents such as infectious organisms. This is the basis for immunity to specific diseases (i.e., production of antibodies). During a period of increased resistance to a specific stressor, resistance to other stressors is decreased. For example, working long hours, eating improperly, and not getting sufficient sleep and recreation add up to stress. A person with such a lifestyle is likely to have lowered resistance and, therefore, to be more susceptible to infection.

The person whose stress reaction is due to invasion by a specific infectious agent, such as a virus, has the physiological response specific to that infectious agent (e.g., a fever and runny nose). At that time, the individual has lowered resistance to other organisms, such as the bacteria or viruses that cause pneumonia. While the body mobilizes its resources to deal with the original virus, only limited resources are available to deal with other threats to health.

Unfortunately, resistance to psychological stressors does not automatically develop, as is the case with immunity to some infectious organisms. Nor does the stress reaction subside as quickly or as completely after a psychological threat is no longer a part of the immediate life situation. Because of mental/emotional/physiological interactions, we can experience stress by remembering a past event, by anticipating some undesirable future event, or even by imagining that something has happened or is happening. When our thoughts are directed to an undesirable event (such as failing a course, being fired, being overworked), the emotional reaction to this *mental activity* triggers the adaptive response.

Another major source of stress for many people is **mental chatter**. This almost continuous stream of thoughts and memories is most likely to occur when an individual is performing routine tasks (such as cooking or folding laundry) that do not require concentrated thought or during quiet times when trying to relax. Mental chatter contributes to insomnia, since the physiological reaction to thoughts can lead to increasing wakefulness. Mental chatter, as used in this discussion, is ongoing, not fully under conscious control, and not purposeful. It is different from conscious use of mental processes for thinking, planning, evaluating, analyzing, and remembering.

Mental chatter that deals with past events may include an embarrassing situation, a failure or an unsatisfactory performance, a disappointment, a lost opportunity for a smart response, or an extensive review of a conversation. But past events cannot be changed; only the present and the future can be altered. This habit of frequently recalling past events that aroused a negative emotion results in a state of chronic stress that can lead to permanent physiological changes—the basis for psychosomatic (*psycho* = mind; *soma* = body) illness.

Mental chatter can also focus on future possible events, rather than memories of past events. These thoughts may involve rehearsal of an expected conversation, something "bad" that could happen to oneself or to a loved one, a loss, or the possibility of abandonment. If worrying about possible future events is habitual, the individual maintains a state of anxiety, and a state of stress exists.

Mental chatter can also include remembering good things that happened or anticipating some type of good experience. Mental chatter concerned with "good" things is satisfying, rather than stress-inducing. Everyone experiences mental chatter, but people vary in the extent to which they react emotionally. Stress management requires learning to control mental chatter so that it does not arouse negative emotions or interfere with sleep.

For Discussion and Reflection

What times of day or during what activities do you experience mental chatter? What types of thoughts or memories go through your mind throughout the day when you are driving, cooking, or completing other routine tasks?

Positive and Negative Emotions

As mentioned at the beginning of this chapter, all emotions are natural parts of the human experience. While emotions are not *good* or *bad* in a moral sense, emotions do contribute to our sense of satisfaction or dissatisfaction, or in other words, whether we *feel* good or bad.

Love

Love is perhaps the strongest positive emotion. There are various types of love and the intensity varies according to type, the object of the love, and circumstances of the moment. Strong feelings of warmth for another person might be thought of as *love*, with milder feelings of the same type being termed *friendliness*. *Affection* implies a feeling less intense than love, but stronger than friendliness. Love implies caring about someone else, being concerned enough to help, understand, and respect the person loved. The capacity for feeling love influences one's outlook on life and attitudes toward people and has a powerful effect on physical and mental health.

Kinds of Love There are many kinds of love: the love of a parent for a child; the child's love, at first self-centered and then extended to others; love for one's playmates; love for material things associated with pleasant memories; love for friends with whom life experiences have been shared; love for people in difficult circumstances, wherever they might be; and love

FIGURE 7-3 **Research has shown a link between gratitude and improved mental and physical health.**

for a patient and their family who are struggling with their stressful situation. Spiritual love is different still and varies according to one's concept of the divine. Each kind of love is expressed in specific ways. Newspaper accounts of some family's misfortune often result in a flood of contributions from strangers, illustrating the capacity of many people to express love for people they have never met. This type of love is an example of **compassion**.

Learning to Love Love is essential to an infant's normal development. Throughout childhood, one gradually learns to extend love to others: parents, siblings, other family members, caretakers, and eventually a widening circle of friends and associates. This learning is basic to the development of such traits as generosity, **altruism**, respect, and courtesy toward others. During adolescence, romantic love becomes a primary concern, and this may extend throughout adulthood. Mature love is a special type of love that evolves through a long-term adult relationship. Each of these types of love can flourish only if the individual's early experiences fostered the development of self-love.

Self-Love Self-love is basic to the experience of love. Without self-love, a person is not able to truly love others. Self-love is not selfish, nor is it egotistic. It is an awareness of "self" as a worthwhile, lovable being who deserves to be cared for. A religious person may experience self-love through the belief "I am a child of God." A similar belief, expressed in nonreligious terms, might be "I am a unique and worthy person." Loving oneself and believing oneself to be lovable are fundamental to a positive self-concept, the best protection one can have against threats to self-esteem as various difficulties of life are experienced.

Self-love enables a person to experience joy and happiness. It also contributes to health and well-being, in part because those who have self-love care enough about themselves to practice habits of safety and health maintenance. They do not abuse their bodies with toxic substances, such as alcohol, nicotine, or other addictive drugs. They eat healthy food, exercise appropriately, get enough sleep, wear seat belts in the car, and do not drive recklessly or otherwise place themselves at needless risk. In other words, a person who has self-love takes responsibility for "self" in all aspects of living.

Unconditional Love Love should be *unconditional*, which means that it is not subject to being withheld whenever one is displeased. Conditional love has an "if/then" basis: *if* you do (or do not do) such and so, *then* I will love you. All too often, conditional love is used as a manipulative tool to control another person. This is destructive to a relationship, but is especially damaging when used by parents to control a child. Conditional love teaches "You're only lovable when you do as I say." This style of parenting can lead to a negative self-concept, the belief that one is lovable only when meeting the demands of another.

Unconditional love, then, not only provides a growing child with a strong, positive self-concept, it also prepares the individual for a more healthful future life. Unconditional love does not mean that one must put up with undesirable behavior from others. It is important to differentiate between the person and that person's behavior. It is also important to realize that you can *love* someone even when you do not *like* them. Unconditional love is available at all times; it survives the ups and downs of a relationship.

Love for a child also includes teaching appropriate behaviors at each stage of development; boundaries must be set in terms of what is acceptable behavior and what is not. Setting boundaries—making it clear that one will not tolerate a specific behavior—is a way of clarifying a relationship; it is not a matter of withholding love.

Gratitude

Gratitude is a thankful appreciation for what we have received or experienced. Research has shown a link between gratitude and improved mental and physical health. Gratitude practices may include writing down what you are thankful for, thanking others who have

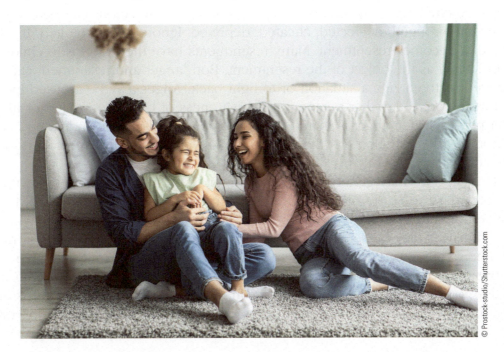

FIGURE 7-4 Cultural and family patterns of emotional expression influence the formation of a child's emotional patterns.

helped you, or simply taking time to stop and appreciate simple moments with an attitude of thankfulness: a sunny day, a hot cup of coffee, a friend's kindness. Positive emotions which are closely associated with gratitude include *appreciation*, *interest*, and *enjoyment*.

Joy

Joy can be described as a feeling of happiness and well-being which may be experienced as a result of a desirable event, such as receiving a promotion or seeing a loved one, or in response to positive thoughts or memories. For example, you might experience joy while looking at pictures of family or of an enjoyable trip you took. Joy may be experienced intensely, or it may be mildly pleasant, as when we say we *enjoy* a certain food or song.

Negative Emotions

Negative emotions are uncomfortable. The intensity of each emotion can range from mild to very strong, causing one to feel a vague restlessness, a feeling of dissatisfaction, or a state of intense agitation. Negative emotions such as anger, fear, guilt, or sadness may occur as a response to the behavior of another person, a specific event or piece of information, or mental chatter. These emotions result in stress and physiological changes.

Anger Anger is aroused by obstacles, threats, or otherwise offensive situations. It is usually short term and directed at a specific object or person, but can be generalized as anger at the world or society. *Hate* may be thought of as intense anger felt toward a specific person or group. *Annoyance* is used to describe a mild form of anger. *Rage* describes intense anger and implies that the anger is expressed through violent physical activity. *Hostility* is a mild form of anger/hate directed to a specific person or group. *Resentment* is chronic anger, which can be a powerful influence on one's behavior.

Anger is the emotional response to one's perception of a situation. The perception usually involves feeling wronged, neglected, cheated, deprived, ignored, or exploited. If the anger is not resolved, it becomes resentment. Many resentments have their origins in childhood, with a parent or sibling as the object of the resentment. Both anger and resentment can arise from feeling powerless to change a situation or to fight back. Anger may be aroused by an unsuccessful effort to control another person, or by awareness of being controlled or manipulated by another person. When anger is shared by a large number of people and control is held by a faceless group ("administration" or "the owners" or "government"), the anger of powerlessness can erupt as rebellion.

As individuals, we may generate our own anger. Some psychologists believe that anger is often secondary to some other emotion. A parent feels fear when a child cannot be found; once the child's safety is assured, anger is directed at the child for having "caused" the situation. Anger may be secondary to other primary feelings, such as embarrassment or disappointment. When one experiences anger toward a friend or family member, it is advisable to consider whether the anger is due to some need of our own not being met. If the anger is due to some type of problem/situation, it is better to state that one is experiencing anger, and then suggest that an effort to solve the problem or situation be undertaken by all parties involved. If the anger is not used constructively, it may develop into smoldering resentment, hostility, or even hatred. **Suppression** of these feelings is likely to eventually result in an explosive verbal outpouring or even destructive physical actions.

One unfortunate example of destructive anger is domestic violence. Violence against another person is an inappropriate expression of anger. Domestic violence involves directing anger toward one's partner or child, usually through physical assault; it also includes verbal assault and any menacing actions that arouse fear in the victim.

The problem of child abuse has received increasing attention over the past two decades. Studies of child abusers reveal that many were themselves abused as children. This is a tragic example of how inappropriate adult behavior influences the child's future patterns for emotional expression. The child who grows up in a home where violent behavior occurs perceives this pattern of family interaction as "normal." Unless that perception is changed through education and counseling, the pattern of violent behavior within the family will continue through succeeding generations.

Fear Fear is aroused by the threat of physical harm or danger to one's sense of security. Fear of physical harm is usually short-lived; the danger passes or the person copes with the dangerous situation. *Terror* and *panic* are terms for describing intense fear; the person who is in a state of terror or panic may flee the situation or may be immobilized by the intensity of the emotional reaction.

Fear is a natural reaction to threat or danger. It mobilizes the body for action—for fighting or fleeing a threatening situation. The body releases adrenaline, which increases the flow of blood, raises the rate of respiration, and stimulates muscle tone. If physical activity does not occur, this readiness for action may be released through "the shakes." Perhaps you have been involved in a dangerous situation, remaining calm until the danger was over and then finding yourself shaking all over or "weak in the knees." Many examples of heroic action involve physical exertion that the individual could not repeat after the excitement had subsided. The outpouring of adrenaline resulted in physical strength far beyond the person's usual abilities.

Fear can also be a reaction to mental chatter. *Worry* is fear based on thoughts about a *possible* event, such as losing one's job, losing a loved one, losing some type of property, or displeasing someone. *Anxiety* involves a higher intensity of fear than worry; it is likely to be a chronic pattern of emotional response to mental chatter. *Apprehension* and *dread* describe fear based on thoughts about some pending event that one perceives as threatening.

Fear is healthful when it is a reaction to a threatening event or situation. When self-generated through mental chatter, fear is pointless and destructive, unless it is used to plan ways to deal effectively with an expected situation. If one is apprehensive about a speech to be delivered on Monday, the best way to deal with the fear is to prepare well, practice the speech until completely comfortable with it, mentally picture oneself delivering the speech effectively, then remember to take several deep breaths before starting to deliver the speech. In the process of preparing for an effective delivery, self-confidence will replace apprehension.

Grief Grief is the emotional response to loss. It can range in intensity from momentary disappointment to deep sorrow that completely absorbs the individual. *Grief* describes intense feelings; *sorrow* implies grief without indicating intensity; *sadness* implies grieving of moderate intensity; and *disappointment* implies a mild form of grief. While fear and anger tend to arouse one physically, grief has the opposite effect. A person who is grieving may find it difficult to perform simple tasks. The body seems to reserve energy at this time for the individual to work through the grief. It is highly desirable, even healthful, to consciously grant oneself time to grieve when loss has been experienced.

Guilt Guilt, as discussed here, refers to self-blaming, rather than to any legal/criminal aspects. A clinical psychology professor once referred to guilt as the "most useless emotion there is." We can feel guilty about many things: something we did or said in the past, something we now wish we had done but did not do at the proper time, words we could have spoken but didn't.

It is impossible to change the past, so it is pointless to stay stuck in guilt about what cannot be changed. Some things can be remedied by doing now what could have been done in the past. Another remedy is forgiveness—of self and others. But forgiveness is not easy; self-forgiveness is especially difficult for people who have been controlled by guilt. Those who try to control others, especially family members or lovers, may use guilt as a manipulative tool.

Striving for self-understanding and learning effective interpersonal skills are one's best protection against the damaging effects of guilt. Anyone who realizes their behavior is strongly influenced by guilt feelings, or that someone is controlling them through guilt, will find professional counseling helpful.

Formation of Emotional Patterns

Emotional patterns are learned through the satisfaction or distress that accompanies various life experiences. Each person's capacity to feel specific emotions may be hereditary, as indicated by the fact that newborn infants show marked differences in their responses to distress. In spite of this hereditary factor, differences in adult emotional patterns are primarily the result of learning.

The people of a baby's world—the social environment—determine to a great degree whether the baby's experiences are pleasing or distressing. Throughout infancy, childhood, and adolescence the formation of emotional patterns is influenced by the emotional expressions and behaviors of others, especially primary caregivers and family members. Later in life, the balance of successes and failures in daily living has great influence on emotional expression. Also, the reactions of other people influence the tendency to show one's feelings or attempt to hide them. Patterns for expressing feelings develop within a framework of various influences on behavior: heredity, environment, basic needs, the consequences of behavior that follow specific life experiences, and interactions with other people.

Cultural and family patterns of emotional expression influence the formation of a child's emotional patterns. Ideally, the child receives loving care from parents and other family members, thereby learning love and trust. However, in many families, work demands limit the amount of time and energy parents have for parenting. So the child may be exposed to a hectic schedule, rushed to the childcare center in the morning and picked up later in the day by an exhausted parent. At times, the balance of emotional expression may be more negative than positive. The behaviors of the adults are the behaviors the child will learn. In addition, the behaviors of childcare personnel and their beliefs about the expression of feelings are important influences on the child's developing emotional patterns.

The community and culture in which a child grows up also significantly influence how the child learns to express emotions. In some cultures, open expression of emotions is accepted and encouraged, while in other cultures, it is considered inappropriate to express strong feelings. Anger, hostility, and aggression may be viewed as signs of strength in some cultures and as indicators of poor self-control in others. Researchers have noted that experiencing positive emotions is correlated across diverse cultures, while other patterns of emotional expression, such as intentionally suppressing negative emotions out of concern for others, is more beneficial in cultures that value interdependence highly (Schunk et. al. 2022).

Although these patterns are learned early in life, they are influenced later through exposure to widening circles of relatives, friends, schoolmates, coworkers, and various peer groups. As you study the remainder of this unit, be aware of your own patterns for expressing each emotion.

For Discussion and Reflection

As you remember specific behaviors you saw in your home as a child, what emotions were likely being expressed? As a child, did you adopt the same behavior? What changes have you made in expressing emotions since your childhood?

Individual Differences in Emotional Patterns

Everyone experiences negative and positive feelings. The tendency to respond to a certain type of situation with a specific emotion, the intensity of our emotional responses, the ways in which we express our feelings, the balance between positive and negative feelings, and the duration of a particular emotion are all characteristic of each person as an individual. People differ, then, in regard to the inner experience (feeling) and in the outward expression (behavior) of emotions.

Sometimes we suppress, or choose not to express, an emotion while in the situation that arouses it, then express it later; this is especially common with anger. If an emotion is extremely intense, and/or the situation that aroused the feeling is painful or unacceptable, then the emotion may be **repressed**. The memory of a traumatic event and the feelings associated with that event may both be repressed, meaning that they are not available to conscious memory. Therapy can help a person access repressed memories/feelings.

Intensity and Frequency Some people have the capacity for very strong feelings, whereas others seem to feel less intensely. Some people react frequently with strong emotion, even to daily annoyances such as traffic slowdowns. Other people react with strong emotion only to situations in which an intense emotional reaction is justified. Some people hide their feelings, which can result in a chronic state of stress.

Temperament The type of emotion (positive or negative) that a person feels most of the time is known as *temperament*. An optimistic person is one whose feelings are primarily positive; a pessimistic person is one whose feelings are primarily negative. Temperament is indicated by the way emotions are expressed: words and tone of voice, facial expression and other nonverbal behavior, and actions.

Most of us prefer the company of people who usually reflect positive emotions. Sometimes people with a pessimistic outlook find mutual satisfaction in each other, which brings to mind the saying "Misery loves company." Some people do not show their feelings readily; their appearance is somewhat the same whether they are feeling good or bad inside. This lack of expressiveness may indicate suppression of emotion, rather than lack of feeling. It is difficult to know how such people feel, and therefore difficult to adapt your own behavior appropriately.

Mood Swings Another difference in individual emotional reactions is the tendency to have mood swings. Each of us has times when we are "blue"; each of us has times when we feel especially good for no apparent reason. This swing from up to down is normal. Some people, however, swing from one extreme to another or remain "down" for long periods and "up" for long periods. Extreme mood swings and/or a prolonged mood at one extreme or the other may indicate a need for professional counsel. Those whose mood swings are within normal range can learn to make full use of the times when they feel good and develop techniques for coping with periods when they feel "low."

The tendency to have long "down" periods can indicate that a person is clinically depressed. Extreme mood swings, down periods alternating with periods of high energy and productivity, may indicate that a person has bipolar disorder. The line between "normal" mood swings and those indicative of a mood disorder is not clear-cut. If the mood swings are serious enough to interfere with work, study, or family relations, then the individual should seek medical evaluation. If destructive or threatening behavior occurs, the individual should have a psychiatric evaluation as soon as possible.

Using Emotions Constructively

Accentuating the Positive

Happiness is determined by how we react to both pleasant and unpleasant experiences in life. Some people use their unhappy experiences for endless conversational material. Others give only short notice to unhappy experiences, rapidly turning their attention to activities that give them satisfaction.

Each of us is free to choose between a negative and a positive outlook. We cannot eliminate all of life's disappointments, but we can refuse to let negative emotions dominate our lives. It is important, however, to consider each negative experience in terms of any lesson that can be learned. By learning from negative experiences, we become more competent for coping with life events.

Open and Honest Communication

Owning your feelings involves stating how a situation is affecting you. Suppose you have a supervisor who frequently changes the schedule for no apparent reason. Some of your coworkers rearrange their personal plans in order to work the changed hours, but criticize the supervisor to other coworkers and the family. One person confronts the supervisor in anger and refuses to accept the changed hours. Still another worker says nothing about the change, but takes sick leave on the day for which the hours were changed. Each of these three approaches has disadvantages. None is likely to alter the supervisor's habit of changing hours on short notice. A cooperative approach is preferable; but first, the supervisor must become aware that there is a problem.

Suppose you approach the supervisor at an appropriate time and calmly state, "I have a problem when my hours are changed. I have to make different arrangements for care of my children." You have made statements of fact, using "I" to describe the effect of the schedule changes. This is "open and honest" communication. No accusation has been made; no blame has been laid on the supervisor. The climate is right for a discussion of the problem and a cooperative approach to finding a solution.

Perhaps there is a good reason for the change in hours. It is easier to accept an undesirable situation if you know that it exists because of unavoidable circumstances, rather than because of someone's poor planning. Perhaps the supervisor was not aware of your childcare needs and therefore was unaware of the inconvenience created by a change in schedule. Regardless of how the supervisor responds, you would have defused any anger that was felt; it will not erupt later in an uncontrolled outburst of feeling. Even more important, the anger will not be displaced onto patients, coworkers, or members of the family who did nothing to cause the anger.

This approach is called an "I-statement," meaning that *feelings* are expressed in a statement beginning with "I," rather than a "you-statement" that accuses or blames the other person. Compare the suggested "I-statement" with an accusative statement: "You are always changing the hours! You are forcing me to change my childcare arrangement! Why can't you make up a schedule and stick to it?" These statements would result in an angry supervisor. Certainly being on the defensive would not put the supervisor in a problem-solving frame of mind.

FIGURE 7-5 Open and honest communication will greatly improve relations with others.

"I-statements" are valuable as a means of expressing both positive and negative feelings. This technique can lead to improved interpersonal relations. Consider the possible effect of the following statements:

- "You always keep me waiting."
- "I really get angry when I have to wait."
- "I was disappointed when I arrived and you were not here yet."
- "You are 15 minutes late."

Obviously, the "you-statements" put the other person on the defensive, may create angry feelings toward you, or may arouse feelings of guilt. On the other hand, the "I-statements" simply state how you feel. The other person cannot deny you your feelings. There is no basis for argument. And you have expressed the feeling verbally and are no longer burdened with anger.

Open and honest communication of positive feelings will greatly improve relations with others. All of us like to hear good things. Open and honest communication is especially important as a means of dealing with negative emotions. The following sections deal with approaches to handling specific negative emotional states.

Dealing with Anger

Negative emotions must be dealt with constructively, or they will have destructive effects. When inner tension builds up from anger, this tension needs to be released. If a patient makes you angry, you cannot throw a bedpan or physically attack the patient. It is not desirable to "blow up" at your supervisor; nor is it fair for you to bottle up your anger until you get home, and then let it loose on your family. (This is called "displaced anger.") Perhaps the tension built up from your anger can help you mow the grass, complete a workout, or chop the vegetables for dinner. In other words, use the energy generated by anger in some type of constructive physical activity. While you are in the situation, use "I-statements" as appropriate or ask questions that will help you understand the other person's views or the circumstances. As you gain understanding, your anger may subside.

Once you are out of the situation in which you became angry, try to understand the reason for your anger. Is the reaction related to old resentments? Do you display a pattern of becoming angry with this person or in this type of situation? Were you frustrated in your efforts to meet some need? Did you have expectations that the other person failed to meet? Were you treated unfairly (in your opinion)?

If you still feel anger, there are several techniques for safely defusing the feelings.

- Talk with someone who knows how to listen. Just talking about the situation—the facts and also your feelings—can provide effective release.

- If you cannot talk to someone about it, write down or record what you would like to say to the person at whom you are angry. Then listen to a playback or read what you have written. Continue until your anger has been released. (Don't forget to erase the recording or destroy the paper!)

- Physical activity, such as riding a bike, walking, or dancing, can also release energy and calm anger. Once you are calm, you can make a rational decision about whether you need to discuss the situation with others or seek a solution.

Many therapists consider that the most effective technique for dealing with anger is forgiveness. It is difficult to forgive someone who has hurt you or cheated you. Yet the anger you carry with you is actually harming *you*—your health and well-being—rather than the one who is the object of your anger. Learning to forgive may be one of life's most difficult lessons. But the power of another person to harm you psychologically is diminished when you are able to forgive. Forgiveness of those who are deceased is just as important as forgiveness of those who are still living.

Self-forgiveness is especially important. It is only human to make mistakes. We all have regrets about things we did or didn't do, about what we said or didn't say. Some matters can be corrected by making amends toward the other person. If the other person is deceased, then the only recourse is self-forgiveness. It is desirable that we learn from the past, however, so that new regrets do not accumulate.

Dealing with Fear

To deal with fear effectively, we must first acknowledge the fear. We all encounter situations that arouse mild fear: a test, an oral report, returning to care for the patient who was critical of you yesterday, reporting to the supervisor that you broke a piece of equipment. In some situations the fear is justified, and the only recourse is to deal with the situation as effectively as possible. Sometimes mentally rehearsing the event in advance as a successful experience prepares you to deal with the situation with less fear.

Sometimes a person's fear is out of proportion to the expected event; fear tends to magnify the dreaded aspects of the situation. Fear can interfere with realistic thinking about a problem, but the problem-solving approach often reveals that there is an acceptable solution. Once a solution is apparent, fear tends to decrease.

Phobias Some people have an intense fear, known as a phobia, regarding something that most people do not find fearful (e.g., heights, being closed up in a small space such as an elevator, flying in an airplane). These fears are "abnormal" when they interfere with daily activities or cause the individual to take extreme measures to avoid the feared experience. Psychotherapy often results in the identification of some past traumatic event that the person had repressed, so that it was not available to conscious memory. In severe cases, the phobia requires a process of systematic desensitization, which may be done by various licensed mental health practitioners.

Post-Traumatic Stress Disorder A more serious example of fear-related memory is known as post-traumatic stress disorder (PTSD). This is manifested by panic attacks, in which the individual relives a traumatic experience through sudden flashbacks or nightmares. This disorder came to the attention of the public after many Vietnam veterans had difficulty adapting to civilian life following discharge from military service. PTSD can have a severe disabling effect if left untreated.

PTSD is experienced by many people who have been involved in a serious accident or have experienced a frightening event such as a flood, hurricane, or tornado. For several weeks or months after such an experience, the individual may relive the experience when trying to go to sleep, or wake up suddenly in a cold sweat with rapid heartbeat, clammy skin, and uncontrollable shaking—a panic attack. Usually, this tendency passes after several weeks, as physical healing occurs. If not, the individual should have professional counseling;

it requires skilled professional intervention to desensitize survivors of traumatic events and free them from recurrent panic attacks.

Dealing with Grief

Grief is an emotion that lasts over a period of time. It may take weeks or months to work through the intense feelings and readjust one's life pattern. Whenever a loss occurs, permit yourself to grieve. When feelings of guilt are associated with grief, professional counseling may be needed to work through both emotions; such a combination is difficult to handle alone.

Emotions and Behavior

Emotions do exist, and they do affect us physically, psychologically, and mentally. To deny these feelings is a form of suppression. Suppressed emotions will have their effects sooner or later, through "blowing up" in an uncontrolled display of emotion, illness, poor coping mechanisms, or poor interpersonal relations.

Self-control is a constructive way of using emotions, rather than not showing emotions. Self-control is a learned behavioral pattern for expressing feelings in socially acceptable ways while dealing with a situation intelligently. The following guidelines can be used to increase self-control:

- Express your feelings at the time they are experienced; if for some reason that is not appropriate, express the feelings as soon as possible in a "safe" setting.
- Own your feelings; use "I-statements" rather than accusative "you-statements" in your interactions with other people.
- Acknowledge (do not deny to yourself or others) that you experienced a particular emotion in a specific situation.
- Ask yourself, "Is this situation important enough to me to justify these feelings?" If the answer is "no," turn your attention to other matters. If "yes," then deal with the situation effectively, perhaps using some of the guidelines that follow.
- Work with others to clarify a problem and find a solution acceptable to all—a "win-win" situation.
- If you begin to experience anger, ask questions about the situation, then *listen* to the answers; better understanding of the other person's point of view may dissipate your anger.
- When you become aware of fear or apprehension, ask yourself whether you are in *real* danger. If the answer is "yes," take appropriate action; if "no," analyze the basis for your feelings and take preventive action if needed.
- Use problem solving to deal with a situation—present or future—so that you feel competent to find a solution and no longer need to feel apprehensive.
- Take responsibility for your feelings and your behavior; avoid blaming others for "causing" your feelings.
- Avoid negative mental chatter. If your thoughts involve future possible events and you become anxious, realize that mental chatter, not a real event, is the source of your anxiety.

- If you have a particular phobia, seek professional help so you can free yourself from this unrealistic fear. Once you have exposed the basis for your phobia, it no longer has the power to control your behavior.

- Use and enjoy humor; be willing to laugh at yourself for getting upset over something trivial. Defuse a tense situation, as appropriate, with a humorous comment or anecdote.

- If you are still "worked up" after a situation that aroused strong emotions, use the energy for some type of constructive physical activity, such as mowing the grass, working out, running, or walking.

- Allow yourself to grieve for any loss you have experienced.

- Become aware of the events of your daily life that give you pleasure and allow time at the end of the day to enjoy thoughts of these good experiences.

- Love yourself. Take credit for your strengths, your competence, your willingness to grow; forgive yourself for being less than perfect.

These suggestions are intended to help you understand yourself and your emotions better. As you become more open and honest with yourself and others about your feelings, you will have a favorable effect on others. As you learn to replace impulsive emotional behavior with actions based on reasoning, you will be free to control situations more effectively. As you develop greater sensitivity to the feelings of others, you are more likely to react appropriately to their behavior.

Emotions are somewhat like a chain reaction. Hostile behavior by one person tends to bring out hostility in others. Aggressive behavior by one person brings about defensive behavior in others. When someone else expresses a negative emotion, do not allow that behavior to arouse a negative emotion in you. Instead, maintain a positive feeling and show your concern with such statements as, "I sense that you are angry" or "I sense that you are really feeling down today." This approach is called "reflecting," meaning that you act as a mirror for the person's feelings. Reflecting indicates that you are "tuned in" to what that person is experiencing, that you care, and that you are giving that person your full attention.

Although you can choose how to express your feelings most of the time, you cannot *control* the feelings or behavior of another person. However, your behavior can *influence* another person's behavior. It requires practice to develop sensitivity to the feelings of others. We can best adapt our own behavior and respond effectively to another person only if we are aware of the other person's emotional state.

As you work with patients and their families, strive to understand their feelings. Notice behavior that may indicate fear, anger, or grief. Avoid adding to such feelings by your own behavior. Take a little more time with the fearful patient, giving effective reassurances as best you can. Acknowledge the grieving person's right to sorrow, recognizing that this emotion needs expression and cannot be worked through quickly. Grant your patient the right to be angry in certain situations; instead of becoming defensive, listen. Then try to resolve the problem that aroused the patient's anger.

Through continuing effort, you can become a health care professional who practices the *art of human relations* along with the technical skills of your field.

Activities

1. Describe how you react when you are angry. What situations typically trigger your anger? How do you express anger—verbally, physically, or both? What is helpful or unhelpful about the way you express anger?

2. Consider the stress you experience in your own life. What percentage of your stress do you estimate results from external events such as work, family responsibilities, or finances? What percentage is the result of inner stressors, such as memories of the past, concerns about the future, thoughts, feelings, and mental chatter? To what extent is each of these stressors within your control? Beyond your control?

3. Consider each of the following emotions one at a time. As you imagine each one, describe the feelings each emotion creates in your body, the mental images it brings to mind, or the actions you imagine taking in response to that emotion: love, happiness, gratitude, pride, fear, anger, sadness, shame.

4. Consider the family, culture, and community in which you grew up. Was free expression of emotions encouraged or discouraged? As an adult, do you continue to express emotions in the way you learned to do as a child, or have you changed the ways that you express emotion?

5. Review the list of strategies given in this chapter for managing emotions effectively. Select one strategy that you would like to implement. Describe why you chose this strategy and how you can use it in your work or personal life.

References and Suggested Readings

Jans-Beken, L., Jacobs, N., Janssens, M., Peeters, S., Reijnders, J., Lechner, L., & Lataster, J. (2020). Gratitude and health: An updated review. *The Journal of Positive Psychology, 15*(6), 743–782. doi:10.1080/17439760.2019.1651888

Schunk, F., Trommsdorff, G., & König-Teshnizi, D. (2022). Regulation of positive and negative emotions across cultures: Does culture moderate associations between emotion regulation and mental health? *Cognition and Emotion, 36*(2), 352–363. doi:10.1080/02699931.2021.1997924

Selye, H. (1987). Stress without distress. *Psychological Bulletin, 131*(6), 925–972.

Adjustment and Patterns of Behavior

Objectives

After completing this chapter, you should be able to:

- Contrast characteristics of a person who is well adjusted with characteristics of a person who is poorly adjusted.
- Describe how one's emotional patterns influence adjustment.
- Explain how the balance between frustration and satisfaction in daily life influences adjustment.
- Discuss strategies for improving adjustment and for adapting to a new situation.
- Give examples of how good adjustment will contribute to your effectiveness as a health care professional.

Key Terms

Adjustment
Burnout

Hassle
Vicious cycle

Adjustment refers to how well an individual has learned to deal with life situations. Each person's adjustment is variable, depending upon circumstances. A person may be well adjusted most of the time, but poorly adjusted during a period when there is a serious problem. Some people are poorly adjusted most of the time. They have not learned to deal with ordinary life situations effectively.

Understanding Adjustment

A person who is well adjusted deals effectively with problems and finds satisfaction in living. A well-adjusted person has developed the habits and skills needed to solve common problems and has developed patterns of behavior that satisfy basic needs. This type of person is well prepared to weather a crisis and reestablish good adjustment within a reasonable period of time.

A person who is poorly adjusted is not living a full life. Such a person feels dissatisfied much of the time. Actually, the poorly adjusted person may not have any more problems than a well-adjusted person. *The difference is that the poorly adjusted person has not learned to cope with obstacles or effectively deal with everyday problems of living.*

The biggest obstacle for the poorly adjusted person is the poor adjustment itself. The habits, attitudes, emotional reactions, and behavior patterns that are a part of poor adjustment create additional problems for the individual. Poor adjustment is a **vicious cycle**. Ineffective behavior often creates additional problems that the individual handles with more ineffective behavior. For example, imagine that you do not budget your money effectively, so you always run short a week or two before the next paycheck. As a result, you use credit cards or borrow money from friends. A portion of the next paycheck goes to pay back what you borrowed, causing you to fall further behind financially the following month. Poor adjustment can be modified only by learning to deal with life situations more effectively.

Effective Behavior versus Ineffective Behavior

The key to adjustment is learning to recognize ineffective behavior and replacing it with another behavior that gets better results. The person who is willing to change can improve adjustment. The person who is unwilling or unable to change behavior patterns will not improve adjustment.

Change is a test of one's ability to adjust. If familiar habits are used in new situations, the results may be quite different from results in the old situation. Change is an opportunity for growth that calls for conscious evaluation of habitual behavior. Ineffective habits should be discarded and new, more effective ones established. To acquire new friends, to fit into a new community, to succeed in a new job, and to do well in a course of study all require that some old habits be discarded and that some new ones be developed.

Larissa and Kay are two high school juniors enrolled in the health occupations course. Both are new in the school, faced with a new and unfamiliar setting. Kay wants desperately to be popular; when her new classmates ignore her, she feels resentment. She becomes critical of the class leaders, looking for opportunities to make uncomplimentary remarks about them. Her classmates soon tire of her negativity. They do not understand that Kay gets some relief from inner discomfort by criticizing those she envies. Kay is using ineffective behavior. Criticizing others makes her feel better momentarily, but it interferes with her forming new friendships.

In the meantime, Larissa decides to broaden her interests. She becomes more active in school affairs, helping with the yearbook and joining several clubs. Each new activity leads to new friends for Larissa. She is also learning new skills and acquiring new outlooks through these various activities. Larissa is using effective behavior to improve her adjustment. She took action to adapt to her new situation and that action proved to be effective. Larissa's goal was to become comfortable in the new situation and broaden her range of interests; gaining many new friends was only one of several benefits.

Julian is a student in the surgical technician program. He knows the procedures must be performed correctly, but his performance often includes errors. The instructor has talked with Julian about his performance. Every error and every problem, according to Julian, was the fault of someone else: the circulating nurse, another student, whoever set up the tray or pack, some member of the surgical team. Julian does not learn from his mistakes or from the instructor/student conference, because he is unable or unwilling to admit that he can make a mistake. He has not learned to take responsibility for his actions, and he denies the consequences of his errors by claiming "It wasn't my fault." Unless Julian changes this pattern of behavior, he will have problems throughout life. He will not be successful as a health care professional because he would not be a safe practitioner.

Emotions and Adjustment

Emotions are a major influence on one's adjustment. A person who experiences positive emotions several times a day is likely to have better adjustment than one who frequently experiences negative emotions. Sometimes the emotion one experiences is a matter of choice. For example, you drop your keys as you try to unlock the car door. You feel annoyed as you pick them up and try again to fit the key into the lock. Somehow the keys slip out of your fingers and fall to the ground a second time. At this point, you can utter a string of four-letter words to express your anger and exasperation. Or you could pick the keys up again, laughingly comment that you seem to have butterfingers today, then pay close attention to getting the key into the lock successfully.

Everyone's daily experiences include some difficulties and some positive experiences. At the end of the day, one person remembers a number of these "good experiences" and gives little thought to the things that did not go well. Another person may finish the day feeling angry about several problem situations that occurred, and have little or no conscious awareness of any good experiences. Each of us may *choose* the type of experience to which we give most of our attention. In most situations, we may either choose to be angry or to deal with a situation unemotionally, working toward a resolution of the difficulty.

Fear is also a powerful influence on adjustment. A person who lives in fear of what "might happen" is expecting bad things to happen. Such expectations influence behavior and also affect how that person perceives events. It is normal to experience fear when faced with a real threat; the well-adjusted person reacts appropriately to such a threat. A person who is chronically anxious, however, is living with fear that

For Discussion and Reflection

Do you know someone who becomes upset about "every little thing"? Do you know someone who is able to handle almost any situation calmly?

arises from negative thinking, rather than any real threat. Habitual negative thinking represents a state of poor adjustment.

Sadness also may be experienced appropriately or inappropriately. Each of us has life experiences that arouse sad feelings. Each of us is exposed to world news revealing terrible things happening, events that we are powerless to change. Someone who is truly grieved by conditions in a third-world country might join the Peace Corps and devote two or more years to try to improve those conditions. Many people address their prayers to such situations; persons who meditate may focus a daily meditation on peaceful resolution of a specific problem, wherever it exists. Others might feel real empathy for the victims of some distant tragedy and send a contribution to an organization that is providing help. Others may feel a brief period of sadness and then shift their attention to their own affairs. These reactions indicate healthful use of sadness.

A person who chooses to focus on tragic events may remain in a sad state, discuss the events frequently, yet take no action to improve the situation. This focus of attention on tragic events allows sadness to interfere with adjustment. As with anger and fear, a person can *choose* the extent to which sadness is allowed to affect one's feelings overall.

The pervasiveness of social media in today's world makes it easier than ever to allow our attention to be drawn to tragic world events; debates over political issues; or other topics which create anger, fear, or sadness without leading to productive action. Most people would agree that staying informed about significant local, national, and global events is worthwhile. However, "staying informed" can easily become an excuse for spending an excessive amount of time and energy reading and debating the details of a situation over which one has no control. Many people have found that limiting their time on social media or curating their social media feed helps them maintain a better attitude and to have more time in the day for family, friends, and hobbies.

FIGURE 8-1 Many people have found that limiting time on social media or curating their social media feed helps them maintain a better attitude.

Frustrations and Satisfactions in Daily Life

Daily Hassles

Hassles are events that cause you to feel irritated, annoyed, frustrated, fearful, or angry. How you cope with daily hassles, or minor frustrations, is a reflection of your adjustment. Hassles are inevitable, but we can choose whether to take them in stride or to become upset about each one:

> *My kids' rooms are a mess.*
> *I can't find the keys.*
> *Traffic was awful.*
> *I had a flat tire.*

How do you typically respond to events like these?

Box 8-1, "Hassles in My Life," is designed to help you identify hassles in your life. Box 8-2, "Satisfactions in My Life," permits you to identify the "good" things that occur. You choose which type of events receive most of your attention, and therefore which type of emotions dominate your daily life.

FIGURE 8-2 Dealing effectively with the hassles of daily life indicates a good level of adjustment.

Box 8-1

Hassles in My Life

Instructions: In the following list circle (1) for each event you experienced yesterday and (2) for each event you experienced during the past week or month. Substitute appropriate words (e.g., "my glasses" for "keys") to adapt a statement to your situation. If a statement just does not apply to you, leave it blank.

1. I couldn't find my keys.	1	2
2. My neighbor's dog barked all night.	1	2
3. My sister called to talk about her problems.	1	2
4. There's no way I can pay all my bills this month.	1	2
5. My partner is thrilled with our new gaming system; I'm not, because our credit card is now "maxed out."	1	2
6. I had to make a difficult decision.	1	2
7. My coworkers take extended breaks and I end up doing more than my share of the work.	1	2
8. One of my clients was especially unpleasant, even though I had given them extra time.	1	2
9. I am having a plumbing problem (again!).	1	2
10. I'm having a really bad hair day.	1	2
11. I tossed and turned all night. (I went to bed really sleepy, then couldn't go to sleep; or, I woke up at 2 A.M. and couldn't get back to sleep.)	1	2
12. My car wouldn't start.	1	2
13. I locked my keys in the car.	1	2
14. Traffic was terrible this morning.	1	2
15. The news is full of crime reports; I just don't feel safe.	1	2
16. There's a rumor that administration plans to "downsize" the patient care staff.	1	2
17. Even on my day off, I just couldn't relax.	1	2
18. Someone (insert name or title) took advantage of me; I'm afraid to confront him or her.	1	2
19. Someone (insert name) smokes too much; I'm afraid he or she will develop lung cancer.	1	2
20. It's harder and harder to please my partner; they complained all through breakfast this morning.	1	2

Total your score for each column. Note that items 1–14 deal primarily with anger and frustration; items 15–20 are more closely related to fear and anxiety.

Now follow the same procedure with Box 8-2 to identify some "good" experiences in your life.

Box 8-2

Satisfactions in My Life

Instructions: In the following list circle (1) for each event you experienced yesterday and (2) for those you experienced during the past week or month. Substitute appropriate words to adapt statements to your situation. If a statement does not apply to you, leave it blank.

1.	I had a good night's sleep.	1	2
2.	My supervisor complimented me on my work.	1	2
3.	I'm looking forward to time off or a trip coming up.	1	2
4.	I found a good buy on my family's favorite food or clothing.	1	2
5.	I enjoyed talking with a new coworker during break.	1	2
6.	One of my patients said, "You are the best!"	1	2
7.	This month I budgeted my money and was able to cover all expenses as well as save a little.	1	2
8.	My energy level has been good lately.	1	2
9.	I ate more fresh fruits and vegetables.	1	2
10.	I exercised two or more days this week.	1	2
11.	I managed my time so that I had free time in the evening.	1	2
12.	I included some recreation in my schedule.	1	2
13.	I spent time with friends and really enjoyed it.	1	2
14.	I confronted (insert name) about (insert issue) and, to my surprise, we had a very satisfying discussion.	1	2
15.	I like the clothes in my closet, and they fit me well.	1	2
16.	I was able to relax and enjoy my day off.	1	2
17.	My neighbor or friend did me a favor.	1	2
18.	My sister called, and we had a good time catching up on news.	1	2
19.	My children are doing well in school.	1	2
20.	I received a favorable work review or a good grade.	1	2

Total the two columns. Now, compare your "hassles" scores with your "satisfaction" scores. Which score is higher? Was it easier to recognize hassles than satisfactions? Or were the satisfactions more recognizable? Do you tend to focus more on your satisfactions or hassles?

Improving Adjustment

How can you improve adjustment? Clinical psychology professor Alan Carr gives the following guidelines for improving happiness and overall well-being:

- Create ways to find meaning and value in life by clarifying your values, setting and working toward goals, and identifying and using your strengths.
- Maintain a healthy lifestyle by eating nutritious foods, exercising, and meditating or practicing mindfulness.

- Take time to enjoy life by savoring experiences and expressing gratitude.
- Take an optimistic, solution-oriented approach to daily problems, telling yourself, "With a little help, I can figure this out or solve this!"
- Strengthen the relationships in your life, including relationships with friends, family, coworkers, and romantic partners.

Each of these strategies requires consistent attention and practice, but over time small steps will create significant changes in your attitude, mood, and physical health.

First, focus on one or two of the strategies until you have made significant progress, then select one or two others. If you attempt to focus on all of the guidelines at the same time, you are likely to become discouraged.

If you can achieve reasonably good adjustment in your usual life situation, then you will be prepared for the challenge of adapting to new situations and dealing with the occasional crisis situations that are an unavoidable part of life.

For Discussion and Reflection

How much time each day do you spend on social media, watching television, or "on your phone"? How much time do you spend each day preparing healthy meals, exercising, and sleeping?

Maintaining a Healthful Lifestyle

The suggestions just listed for improving your state of adjustment are somewhat broad and require conscious effort over a period of time. Steps for improving your daily habits can be taken immediately, and these daily habits definitely contribute to one's state of adjustment. A diet that consists largely of junk food, the use of addictive substances, lack of balance in work and play, lack of exercise, and inadequate sleep can all interfere with good adjustment. To feel and function at your best, include the following habits in your lifestyle:

- Eat several servings each day of fresh vegetables and fruit, some eaten raw.
- Drink at least eight cups of water each day.
- Exercise regularly.
- Avoid harmful and addictive substances.
- Participate regularly in recreational activities that help you release stress and regenerate your energies.
- Allow adequate time for sleep.

It is tempting to dismiss these habits by saying "With my schedule, I don't have time to cook fresh food, exercise, or sleep a full eight hours." However, most people find that when they make self-care a higher priority than television, social media, or talking and texting on the phone, they are able to make small, positive changes that increase their sense of well-being and their ability to maintain a state of good adjustment.

The Role of Joy and Laughter

The therapeutic effects of laughter came to the attention of the public and the health community with the publication in 1979 of Norman Cousins's book, *Anatomy of an Illness as Perceived by the Patient.* Cousins described how laughter had helped him recover from a debilitating illness for which there was no known cure. Since Cousins was an internationally famous journalist, his story had such a high level of credibility that it had an impact on health care delivery. Within a year or two, conferences were being held to teach health care professionals about the value of humor and laughter.

Research since that time has revealed that there are physical, mental, and emotional benefits of laughter and joyous experiences. The physical benefits include improved circulation, higher oxygen levels, enhanced immune functions, and increased levels of hormones that influence how one copes with stress. Laughter is now acknowledged as a factor in health, whether for the purpose of maintaining health, managing stress, or coping with illness. Some simple techniques for purposely putting more laughter into your day include:

- Look in the mirror at least once a day and tell the image you see there to laugh with you; even that moment of forced laughter will be beneficial.

- At least once a day, remember some funny incident or joyful experience; take a few minutes to laugh or experience joyful feelings.

- Place a keepsake from some fun or joyful experience where you can see it and enjoy a laugh or feelings of joy, even if only for a moment.

- Share funny experiences with other people; when you make them laugh, you also laugh and everyone benefits.

- Choose friends who like to laugh; it is hard to be "down" when you are around people who laugh often.

- Seek out humor that you can share with others.

Avoiding Burnout

Every health care professional is at risk for developing burnout syndrome. **Burnout** is a state of deterioration that affects an individual physically, mentally, and emotionally. It develops gradually over a period of weeks, months, or years of living or working in a high-stress situation, during which the individual may not eat properly, gets minimal rest, has few opportunities for recreation and self-renewal, experiences much frustration, receives little emotional support from others, and/or ignores signs of illness in order to keep going. Anyone with a tendency to be a "workaholic" is risking burnout. Some common signs of burnout include the following:

- A conscientious worker begins to make errors, take longer to perform tasks, or fail to complete assigned work.

- The worker feels increasing frustration and loss of interest in work.

- The worker may believe that his or her efforts are unappreciated and develop a negative attitude about the job.

- Fulfilling job responsibilities becomes increasingly difficult.

- Coworkers may notice increased irritability or complaints.

- Physical symptoms include fatigue, frequent minor illnesses, gastrointestinal disorders, headaches, or various aches and pains.

- There may be increased consumption of caffeine, tobacco, or alcohol or a tendency to seek relief through drugs, either legal or illegal.

For Discussion and Reflection

Have you experienced the symptoms of burnout described? To what extent did your working conditions contribute to your experience? Your personal habits?

The causes of burnout may lie within the individual—unhealthful life habits, failure to take responsibility for one's own well-being, a dedication to the job that results in too much work and not enough self-care, and failure to use effective stress management strategies. Often the causes of burnout are within the work environment—stressors such as uncomfortable physical conditions, unpleasant working relations, supervisor or management behavior, lack of encouragement and emotional support, and lack of recognition or reward for work done well. In many cases, the causes of burnout may be a combination of personal habits and working conditions.

The best protection is a lifestyle that includes all of the above suggestions for improving adjustment plus the regular use of effective stress management techniques. If the stressors of the work setting affect numerous workers, management should eliminate as many stressful conditions as possible. If work conditions cannot be improved and the worker is not able to deal effectively with the resulting stress, then it is time to seek employment elsewhere!

Adapting to New Situations

When a change occurs in your life situation—for better or worse—modify some of your patterns of behavior in order to achieve a state of good adjustment in the new situation. If the change is minor, you may adapt with little awareness of stress. If the change is great, however, you may go through a stressful period before you achieve adjustment. You may even be very unhappy at first, wishing that you could return to the old situation. As you successfully adapt, you will gradually begin to feel comfortable in the new situation.

The degree of disruption a change causes in one's usual pattern of living is dependent upon the type of change. Some changes you are likely to encounter include job changes, moving to a new neighborhood, a change of supervisors, a new administration in your place of employment, and changes in operational procedures and policies. A major change all of us have to face at some time is the loss of relatives and friends.

In general, adapting to change requires acceptance of the new situation and a conscious effort to adapt. If the change involves new tasks and new people:

1. Study the situation carefully.

2. Observe the behavior of others.

3. Learn the policies and regulations of the new situation.

4. Consciously adopt behaviors that are appropriate for that situation.

If you find that the new situation requires you to follow procedures that are unsafe (for you or your patients) or are unethical, you have a conflict: you can lower your standards and console yourself with the thought, "I'm just doing what everybody else is doing"; you can use appropriate procedures to try to change practices, a risky approach for a new employee; or you can leave the situation.

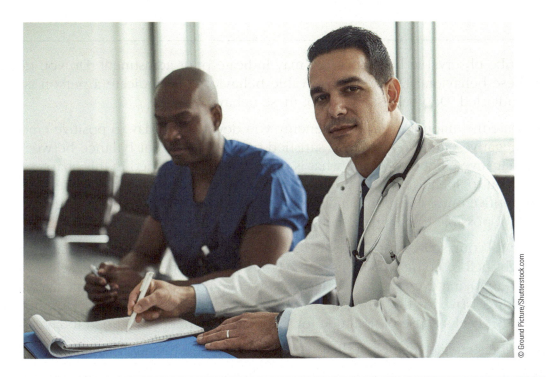

© Ground Picture/Shutterstock.com

FIGURE 8-3 To adapt to a new work environment, you will need to adjust to the regulations and procedures of the new workplace.

There is also the possibility that the new situation has more rigorous standards than your previous position. In that case, you have a challenge: to improve your performance in order to be acceptable to your new coworkers and supervisors. Willingness to learn and to improve performance will earn favorable evaluations for you; rebelling against the higher standards will mark you as an unsatisfactory employee.

A behavior that interferes with adapting to a new situation is clinging to the old situation. Comparing the old situation to the new, especially when you indicate your preference for the old, reveals that you do not yet accept the present situation. One sure way to antagonize new coworkers is to tell them repeatedly how you did things on your previous job. This behavior indicates poor adjustment to one's present job situation.

Adapting to the Role of Health Care Professional

You are already aware that becoming a health care professional requires certain modifications in behavior. Perhaps you have had a job in which you were allowed to do many different tasks and accept as much responsibility as you were able to handle. As a health care professional you will have a well-defined role. You may find it annoying to have limitations placed on your role, especially if others perform tasks you believe you can do. Performance within one's defined role is necessary within the health field; to exceed that role may endanger a patient and also may have legal implications. You are already aware of the change you must make in giving health care suggestions to your friends. Refrain from any advice or actions that appear to be efforts to diagnose or prescribe. Essentially, adjustment to being a health care professional requires knowing one's role and performing within it, while also accepting and abiding by the code of ethics appropriate to that role.

Activities

1. Describe observable behaviors that may indicate poor adjustment. Do you display any of these behaviors? Describe observable behaviors that indicate a person is relatively well adjusted. Do you display any of these behaviors?

2. Estimate the amount of time and energy you devote each day to positive emotions versus negative emotions. Are you satisfied with your current balance between positive and negative emotions? If not, what is one strategy mentioned in this chapter that might help you to spend less time focusing on negative emotions and more time experiencing positive ones? (Keep in mind, negative experiences and emotions are part of life, so it is not possible to eliminate them entirely.)

3. Refer to your scores for Boxes 8-1 and 8-2 and review the items that you marked. Tonight before going to bed, list the hassles you experienced today; select one particularly annoying event and consider ways you could prevent that particular hassle from recurring. Now, list the satisfying events of the day and consciously experience "good feelings." Feel a sense of gratitude for the good experiences you had today.

4. Describe strategies that could help you adapt to a new situation.

5. Explain how your ability to adjust to new situations will contribute to your success as a health care provider.

References and Suggested Reading

Carr, A. (2020). *Positive psychology and you: A self-development guide.* Routledge.

Carr, A., Cullen, K., Keeney, C., Canning, C., Mooney, O., Chinseallaigh, E., & O'Dowd, A. (2021). Effectiveness of positive psychology interventions: A systematic review and meta-analysis. *The Journal of Positive Psychology, 16*(6), 749–769. doi:10.1080/17439760.2020.1818807

Mbiriri, M. (2020). Laughter therapy as an intervention to promote psychological well-being. *Journal of Humanities and Social Policy 6*(1): 1–7.

Udayar, S., Urbanaviciute, I., Morselli, D., Bollmann, G., Rossier, J., & Spini, D. (2021). The LIVES Daily Hassles Scale and its relation to life satisfaction. *Assessment.* https://doi.org/10.1177/10731911211047894

Behavior and Problems in Living

Life does not always flow smoothly. There are many problems in daily living. Anyone with a health need has new problems in addition to those of the usual life situation. Health care professionals must be aware that many patients are reacting to threat and, possibly, overwhelming problems. The patient needs acceptance, understanding, and caring from those who provide health care.

Section III is designed to help you understand some types of behavior likely to result from threat. By learning to cope effectively with personal threat and its effects, the health care professional prepares to understand and accept the behavior of others who are reacting in their own way to threats in their life situations.

Common Threats to Adjustment

Objectives

After completing this chapter, you should be able to:

- Describe how each stage of life presents developmental tasks that contribute to adjustment.
- Explain how major life changes can challenge adjustment.
- Discuss how social and cultural stressors impact adjustment.
- Give examples of chronic stressors and how they affect adjustment.
- Define resilience and list coping skills that can improve a person's resilience.

Key Terms

Attention deficit
  disorder (ADD)
Attention deficit
  hyperactivity
  disorder (ADHD)

Autism spectrum
  disorders
Coping skills
Developmental disorders
Discrimination

Dyslexia
Family dynamics
Resilience
Separation anxiety

The adjustment of any one person can be very poor, very good, or anywhere in between. Each person has a relative state of adjustment that characterizes that person most of the time. Adjustment, however, is always subject to change. Life experiences require changes in behavior to adapt to new situations and cope with new problems. Our state of adjustment can always be threatened by difficult situations.

A state of good adjustment *most of the time* is the best protection a person can have against the difficulties of life. Chapter 8 discussed strategies for maintaining good adjustment while dealing with typical situations in daily life. By developing skills that help us deal effectively with our daily life problems, we prepare ourselves for dealing with more intense challenges that we may face.

Adjustment Through Stages of Life

As human beings, we are designed to grow, change, and develop throughout our lives. Each stage of life brings new opportunities but also presents new challenges. Sometimes these normal changes threaten our adjustment and require us to learn new behaviors or **coping skills** if we are to remain well-adjusted. Psychologist Erik Erikson created a theory of development that describes eight stages of life that humans experience. Each stage provides the opportunity to develop certain qualities or skills that strengthen the individual's sense of self and ability to interact with their environment. If a child is not able to develop these skills due to an unsupportive environment, developmental disabilities, or other reasons, they will have difficulty mastering the skills that come at later stages.

Early Childhood

Children develop most rapidly during the first few years of their lives. They develop gross motor skills such as walking, running, and jumping and fine motor skills such as holding a pencil or fork. They learn to use language to communicate their wants and needs, and they practice basic social skills such as table manners and sharing.

Children are constantly learning about the world around them. They feel secure when they know what to expect from others, but they often find new people and places frightening. A predictable routine provides security, while chaos or unexpected changes can cause anxiety. Changes in family schedule, bedtime routine, or child care should be introduced gently and gradually.

According to Erikson, three key stages occur in early childhood. Between birth and about age 18 months, infants learn to trust their caregivers, and by extension, other people generally, to provide for their needs. If caregivers are angry, hostile, neglectful, or absent, infants develop mistrust, learning not to depend upon others to meet their needs. At age 2 to 3 years, young children become more independent, mastering skills such as toilet training, feeding themselves, and dressing themselves. If they are successful, they begin to develop a sense of autonomy, of being able to take care of themselves. If they struggle with these skills due to lack of support from adults, developmental delays, or other reasons, they may develop self-doubt or shame, believing they cannot do tasks correctly. Between ages 3 and 5, young children continue to become more independent, developing a sense of purpose and control over their surroundings and activities. Children who have difficulty mastering independent activities may develop a sense of self-doubt, becoming reluctant to try new things for fear of failure or embarrassment.

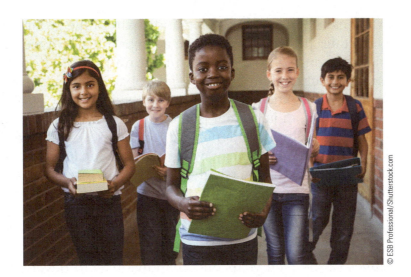

FIGURE 9-1 For children who have developed physical, intellectual, and social skills during the early years, facing new situations becomes easier as they progress through elementary school.

Young children may also experience **separation anxiety** when they enter a new day care or school. For days or even weeks, they may cry, claim to be sick, or beg to go home. Some elementary-school students experience anxiety when coming to a new school or returning after a long vacation. To resolve separation anxiety, parents, childcare providers, and health professionals should work together to help the child get used to the new situation and should be understanding of the child's feelings without giving in to demands to go home.

Middle Childhood

For children who have developed physical, intellectual, and social skills during the early years, facing new situations becomes easier as they enter and progress through elementary school. Each year brings a new class, new friends, and new experiences. According to Erikson, between the ages of 5 and 11, children who are academically and socially successful will develop confidence and a sense of competence. Students who are not able to succeed in school and in peer relationships can develop a sense of inferiority and a lack of confidence.

For students who lack basic skills or are developmentally delayed, entering school can create additional fears and problems. For many students, difficulties in school can be traced to a lack of school readiness skills. Poor social skills may lead to conflicts with classmates, while delayed intellectual development can create a pattern of school failure. Daily situations such as school assignments and interacting with peers can pose major threats to a child who is already poorly adjusted. The earlier parents, educators, and health care professionals can intervene to help such children develop needed skills, the more likely the child will be successful.

Adolescence

As young people enter the teen years, they struggle to establish an identity separate from that of their parents. Adolescents are inclined to worry about appearance, self-worth as a person, the future, and—very important—the opinions of others. Relationships with peers become extremely important. Teens need to feel accepted and a part of the group; disappointment or rejection by members of their peer group can pose a major threat to a teen's adjustment. Peer pressure—the feeling of having to go along with the group in order to be accepted—can influence teens' choices about clothing, about using tobacco and alcohol, or about sexual relationships. Mood swings and variable adjustment are typical of the adolescent period.

Romantic relationships form an important part of many teens' lives. Because many young people choose to become sexually active during the teen years, sexual relationships and pressures can create additional stress. Teens may worry about pregnancy or sexually transmitted diseases. Teens may also become increasingly aware of their gender identity and sexual preferences. Health care professionals may find that teens turn to them with questions the teens are uncomfortable asking a parent, particularly if parents are not supportive.

The teenager who has a positive self-concept and relatively good adjustment is likely to adapt to the challenges of the adolescent period. According to Erikson, successfully adapting to the changes of the teen years allows individuals to develop a strong identity, or sense of self. On the other hand, if an individual enters adolescence with a negative self-concept, poor interpersonal skills, ineffective behavior patterns, and/or a lack of support from family members, they may experience confusion and a lack of confidence about their identity, or "who I really am." If adolescence proceeds at a favorable pace, childhood patterns are gradually replaced by more mature patterns of behavior. If such growth does not occur, then childish patterns of behavior may continue into adulthood.

Young Adulthood

Young adults face many changes as they establish their independence from their parents. Common changes include completing high school and beginning college or a job, setting up a home of one's own, and for some, starting a family. Each of these changes brings new experiences and responsibilities. Young people who have already developed good coping skills will usually adapt to each of these changes. However, young adults with a pattern of school and family problems may see similar problems develop in their jobs or their own families unless they learn more effective ways of coping. Erikson describes the ages of 18 to 40 as a time of finding love and relationships, including romantic relationships and friendships.

FIGURE 9-2 Relationships with peers are extremely important to teens.

Individuals who create a sense of connection with others during these years experience intimacy and emotional satisfaction. For those who are unable to create strong relationships with others, a sense of isolation can result.

Middle Adulthood

According to Erikson, during the ages of 40 to 65, people begin to reflect on their accomplishments thus far. Individuals may build on past successes as they remain active in their careers and communities or change direction and start a new career. On the other hand, some individuals feel discouraged about lost opportunities or lack of success, causing them to give up on earlier aspirations, become fixated on telling stories about "the good old days," or develop rigid daily routines that offer little opportunity for change and growth.

Middle-aged adults may become painfully aware of the passing of time. Children are growing up and leaving home, leaving parents with an "empty nest." Physical changes can affect one's moods and emotions. Many adults have difficulty accepting these signs of disappearing youth. The popular term "midlife crisis" describes an adult who is having trouble adjusting to the changes of middle age.

Older Adulthood

Older adulthood, according to Erikson, is a time of looking back and assessing life. Individuals who are satisfied with their work and relationships develop a sense of fulfillment and wisdom, while individuals who have not found satisfaction in these areas may develop feelings of regret, sadness, and fear.

Older adulthood brings many changes. Losses of friends and relatives require frequent funeral attendance. Retiring from work that has been a major part of life for many years can provide free time for travel and hobbies, but for some, it creates a lack of purpose. Older adults may face a number of fears: losing their independence, not having enough money, becoming physically or financially dependent upon others, becoming ill, or dying. The uncertainties of these years can affect attitudes, feelings, relationships, and total behavior. Some older adults view the future as dismal, offering only the prospect of increasing losses and, eventually, death.

On the other hand, some older adults experience this portion of life as "the golden years." For those who are financially secure, remain in reasonably good health, and enjoy close ties to friends and family, the later years can be rewarding. These adults enjoy opportunities such as retirement, travel, socializing, and spending time with grandchildren. As with every other age, effective coping skills and supportive relationships help a person deal with life changes and maintain a good state of adjustment.

For Discussion and Reflection

Consider your own journey through several of the life stages described. What changes did each stage bring? Did you find it easy or difficult to adjust to these changes?

Adjusting to Life Changes

In addition to facing developmental changes and societal pressures, people of all ages must occasionally cope with major changes such as new experiences, illness, divorce, or death.

These changes may require a person to give up old behaviors and learn new ones. Some changes considered particularly stressful include:

- Change in marital status (marriage, separation, divorce, or reconciliation)
- Change in employment status (being fired, retiring, or starting a new job)
- Death of a spouse or partner, family member, or close friend
- Injury or illness (one's own or that of a family member)

Each of these changes can threaten a person's adjustment for a time while new behaviors are being learned.

New Experiences

Even when they are positive, new experiences can be stressful. An adult beginning a new job must learn how to function in a new environment and get to know new coworkers. A student who graduates from high school and begins college must adapt to living away from home and assuming a greater amount of responsibility. A new parent may become exhausted and overwhelmed by the demands of caring for a young child. Adapting successfully to a new situation requires patience and often the support of family and friends. Any life event can become a crisis that creates anxiety and unhappiness for one who has not learned to deal with change.

For Discussion and Reflection

What new experiences have you encountered that required you to make major adjustments to your daily habits? Examples include getting married or divorced, having a child, getting a new job, or going back to school.

Illness

Illness is always a threat to adjustment. It interferes with the usual pattern of living, is accompanied by discomfort, may involve doubt as to the outcome, and often creates financial problems. Patients and their families react to illness according to the degree of threat it represents. Adjustment is always poorer during illness. Sometimes behavior patterns that are not typical of a person appear during illness. Someone who is usually easy to please, for example, may be very difficult to please during an illness. A person who is usually quite well adjusted may show signs of poor adjustment during the period of illness. The patient may react with anger or fear to feelings of helplessness or being dependent on others. Interestingly, the poorly adjusted person may react with positive feelings if the illness provides an escape from having to deal with daily problems.

The person who is self-reliant and has learned to deal with life problems usually finds illness frustrating. Familiar techniques for solving problems do not cure the illness. Perhaps the patient is accustomed to giving orders; now, the physician, nurse, laboratory assistant, radiology technician, and other personnel seem to be in charge. The shift from being independent to a state of dependency seriously threatens adjustment. The behavior of a patient may be markedly different from that person's usual behavior.

Divorce

Divorce is almost always a traumatic experience for everyone involved, especially the children. Even if both parents agree that divorce is preferable to continuing the marriage, children are affected emotionally as they see their home and family breaking apart. Their daily life changes in many significant ways. The adults are dealing with their own emotional reactions to the trauma of marital discord. They may be unaware of the child's reactions: anger toward one or both parents, belief that the parent who is moving out "doesn't love me anymore," or possibly guilt, believing that they are the cause of the family breakup. If the divorce is hostile, there may be a custody battle. Then the child has a serious conflict of loyalties and may witness numerous hostile encounters between the parents. The child experiences emotional turmoil: a mixture of love and hate, anger and grief, guilt about divided loyalty, and negative feelings toward one or both parents.

When either parent remarries, a stepparent enters the picture, further complicating the child's emotional life. If the parent who remarries is the custodial parent, and the new stepparent also has children, the result is a "blended family." A period of turmoil may last for months because each person must adapt to new family relationships and establish new patterns of interaction. Ideally, these adaptations occur with minimal trauma, and family dynamics eventually become positive. It is unrealistic to expect this to happen immediately. Family counseling can assist blended families in making these adaptations.

Death

The death of a family member or friend can be very traumatic. Children especially need help in understanding death, accepting the permanence of death, dealing with feelings associated with the deceased, and coping with the sense of loss or abandonment. Effective grieving is very important. If grief is not processed, the suppressed emotions can affect future attitudes, emotional expression, and behavior when another loss is experienced. Chapter 16 discusses the effects of grief in greater detail.

Social and Cultural Stressors

As an individual grows up and grows older, they must also cope with the pressures of society. Stressors such as peer pressure, drugs, and **discrimination** can become serious threats to a person's adjustment.

Stressors of Childhood

Many children feel tremendous pressure to do well in school and/or sports and to be accepted by peers. For some children, success in these areas seems to come naturally. For slow learners, shy children, or those with behavioral difficulties, school becomes a major source of stress. Some children may also have difficulty fitting in with others and making friends. As a child moves into the older elementary and middle school years, peer relationships become increasingly important.

Stressors of Adolescence

All the sources of childhood stress continue through adolescence—accompanied by additional sources of stress: the pressure of competition (athletics, extracurricular activities, school politics), pressure to excel (especially if college-bound), the need to belong, the need to be attractive to potential romantic partners, eagerness to finish driver education and get one's own car. These are the familiar pressures of adolescence.

There is also the threat of school violence. Gangs exist in many schools; by belonging, there is safety in numbers, but one must conform to the gang's practices and beliefs. School shootings are increasingly reported in the media, and public schools conduct regular lockdown and evacuation drills to prepare students and staff for the possibility of an armed intruder.

Peer Pressure Adolescence is a period when peer approval is extremely important. It is a time of life when family influence is challenged by the peer group because of the individual's need to belong. For that reason, each adolescent must choose between participating in certain practices that are widespread through the student body and the risk of being the outsider. Peer pressure can be external, such as when peers urge an individual to join them in a potentially harmful activity, or internal, such as when the individual feels that they must participate in the activity that others are doing to be accepted, even if others have not specifically told them to do so.

Drugs Drugs are a major problem, sometimes being sold and used in school restrooms and parking lots. At social events there is peer pressure to use drugs such as marijuana, crack, cocaine, heroin, methamphetamines ("meth"), and others. "Just say 'No!'" is not easy advice to follow; by saying, "No," the student risks disapproval of the peer group. According to the National Institute on Drug Abuse (2021), the percent of teens using illegal drugs in the United States has declined in recent years. However, in many communities, drug use remains a serious problem among teens.

Sexual Activity When the adolescent begins to date, there may be pressure almost immediately to engage in sexual activity. This may conflict with beliefs about morality the adolescent has learned in the home and through religious or spiritual practices. The adolescent experiences an internal conflict: the need for acceptance by the peer group and the need to uphold one's standards and maintain self-esteem. Today's trend of becoming sexually active during the teens has significant health implications: pregnancy, sexually transmitted diseases, and the emotional effects of abandonment by a partner to whom one has become emotionally attached. In many communities, sex education remains a controversial subject. Providing information on self-protection or distributing prophylactic materials through a school program is emphatically opposed by many adults. A health care professional is very likely to be approached by a teenager who needs information or help in regard to sexual activity.

Fortunately, not every adolescent is exposed to these stressors, but many are exposed to all of them. Numerous stressors experienced by adolescents today were less prevalent when their parents were in high school. Many parents therefore do not understand or accept the problems today's adolescents face at school. Every adolescent needs to be able to discuss these problems regularly with an adult who understands the problems, encourages the expression of feelings, and helps identify appropriate ways to deal with these difficult situations.

Stressors of Adulthood

Many of the stressors and serious traumas of childhood and adolescence continue into adulthood. Some that are discussed below also occur during childhood or adolescence. But certain stressors, such as discrimination and domestic violence, seem more appropriate for discussion within the framework of adulthood.

Discrimination Members of minority groups in all cultures and throughout time have experienced discrimination. There seems to be an innate human need for perceiving people in "us/them" terms, favoring those who are members of the "us" group. But this tendency does not excuse discrimination that violates the rights of others because of sex, gender identity, sexual preference, race, nationality, ethnic group, age, or religion.

Federal laws protect equal employment opportunities and prohibit discrimination on the basis of race, sex, and age. But laws do not change attitudes or beliefs. Discriminatory practices still exist, in educational settings as well as in the marketplace. Discrimination may be practiced against anyone because of a specific attribute, such as race, sex, gender identification, sexual preference, religion, age, weight, or other attributes.

Sexual Harassment Sexual harassment is one of the most frequently reported complaints in the workplace today. It may also occur in an educational setting. Usually the victim is someone with limited power (student, secretary), whereas the perpetrator (teacher, supervisor, customer) has some degree of power over the victim. The harassment may be verbal, may consist of inappropriate touching, or may involve requests or demands for sexual acts. Sometimes the victim perceives the harassment as including the threat of being fired; sometimes the promise of favorable treatment (a good grade, a promotion, a "business" trip) is implied or stated directly. Some individuals enjoy the attention and use these "offers" as opportunities for self-advancement. Most people, however, consider these unwanted sexual advances as harassment and see themselves as victims. Anyone who believes that they are being harassed should consider several questions:

- What can I do about this situation?
- How can I protect myself?
- What options are available to me?
- What is the best way to stop these unwanted advances?

Emotional reactions to sexual harassment include anger, fear, and guilt; the threat to self-esteem is obvious. The individual who is accused of sexual harassment usually either denies that it occurred or blames the victim. At one time the victim of sexual harassment had no recourse. Reporting the incident to a supervisor carried a risk of being fired, accused of lying, or worse. All too often, the perpetrator would be the supervisor. Today, however, it is possible to take legal action, since sexual harassment is covered by federal laws against discrimination. An individual who chooses to file a complaint should have some type of evidence, other victims who are willing to join the complaint, and/or witnesses who have heard or seen examples of harassment. The complaint probably will not be handled in the victim's favor if it becomes a matter of "one person's word against another's."

The best approach is to stop harassment when the first incident occurs. Using "I-statements," the victim can express feelings and then in a matter-of-fact way establish limits on behavior. If this does not stop the harassment, then the employer's procedure for filing a complaint should be followed. A complaint can be filed with the proper federal agency if the employer does not take action to stop the harassment. If the victim does decide to file a complaint, they should be aware that there is risk of reprisal from the accused, from the employer, or even from colleagues who choose to side with the accused.

National and World Events

Some national and world events can be considered traumas in the life of the individuals affected. Trauma is discussed in greater detail in Chapter 10. However, even individuals who do not experience a traumatic loss directly may have to make significant adjustments to their daily lives. The global COVID-19 pandemic of 2020 and the following years offers a key example. Many communities issued lockdown orders, closing businesses and requiring individuals to remain at home in order to limit the spread of COVID-19. Remaining at home for weeks or months with limited social contact, fewer opportunities for physical activity, and—in some areas—limited access to fresh, healthy foods, had a significant impact on the mental and physical health of many individuals. The World Health Organization reported that during the first year of the pandemic, rates of anxiety and depression around the world rose by 25% (2022).

During lockdown, individuals' responses to this threat to their adjustment varied: Some individuals became fearful, isolated, and depressed, checking social media for the latest death rates and watching television news reports for hours. Others decided to use their time in lockdown to learn a new language, read books, or grow a garden. Some people looked for ways to help others, such as contributing financially to community members who lost jobs during the pandemic or regularly contacting friends and family who lived alone to cheer them up.

© Cryptographer/Shutterstock.com

FIGURE 9-3 The COVID-19 pandemic of 2020 and the following years had a significant impact on physical and mental health worldwide.

The example of the COVID-19 pandemic illustrates both the impact of events beyond our control and our ability to choose our response to difficulties. Events of national or global magnitude require individuals to adapt to circumstances they did not choose and cannot control. Physical health, mental health, finances, and most other areas of life may be impacted. Individuals who have previously learned good coping skills, who have a good level of adjustment, and who have support from friends, family, and community resources will be better equipped to "make the best of a difficult situation." On the other hand, individuals who lack coping skills in daily life or who lack access to friends, family, and community support are likely to experience greater difficulties.

Chronic Stressors

A chronic stressor refers to a situation that develops gradually and persists for a long time. A person with ongoing financial problems, family difficulties, or learning disorders may find it especially difficult to remain well adjusted. Often, difficulty in one of these areas affects an individual's performance in other areas of life. For example, an individual in an unhappy relationship may find it difficult to concentrate at work. A child whose parents fight constantly may misbehave at school. A parent who is struggling to make ends meet may snap at the children. Health care professionals may be able to refer patients to appropriate community agencies for financial help, counseling, or educational evaluation.

Financial Problems

Financial problems have many causes. Some individuals may be unemployed or lack the skills needed to earn a comfortable living. Others may have a reasonably good income but find themselves faced with overwhelming medical or legal expenses. Many people lack money management skills and find themselves in financial trouble because they do not know how to budget and set priorities. One family could not afford a car but spent $50 per week on a rent-to-own large-screen TV. A young parent who could barely pay the rent spent about $8 per day on prepackaged lunchbox items for the children even though they were eligible to receive free lunch at school.

Other individuals face overwhelming credit card debts. Many community agencies offer free financial counseling. Health care professionals should also be aware that out-of-control spending sprees are one symptom of bipolar disorder. For their own protection, individuals diagnosed with this disorder should not have access to checks or credit cards.

Family Difficulties

Family is an important part of most people's lives. Healthy families provide emotional support, unhealthy or dysfunctional families can create anxiety and distress in a person's life. Put simply, a healthy family is one in which all family members are kind, caring, and respectful toward one another. Effective families function like a team, each person doing his or her part but also helping other members when needed. All families have conflicts and disagreements, but healthy families work to resolve their problems in a way that protects each family member's dignity.

A dysfunctional family may fight often or just not communicate at all. Members of an unhealthy family may not trust one another and may feel that other family members do not respect or care for them. Winning and being "right" become more important than working together. For adults, unhealthy **family dynamics** often lead to separation and divorce.

FIGURE 9-4 Healthy family relationships help children become well-adjusted and able to adapt to new situations.

What begins as poor communication and unhealthy dynamics often grows into feelings of unhappiness with the relationship, a lack of love for the spouse, and the desire to be with someone else. Some children in dysfunctional families misbehave or do poorly at school. Some use drugs or alcohol. Still others turn to relatives and friends for support and understanding. Unfortunately, unhealthy family dynamics are often learned and passed on to the next generation.

Being part of an unhealthy family is a tremendous threat to one's adjustment. Unfortunately, many of the families depicted in movies and on television are dysfunctional. Because the media portrays family difficulties as humorous and commonplace, viewers may come to accept fighting, insults, and infidelity as normal. In reality, these behaviors are symptoms of an unhealthy family. Counseling is available in most communities and can help families learn more appropriate ways to interact with one another.

Learning Problems

In recent years it has become common for parents to seek medical advice when their child has difficulty in school. These difficulties may include poor grades, failure to learn new concepts, trouble completing assignments, or behavior problems. Today attention, learning, and behavioral disorders are most often diagnosed during the elementary school years. However, older students and even adults may suffer from undiagnosed disorders. These disorders can pose a threat to a person's adjustment at any age. Health care professionals should be aware of the signs of some common disorders and should encourage the child's parents or affected adult to seek professional evaluation. Warning signs of learning problems include:

- Slow development in speaking and writing
- Difficulty expressing ideas or understanding directions
- Difficulty with forming letters, writing, and spelling

- Difficulty memorizing and remembering information
- Clumsiness, poor handwriting, or poor coordination
- Difficulty paying attention and completing tasks
- Sloppiness, carelessness, or lack of organization
- Tendency to misinterpret others' behavior and become upset
- Sudden mood changes, frequent frustration

These behaviors may indicate a variety of learning problems. Some of the more common are described in the following sections.

Attention Deficit Disorder and Attention Deficit Hyperactivity Disorder **Attention deficit disorder (ADD)** and **attention deficit hyperactivity disorder (ADHD)** describe a pattern of inattentive, impulsive, and hyperactive behaviors. Students with ADD/ADHD may appear disorganized and have difficulty remembering information and completing tasks. They may show aggression and have poor relationships with their peers. Other common behaviors include daydreaming, staring into space, constantly moving or getting up, and blurting out. ADD/ADHD is a medical diagnosis, but health care professionals often seek input from a student's parents and teachers before making a diagnosis. Treatment of ADD/ADHD usually includes behavior modification and medication. Treatments such as hypnotherapy and neurofeedback have also proven successful for some individuals.

Learning Disorders When a student's academic achievement is significantly lower than one would expect given the student's level of intelligence, they may have a learning disorder. The three primary types of learning disorders are reading disorders (also called **dyslexia**), mathematics disorders, and writing disorders. A student with a learning disorder isn't "dumb" but has difficulty with a particular subject area. Students with identified learning disorders are entitled by federal law to receive special educational services, so health care professionals should encourage parents to have their child evaluated if a learning disorder is suspected.

Developmental Disorders

As their name suggests, **developmental disorders** affect an individual's mental or physical development. The two most prevalent developmental disorders in the United States are mental disabilities and autism spectrum disorders. These disorders are usually diagnosed in the preschool or elementary school years.

Intellectual Disabilities When most people hear the term *intellectual disability*, they imagine an individual who is severely disabled. In fact, intellectual disabilities can be mild, moderate, severe, or profound. An intellectual disability is typically identified through tests of intelligence and adaptive behavior skills, or skills needed to care for oneself and function in everyday situations. Mild disabilities may not be identified until the school years, when it becomes clear that a child is learning at a rate slower than that of classmates. In older adults, a mild intellectual disability may never have been formally identified. Like individuals with learning disorders or physical disabilities, individuals with intellectual disabilities are protected against discrimination by federal law.

Autism Spectrum Disorders **Autism spectrum disorders** include the disorders which have previously been referred to as classic autism, pervasive developmental order—not otherwise specified (PDD-NOS), and Asperger syndrome. Individuals with these disorders process and respond to information differently than typical individuals, causing difficulty with communication, behavior, and social interactions.

Autism affects each individual differently, and the degree to which daily functioning is impaired can be mild to severe. Persons with autism can have low, average, or high levels of intellectual functioning. Over the past few years, more and more children are being diagnosed with autism spectrum disorders. Treatments include special educational programs, occupational therapy, speech therapy, medication, and modified diet. In 2018, the Centers for Disease Control and Prevention reported 1 out of 44 eight-year-old children in the United States is diagnosed with an autism spectrum disorder.

For Discussion and Reflection

What experiences have you, a friend, or a relative had with one of the learning or development disorders described? What challenges did the individual have to overcome as a result of the disorder?

Behavior Disorders

While most children misbehave at times, some develop a pattern of problem behaviors that can severely disrupt the school or home environment. Students with oppositional defiant disorder routinely defy the authority of parents or teachers. When told to do something, they may intentionally do the opposite. Students with a conduct disorder may not only disobey parents and teachers but also threaten or harm others, steal, or vandalize school or public property. These students may be treated with behavioral modification, therapy, and/or medication. Whenever possible, families of affected students should also seek counseling, since living with a family member's disorder is stressful. Likewise, many experts believe that family dynamics influence or even create behavior disorders. Improving family interactions can improve the problem behaviors.

Discipline and Home Environment While it is important to detect and treat legitimate disorders, families often find that children's behavior and academic performance improve when parents learn more effective discipline techniques. Contrary to popular opinion, *discipline* does not mean *punishment*. Discipline means teaching children the difference between appropriate and inappropriate behaviors and guiding them to choose behavior that is appropriate to the situation. Effective discipline includes the following techniques:

• Develop a warm, caring relationship with children.
• Explain and model socially appropriate behavior.
• Keep rules and expectations clear, simple, and age-appropriate.
• Enforce rules calmly and consistently.
• When necessary, discipline a child with time out or loss of a privilege, not by hitting or yelling.

In addition, children learn and behave better when they receive good nutrition and when parents monitor television and video games. Exposure to violent TV programs and video games has been linked to aggressive behavior.

Resolving a negative family situation can also improve behavior. One second grader developed a serious problem with aggressive and defiant behavior at school. Upon investigation, it was found that her mother used harsh punishments and often told the girl, "You're no good." Shortly after her father gained custody, the girl began to behave appropriately at school.

Coping Skills and Resilience

Surprisingly, well-adjusted people are not always those who have led lives free of difficulty or trauma. Ultimately, it is not what happens to us that determines our level of adjustment, but how we cope with it. Good coping skills and resources can help a person regain a good level of adjustment even when faced with difficult circumstances. The following coping skills and resources help individuals deal with problems as they occur:

- Eat a healthful diet and exercise regularly.
- Get a full night's rest.
- Talk to a friend or family member about emotions and problems.
- Set goals and work toward them one step at a time.

A similar concept is **resilience**, the ability to bounce back or recover from problems. Factors associated with resilience include having a positive attitude, believing one has the power to change one's circumstances, and developing strategies to reduce stress. Being part of a support network such as a caring family or community group can also help a person recover from difficulty.

Coping with a difficult situation takes time. During the period of readjustment, a person may find counseling or a support group helpful. These resources are especially important for a person who has experienced a trauma. Chapter 10 examines different types of trauma and the reactions a victim of trauma is likely to experience.

Activities

1. Consider your own life up until the present. Which of the life stages below have you experienced so far? What challenges and opportunities stand out as most significant for you? Now consider a friend or relative at a later stage of life than you are. What challenges or opportunities have they experienced?

   Early childhood

   Middle childhood

   Adolescence

   Young adulthood

   Middle adulthood

   Older adulthood

2. Consider several of your life experiences that involved new situations. Try to recall how you felt during the early days in the new situation. Which of your familiar behaviors were inappropriate in the new situation? What changes did you make in your behavior patterns as you adapted to the new situation?

3. Describe your experience during the COVID-19 pandemic of 2020 and the following years. What changes did you experience in your daily life, school or job, and relationships with others? How did you adjust to these changes?

4. With a classmate, discuss how you might respond to the following situations in your role as a health care professional.

   a. A parent consults you about Luis, a second grader. They tell you that Luis has trouble remembering what his teacher said in class. Homework takes him hours to complete, and he often cries with frustration because he doesn't understand. The parent says, "One day Luis can do the work, and the next day it's like he's forgotten everything." What might you suggest?

   b. Deja, a fourth grader, has developed a behavior problem at school. She blurts out comments in class, hits others, and occasionally steals pencils and other small items. Her parents ask you what they should do to help Deja. What factors might you consider in discussing Deja's behavior with her parents?

5. Review the discussion of coping skills and resilience in this chapter. How would you rate your current level of resilience on a scale of 1 to 10 (1 = not effective; 10 = very effective)? What's one action you could take to improve your coping skills and resilience when faced with difficult circumstances?

References and Suggested Readings

Centers for Disease Control and Prevention. (2022). Autism spectrum disorder. https:///www.cdc.gov/ncbddd/autism/facts.html

Centers for Disease Control and Prevention. (2022). Developmental disabilities. https://www.cdc.gov/ncbddd/developmentaldisabilities/index.html

National Institute on Drug Use. (2021). Percentage of adolescents reporting drug use decreased significantly in 2021 as the COVID-19 pandemic endured. https://nida.nih.gov/news-releases/2021/12/percentage-of-adolescents-reporting-drug-use-decreased-significantly-in-2021-as-the-COVID-19-pandemic-endured

World Health Organization. (2022). COVID-19 pandemic triggers 25% increase in prevalence of anxiety and depression worldwide. https://www.who.int/news/item/02-03-2022-covid-19-pandemic-triggers-25-increease-in-prevalence-of-anxiety-and-depression-worldwide

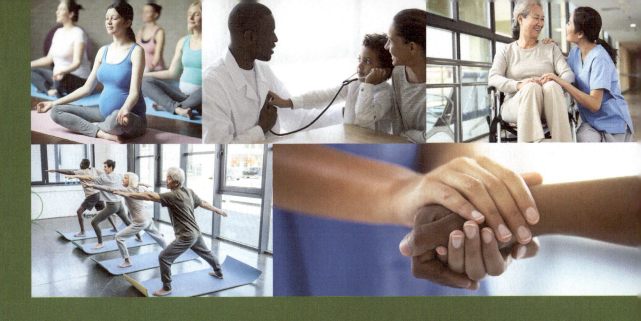

Effects of Trauma

Objectives

After completing this chapter, you should be able to:

- Define trauma.
- List traumatic effects of each of the following: natural disasters, war or terrorism, rape, and child abuse.
- Describe the cycle of domestic violence and the types of help needed by victims of domestic violence.
- Describe normal reactions to traumatic events as well as the symptoms of the following psychological disorders: anxiety disorder, panic disorder, post-traumatic stress disorder (PTSD), phobias, and depression.
- Describe how health care professionals can provide trauma-informed care.

Key Terms

Abuse	Pedophilia	Sexually transmitted
Incest	Perpetrators	disease (STD)
Neglect		Trauma-informed care

Chapter 9 describes threats to adjustment that everyone experiences. Some people are fortunate in that they have never experienced severe trauma, but today more and more people, of all ages and from all walks of life, experience some type of trauma. Health care professionals need to be aware that these experiences are serious threats to adjustment and have implications for the physical, mental, and emotional health of victims.

You, as a health care professional, are more likely to encounter victims than perpetrators. You also need to be aware that any given patient may be a victim, even if the patient does not volunteer information to that effect. Any suspicion that you have should be reported to your supervisor and/or the physician for further evaluation and possible legal action. *Follow the policies and procedures of your employing agency; do not attempt to handle such a matter yourself.* Just as important, *do not ignore the indications that aroused your suspicion.*

What Is Trauma?

A trauma is an event that poses a serious threat to one's life or well-being. Trauma includes experiencing, witnessing, or learning of a crime, act of aggression, accident, natural disaster, or act of war. Physical, emotional, and sexual abuse are also considered traumas. Experiencing a trauma poses a serious threat to a person's adjustment. Even people who are normally well adjusted will develop physical and emotional reactions following a traumatic event.

A traumatized person may require medical attention immediately after the event. In other cases, the person may seek medical advice days or weeks later when secondary symptoms develop. In addition to treating physical injuries, health care professionals should inform patients about normal reactions to trauma and refer them to a mental health professional if these reactions become severe.

Traumatic Experiences

While any difficult situation may be perceived as a trauma by the person who experiences it, the following discussion focuses on events that are commonly recognized as traumatic. By understanding the most common types of trauma, health care professionals will be better equipped to assist trauma victims in understanding their own reactions and seeking the help they need.

Victims of a single event, such as a mugging, experience intense emotional reactions in addition to their physical injuries. After the physical injuries have healed, professional counseling may be needed for processing the emotional trauma. Victims of recurrent trauma, such as long-standing **abuse**, need help in escaping their situation; these victims benefit from professional counseling—to develop new insights and resolve deeply rooted emotional trauma.

The Perpetrator

In reading the following paragraphs, remember that there are traumatic *events* (such as accidents), there are **perpetrators** (persons who inflict the trauma), and there are persons suffering from the event, who may refer to themselves either as *victims* or *survivors*, depending upon their preference. The perpetrator's behavior may result from behavior patterns learned at home or on the street, cultural patterns, uncontrolled emotional expression, criminal tendencies, or a psychiatric disorder. The perpetrator's behavior may be considered acceptable within that particular culture or may fall into the category of psychiatric disorder or criminal behavior. Discussion of the causes of a perpetrator's behavior is beyond the scope of this book; the study of such behavior falls within the disciplines of sociology, psychology, psychiatry, and criminology.

Blaming the Victim

The trauma experienced by the victim is magnified when others choose to blame the victim. Those who would defend a rapist are likely to claim the victim "was asking for it," citing manner of dress or presence in a particular location.

This tendency to blame the victim sometimes extends even to those who are the victim of a criminal act or are involved in an accident:

Why were you out at that time of night?

Why did you go to that place? You should have known better!

How many times have I told you not to drive so fast?

Being blamed for what happened adds to a victim's emotional trauma. It is only natural to feel anger when being blamed at a time when one's need is for expressions of caring and emotional support. Although blaming may actually be a friend's or relative's expression of concern, it is inappropriate and not what a victim needs to hear. Also, blaming may be an example of displaced anger, from the cause of the event or the perpetrator, to the victim; this too is inappropriate. The health care professional sometimes has an opportunity to point out to relatives a victim's need for expressions of caring, emotional support, and protection from being blamed. The following statements show caring and support, rather than blame:

I know this is hard to talk about. Thank you for trusting me with this information.

I'm sorry that happened to you.

I'm here to listen if you'd like to talk.

Everything you're feeling right now is valid.

How can I support you right now?

Crimes and Accidents

Muggings, carjackings, burglaries, gang beatings, and other types of violence are all too prevalent. Some groups of people are targeted disproportionately. For example, the U.S. Department of Justice reported that between 2017 and 2020, individuals who identified as gay, lesbian, and transgender were more than twice as likely to be the victims of violent crimes as cisgender persons (2022). Experiencing or witnessing crime or acts of violence can have traumatic effects.

Unintentional injuries, whether by automobile accident, workplace injury, or other forms of accidents, are a leading cause of death, especially for men under the age of 25. In addition, thousands of people each year sustain disabling injuries.

Anyone who is the victim of a crime or who survives a serious accident has emotional trauma in addition to any physical injuries sustained. The health care system tends to focus on physical injuries, however. Once victims have been treated in the emergency room or discharged from the hospital, they usually receive follow-up treatment primarily for their physical injuries.

Fear and anger usually accompany the physical trauma of crimes and accidents. Some people can process these feelings over time; others need professional counseling to deal with the intensity of the feelings and any disabling effects, such as panic attacks or chronic anxiety. It is appropriate, within the role of some health care professionals, to suggest to victims that they may benefit from counseling to deal with the emotional effects of their traumatic experience.

Natural Disasters, War, and Terrorism

We often hear news reports of floods, hurricanes, tornadoes, and earthquakes that have taken lives and left many people without homes. A natural disaster can be devastating for both the community and the individuals affected. Damage to or loss of one's home, school, or workplace threatens one's sense of security and normalcy. An individual who has experienced a natural disaster may experience any of the reactions to trauma described earlier. In addition, some people may develop anxiety or phobias related to the experience. For example, a person who lived through a hurricane or tornado may become distressed during thunderstorms or high winds.

Experiencing or witnessing war or terrorist acts also causes trauma. Individuals often feel overwhelmed by fear, helplessness, and vulnerability. They struggle to understand what has happened and why. Scenes of destruction or suffering may play through a person's mind over and over. For those who lose friends, family, or homes, there is a tremendous sense of grief as well. War and terrorist acts can breed distrust among different nations or ethnic groups, planting the seeds for further aggression in the future.

Military personnel in combat face traumatic situations constantly. For some, the psychological effects are so devastating that they never regain their previous level of adjustment even after returning to civilian life. Many veterans find themselves unable to function after returning home. These veterans suffer from post-traumatic stress disorder.

FIGURE 10-1 A natural disaster can be devastating for both the community and the individuals affected.

Natural disasters, war, and terrorism affect not only individuals, but also entire communities. These large-scale traumas provoke many of the same reactions as other traumas. However, a trauma experienced by many has some noteworthy differences. Because many people have been affected, finding someone to talk to about the experience may be easier. Some survivors may find comfort in the feeling that, "We're in this together. I'm not alone." On the other hand, friends and family who are also traumatized may not be able to provide much emotional support. Ongoing media coverage and community discussion become constant reminders of the event.

For some individuals, the COVID-19 pandemic of 2020 and the following years was a traumatic experience. Many people lost friends and family members to COVID-19. Others lost jobs, businesses, and even their homes due to the economic impact of lockdowns. Some people became extremely sick after contracting the virus and continued to suffer long-term effects for months or years afterward. Any serious illness can potentially be experienced as a trauma by the sick person and those close to them. Because it was global in magnitude, the COVID-19 pandemic is one of the most dramatic examples in history of a shared traumatic experience.

Bullying

Many children experience teasing and bullying in the home, on the playground, and at school. The child who is noticeably different (has a physical disability or a tendency to stutter, for example) is especially at risk for teasing by the peer group or bullying by larger children. School policies regarding children with behavioral disorders or learning difficulties set these children apart, a practice that often results in a child being labeled and possibly rejected by classmates. Bullying, however, is a more serious problem.

Bullying includes several aggressive behaviors, including name-calling, put-downs, threats, taunting, physical assault, taking or damaging property, and forcing a person to do something he or she does not want to do. A bully may be aggressive or passive. Aggressive bullies may instigate a bullying situation, while passive bullies rarely "start the fight" but join in once an aggressive bully has set the stage. Bullying can be described as follows:

- The behavior is intended to harm or disturb less powerful victims, who are smaller, weaker, or unable to defend themselves.

- The behavior occurs repeatedly over a period of time.

- The bully chooses a time when winning is almost certain, such as when there is no one present with the authority to intervene.

- The bully often has one or more allies present.

By choosing a weaker victim and surrounding themselves with allies, the bully, who lacks real courage, gains a sense of power by overpowering the victim.

Many parents and teachers view bullying as a normal part of growing up and therefore do little to intervene. Children who fight are often described as "tough" or "standing up for themselves." Some parents of aggressive bullies are secretly proud of their child's tough reputation or blame other children for starting the fight.

Unfortunately, bullying often occurs more in schools than in any other single place. Research suggests that much bullying could be prevented by clear and consistent school discipline policies and close adult supervision on playgrounds before and after school. All students who report bullying should be taken seriously, and their anonymity should be protected.

Children who bully others need both firm discipline and understanding. Bullying behavior is often an indicator that a child comes from an unhealthy family. Researchers suggest that failure to bond with parents in the early years, lack of love, and ineffective discipline increase the likelihood of bullying. Some aggressive children are copying aggressive behavior they have learned from parents. For example, a parent might tell a child, "Don't let anyone walk all over you." While bullying behavior should not be excused on the grounds that a child came from a difficult home, attempting to change the behavior without addressing its cause is unlikely to stop bullying. Many community mental health centers offer family counseling, parenting classes, and anger management sessions that can help bullies and their families learn more acceptable behaviors.

Victims of bullying require help in several areas:

- They need adult intervention to end the bullying or at least avoid bullying situations.
- Victims of bullying often need help to address the low self-esteem and feelings of powerlessness as a result of being repeatedly threatened or overpowered.
- They also need to learn how to protect themselves physically and emotionally in the future.

When bullying is not adequately addressed, the effects can be devastating for the individuals involved and their community. Young people who have been threatened, taunted, and assaulted can develop the attitude, "No one cares about me. Everyone's against me." For some, this attitude leads to depression; for others, it creates a desire to strike back. Investigations into several school shootings in recent years revealed that the shooters had been the targets of bullying or felt rejected by their peers.

Adults may experience bullying in the workplace, the community, or in personal relationships. Anyone who routinely uses intimidation and manipulation to get his or her way at the expense of the rights of others is a bully. Standing up to a bully takes strength and courage. It is important to set limits and let the bully know in no uncertain terms when they have crossed the line. The bully must be told that the behavior is unacceptable and will not be tolerated.

With the popularity of the Internet, text messaging, and other technological forms of communication, *cyberbullying* has increased. Examples of cyberbullying include spreading vicious rumors, insults, threats, or hate messages through electronic messages. Cyberbullying occurs most often, though not exclusively, among adolescents. Victims of cyberbullying may experience fear, depression, lowered self-esteem, or even become suicidal.

For Discussion and Reflection

Did you or someone you know experience or observe bullying in school? What was that experience like?

The child who has positive emotional support in the home survives teasing and some degree of bullying without serious damage. The child who does not have opportunities for processing feelings about these experiences is likely to suppress anger and fear, develop a negative self-concept, and have problems with interpersonal relations. These experiences, though not as dramatic as some types of trauma, can have lifelong effects.

Child Abuse

Child neglect and abuse are serious problems today and can take several forms:

- **Neglect** includes leaving young children unsupervised or failing to provide adequate food, clothing, shelter, hygiene, and medical care.
- Abuse includes harming a child emotionally or physically. Verbal abuse consists of put-downs, cursing, or making repeated comments like "You're no good. I wish you'd never been born. You're going to end up in jail just like your father (or mother)."
- Emotional abuse includes "mind games," manipulation, or using fear to control the child.
- Physical abuse can include inappropriate discipline such as harsh beatings or locking a child in a closet. Any physical assault upon a child can be considered abusive, particularly if marks or bruises are visible afterward.
- Sexual abuse occurs when an adult or older child forces a child to take off his or her clothes or perform any sexual act. While the act itself is physical, the damage to the victim is emotional, mental, and physical.

Both boys and girls can be victims of sexual abuse. The perpetrator is most often a close family member, but may be a family friend or authority figure. If the perpetrator is a parent or sibling, the sexual encounter is **incest**. If the child is under 13 years old and the perpetrator is 5 to 10 years older than the child, it is **pedophilia**; the abuser is a *pedophile*. Studies of pedophiles indicate that many were themselves sexually abused as children.

With the rise of the Internet, there has been increasing public concern about "sexual predators" who meet young people online and engage them in inappropriate online or in-person sexual activities. Many schools now teach Internet safety guidelines. Parents should also monitor teens' online activity and maintain open communication to encourage teens to discuss any inappropriate online experiences. When teens are unsupervised, lack a supportive and caring family, or have a history of trauma or abuse, they are more vulnerable to sexual predators as well as more likely to engage in other high-risk behaviors.

Health care professionals, teachers, law enforcement officers, and other professionals are legally required to report suspected cases of abuse and neglect to their local Child Protective Services office. Community members and relatives may also make reports. The U.S. Department of Health and Human Services reports that in 2020, over 618,000 cases of child abuse and neglect were substantiated. Many professionals believe that for each case that is reported and substantiated, there are many more that are never reported or that would be difficult to prove.

> **For Discussion and Reflection**
>
> Based on your own knowledge and experiences online, what advice would you give to teens regarding Internet safety?

Traumatic Effects The effects of sexual abuse on a child can affect adjustment throughout life. Sexual abuse includes mental and emotional abuse as well as physical acts. The perpetrator uses various devices to keep the child from exposing him. The act may be presented as "our secret" and the child made to feel that they are being given very special attention. If the child reacts negatively, the perpetrator may use threats to keep the child from telling anyone. Some perpetrators convince their victims that they are to blame, thus using shame and guilt to control the child. This enforced silence results in suppression of intense feelings: anger, fear, grief, and guilt.

Unfortunately, many adults refuse to believe a child who does try to tell them about being sexually abused. It is especially difficult for parents to believe that a respected authority figure, such as a teacher, coach, or member of the clergy, would sexually abuse their child. Many adult survivors of child sexual abuse tell of seeking help from an adult, only to encounter disbelief and accusations of lying. Parents, teachers, ministers, adult friends and neighbors, and especially health care professionals must *listen* when a child tries to tell what some adult did to them. Although the child may not have the vocabulary to describe the event in adult terms, it is important to *let the child tell what happened in his or her own words*. Do not suggest words you think might help the child's description, since that could be construed legally as having "planted the idea in the child's mind."

Sexual abuse can cause physical, mental, and emotional damage:

- Victims grow up with low self-esteem, suppressed anger and fear, feelings of guilt and distrust, and perceptions of the world as a hostile place.
- They may contract a **sexually transmitted disease (STD)** or sustain other physical injuries.
- As adults, many survivors of childhood sexual abuse have difficulty forming an intimate relationship. Many have one relationship after another; others avoid intimacy altogether.

The lifelong effects of child sexual abuse are now acknowledged by the mental health community. Through psychotherapy and techniques such as hypnosis, many adults have been able to bring repressed memories to the conscious level, a necessary step in order for therapy to proceed. Support groups for survivors of abuse and incest have been established in many communities.

While enduring abuse is traumatic for a child, reporting the abuse and ending the situation can be traumatic as well. One 10-year-old girl told her mother that her stepfather had sexually abused her. As a result, the mother took the children and moved out. The abuse had ended, but now the girl faced the trauma of losing her stepfather and stepgrandparents. She had to adjust to a new home, a new neighborhood, and a new school. Some abused children who are "wise to the system" choose not to report being abused because they fear being taken from their parents. Enduring abuse is the price they pay to protect their families and avoid confrontation.

Appropriate action depends on the situation. Criminal charges may be filed against the perpetrator, but adults should not let that possibility prevent them from protecting the child against further molestation. Pedophiles tend to repeat their behavior, so every child within range of a pedophile is at risk.

The sexually abused child enters the adolescent period having already experienced some type of sexual activity. Some behaviors, emotional patterns, attitudes toward sex, levels of trust in others, and interpersonal relations differ from those of their sexually inexperienced classmates. Some children try various forms of escape: alcohol, drugs, food, sleep, or withdrawal. Those who have strong guilty feelings may inflict physical pain on themselves by head banging, beating hard objects with the fists, cutting or mutilating themselves, or even attempting suicide. These behaviors may be exhibited during adolescence or adulthood, years after the sexual abuse stopped or the individual escaped from the abuser.

Rape

The use of threats or force in order to engage in a sexual act is *rape*. It is a crime and should be reported, even if the perpetrator is a relative, friend, date, or coworker. *Rape is an act of aggression that violates the victim physically and emotionally.* Rapists tend to have a hostile attitude toward women. They may also have an intense need to experience a feeling of power over others. Some rapists want to inflict pain and enjoy the woman's fear. Because the experience satisfies the rapist's need for power and control, he is likely to rape repeatedly and to have more than one victim. The rapist who does not feel powerful enough to force himself on an adult woman may choose a child as victim. Rape is one of a number of acts included in the legal term "sex offender."

The rape victim often is victimized further by family members and/or "the system." If the rapist is a relative, family members may not believe the victim's report; some may actually side with the accused rapist. If the victim reports the rape to police, she may be subjected to dehumanizing procedures by officers who do not understand the significance of rape. Comments made about a rape or a rape victim often show total lack of understanding that *rape is a violent act of aggression.*

In many communities, the concerns of rape survivors, health care professionals, and law enforcement personnel have led to educational efforts to sensitize officials to the needs of a rape victim. Every rape victim should have professional counseling to help deal with intense emotions and the serious threat to self-esteem. Counseling and a support group can help the victim regain confidence in her ability to go about her daily routine without fear.

Stalking

Stalking may take the form of unwanted letters, phone calls, emails, or gifts, or it may include following or spying on the victim. One in 10 women and 1 in 50 men experience stalking at some point (NCADV, 2020). Posting inappropriate or negative information online or in a public place can also be considered stalking. While many people occasionally find themselves the object of unwanted attention, these behaviors can be considered stalking if they cause victims to fear for the safety of themselves or their family members.

Adult Abuse

Adult abuse has received growing media attention. Adult abuse occurs when older adults or adults with disabilities are neglected or mistreated by adult children, spouses, or other caretakers. For adults with developmental disabilities, the risk of being physically or sexually assaulted may be significantly greater than it is for other adults. Women who are disabled are assaulted, raped, and abused more often than women who are not disabled. Older adults are also at risk for neglect, emotional abuse, and physical abuse. Abusers may include nursing home staff, adult children, spouses, or other relatives. Just as health care professionals have a legal duty to report suspected cases of child abuse, they have an ethical duty to report suspected adult abuse to the authorities.

Domestic Violence

Abuse by one's spouse or partner is now recognized as a public health problem in the United States. According to the National Coalition against Domestic Violence (2020), one in four women and one in ten men will experience domestic violence at some point in their lives. Spousal abuse is found in all cultures, races, occupations, income levels, and ages.

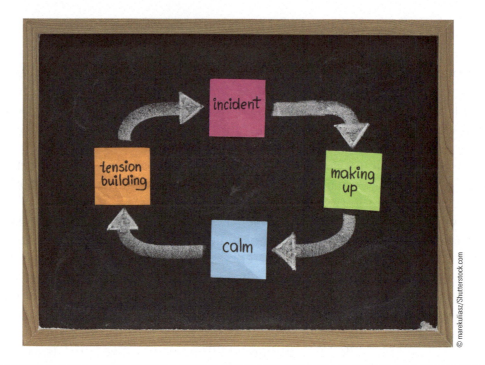

FIGURE 10-2 In an abusive relationship, the cycle of abuse alternates between periods of calm and periods of abuse.

Spousal abuse can take various forms, including physical aggression (assault), emotional trauma, "mind games," deprivation of needs (including access to money), and isolation from relatives and friends. Employers lose billions of dollars every year because of lost workdays, medical costs, and other problems associated with domestic violence.

The Abuser Personality

Abusers have two personalities: the public personality, that of "a really nice person," and the private personality, controlling and demanding. Few people would enter knowingly into an abusive relationship. The abuser initially is charming and shows care and concern, so the partner enters the relationship expecting romantic love and warmth. Gradually the abuser begins to make demands that lead up to isolating the victim from family and friends, getting control of the victim's money, controlling the couple's activities (eliminating the victim's activities and interests), requiring explanations for the victim's behavior or comments, demanding a report on any time spent away from the abuser, and making decisions for the victim. These demands are first made within an acceptable, and possibly flattering, context:

- I can't stand to be away from you.
- I want you to spend more time with me.
- You spent all afternoon with your friend when I needed you to be with me.
- I want you to be here while I watch TV.
- I want you to be home when I get back.
- You know how important you are to me.

Initially the abuser makes the victim feel important and loved, but comments such as the above are leading up to controlling not only the relationship, but also all aspects of the victim's life. The abuser's objective is *power*—total control over the other person.

The following statements illustrate the increasing degree of control:

- What did you and your friend talk about all afternoon?
- What did you do while I was away?
- I'll take care of paying the bills; I handle money better than you do.
- Wear that outfit; you really look great in it.
- Don't wear that to the party.
- What were you and Joe laughing about?
- Why did you stay in the kitchen with Amy so long?
- What did you mean when you said . . . ?

Next, the abuser begins to chip away at the victim's self-esteem:

- Why did you say . . . ? That was stupid!
- Why can't you be more fun when we party?
- Why can't you be a better parent/spouse?
- You can't do anything right.
- You made me angry (jealous).
- You caused us to run out of money.
- You had me so upset I ran a red light; it's your fault I got this ticket.
- Yes, I drink too much, but it's because you make me so . . . .
- I didn't get the promotion; you should have been nicer to my boss at the Christmas party.

Effects on the Victim

Once the victim begins to believe that they really are the cause of the couple's problems, the abuser has tremendous power. With low self-esteem and overwhelming feelings of guilt, the victim is less able to evaluate the relationship and definitely less able to leave it. Once the abuser's power is established, the abuse may include physical aggression. The physical abuse may escalate until the victim sustains serious injuries or is killed.

Individuals who grew up in a home where domestic violence was a way of life may simply accept abuse as part of a relationship. At some point, the victim may realize they do not have to submit to abuse. The victim may seek escape, but escape may require help from family, friends, or a community agency. Some victims choose to stay in an abusive relationship rather than risk the uncertainties of being alone.

Escaping Abuse

Most victims of domestic violence need outside help to escape the abusive relationship. Since an abuser takes control of the family's finances, the victim has no financial resources to aid in escape. Sometimes the abuser tries to ensure that the victim remain financially dependent.

Personnel in domestic violence shelters report that many victims who appear ready to become self-reliant actually go back to the abuser. Sometimes it takes several attempts before the victim finally escapes permanently. Many of these victims need several types of help:

- The belief that they do not have to submit to abuse
- Financial assistance
- A separate place to live
- Childcare
- Job and/or job training
- Child support
- Legal protection

As soon as arrangements are made for physical survival, it is important that the victim receive counseling to counteract the destructive effects of the abusive relationship. The damage to self-esteem may take years to overcome. Processing fear, anger, and guilt may require many months. Without effective counseling, the victim may not be able to trust another partner or establish an intimate relationship based on equality.

Hopeful Signs

The problem of domestic violence in American society has finally gained legal recognition. In 1995, the U.S. Congress passed the Violence Against Women Act (VAWA). The VAWA has been reauthorized several times, most recently in 2022, providing funding for sexual assault treatment, education, and prevention programs. This is the first federal law that recognizes and attempts to stop violence against women. The VAWA contains a civil rights remedy for victims of violence to file charges through a federal court and seek monetary compensation, court-ordered protection, and costs of legal expenses.

Reactions to Trauma

Normal reactions to a traumatic experience vary by individual. Immediately following the event, an individual may experience any of the following:

- Shock, a feeling of being stunned or dazed
- Denial, or not accepting what has happened
- Numbness, or feeling disconnected from the world around them

Once these initial reactions pass, individuals may experience ongoing symptoms:

- They may become moody, irritable, or anxious.
- They have physical symptoms such as sweating or a rapid heartbeat.
- Sleep and eating patterns can change.
- Individuals may have repeated memories of or dreams about the traumatic event.

These reactions can develop immediately after the traumatic event, or they can be delayed for months or years.

Some people recover quite quickly from trauma, while others suffer for a long time. Friends may tell an individual, "Just get over it, stop dwelling on the past." But some trauma survivors are not able to return to their prior level of adjustment on their own. Health care professionals can assist these individuals by assuring them that their feelings are normal reactions to trauma and that they aren't "crazy." Counseling or a support group may be particularly helpful for these individuals.

The severity of reactions can also vary. For some individuals, reactions can be so powerful that they appear similar to mental illness. Health care professionals should be familiar with common reactions to trauma so that a traumatized person will receive an appropriate diagnosis and referral for help. The sooner after a trauma a person can talk about the event and receive emotional support, the less likely it is that long-term problems will develop.

Anxiety

A person experiencing generalized anxiety may worry most of the time, have trouble sleeping, and appear shaky or nervous. A patient with anxiety may say, "Doctor, I need something for my nerves." The anxious person may or may not recognize a connection between the trauma and the anxiety. More specific conditions associated with anxiety include panic disorder, post-traumatic stress disorder, and phobias.

> **For Discussion and Reflection**
>
> Have you or someone you know experienced a traumatic event? Did you or that individual experience any of the immediate or ongoing effects described?

Panic Disorder Some individuals experience recurring, unexpected anxiety or panic attacks. During these attacks, the person can have a pounding heart, chest pain, difficulty breathing, numbness or tingling, and a dizzy or faint feeling. The skin may become pale and cold. A patient may say, "I thought I was dying" or "I thought I was having a heart attack." While a single panic attack does not necessarily indicate panic disorder, recurring panic attacks or fears of having more attacks are signs that a patient needs treatment.

Post-Traumatic Stress Disorder When a person continues to re-experience a trauma for weeks or months after it occurs, he or she may be experiencing post-traumatic stress disorder (PTSD). The term *PTSD* was coined following the Vietnam War when large numbers of soldiers returning from combat were unable to recover from the horrifying situations they had witnessed. Some were unable to function in jobs or in their families, and they felt they had no one to talk to since friends and family back home could not imagine the traumas they had endured. Soldiers in other wars had had similar reactions, referred to as "shell shock" or "battle fatigue" in World War I and World War II. After the Vietnam War, PTSD was recognized as a serious psychological disorder that could result not only from war, but also from almost any trauma.

Symptoms of PTSD include reliving the event through nightmares or flashbacks. The person may have strong reactions to or avoid anything that serves as a reminder of the event. She may be irritable or jumpy, feel in danger, or need to be "on guard" at all times. On the other hand, some people experiencing PTSD may feel numb, have difficulty remembering details of the event, and show a lack of interest in work or leisure activities.

Phobias A phobia is an intense, irrational fear that lasts for six months or more. Phobias may develop in response to a traumatic experience, or they may develop spontaneously. For example, one young girl developed a fear of the dark after her mother's car hit and killed an animal while driving at night. The girl feared that she would see a wounded animal if she looked out the window when it was dark. Some common phobias include fear of snakes, lightning, or speaking in public. A person with a phobia usually avoids the feared situation and experiences extreme anxiety if forced to enter it. Some individuals are unable to leave home because of their phobias. Treatments include therapy, hypnosis, and desensitization, in which the person is gradually exposed to the feared situation while in a state of relaxation. Ultimately, overcoming a phobia involves helping the person lower her anxiety until she is able to enter the feared situation more calmly.

Depression

Depression is characterized by a feeling of sadness that won't go away. A depressed person may feel tired all the time and show a lack of interest in work, school, or leisure activities. She may have trouble concentrating and making decisions. Low self-esteem or even thoughts of suicide may be present. Additional symptoms of depression include restlessness, trouble sleeping, and sudden changes in appetite or weight. A person experiencing depression may appear to be very emotional, negative, or pessimistic, making comments like, "Nothing seems to matter anymore," or "It doesn't matter what I do. Nothing will help anyway." He or she may withdraw from social activities and avoid interactions with others. Trauma is only one cause of depression; other possible causes include genetics, poor coping skills, or ongoing conditions in a person's life, such as an unhappy relationship.

The Survivor Role

Each victim reacts to trauma in accordance with their established patterns of behavior. For some, the role of victim provides certain benefits that they do not want to give up, and so "I am a victim" becomes part of the self-concept. Some refuse to work through the emotional effects, choosing instead to hold onto their anger, fear, or hatred. For these individuals, sharing their traumatic experience becomes a way to gain sympathy and support from others. Others find valuable lessons in their traumatic experience and make significant lifestyle changes to improve the quality of their lives.

One woman who was the victim of sexual harassment filed complaints through appropriate channels, with no results. She later filed a lawsuit and eventually received a substantial financial settlement. Instead of simply enjoying her financial gain, she chose to set up a nonprofit organization to provide assistance to others in dealing with sexual harassment. She also serves as a consultant to businesses and provides on-site seminars to help employers establish safeguards against sexual harassment in the workplace. This is an example of how a person can learn from a bad experience and eventually use that learning for a constructive purpose.

Trauma-Informed Care

As a health care professional, you will likely meet many individuals who have experienced some type of trauma. Many health care agencies provide training for their staff in how to address the effects of trauma, both immediate and long term. There are various treatment models for **trauma-informed care**, but most address these common themes:

- Safety: Developing a plan to keep oneself physically and emotionally safe
- Managing emotions: Learning to cope with fear, anger, worry, and other emotions; learning to make decisions rationally; regaining the ability to trust other people
- Loss: Acknowledging and coping with lost loved ones, relationships, or opportunities
- Planning for the future: Developing a positive vision for life in the future and planning achievable step-by-step goals to get there

Health care professionals should encourage victims and relatives to understand the serious nature of psychological trauma and help them recognize the need for professional assistance. Although the disabling effects of physical trauma are obvious, psychological trauma is less likely to be understood or acknowledged. With encouragement from a health care professional, the victim may accept that he or she needs professional assistance in dealing with the psychological effects of the traumatic experience. Research indicates that most patients want to be asked about traumatic experiences by their health care provider, and that doing so can lead to improved health outcomes (Tomaz & Castro-Vale, 2020). With therapy, the victim may regain a healthy state of adjustment within a few weeks or months. Without therapy, the victim may remain in a state of poor adjustment for months or years.

FIGURE 10-3 Research indicates that most patients want to be asked about traumatic experiences by their health care provider.

Activities

1. Define *trauma* and give examples of experiences that are typically considered traumatic.

2. Consider any life experience that was emotionally traumatic for you. Did you receive any encouragement and support from friends and relatives? Did any health care personnel who cared for you show concern about the emotional effects of your experience? Do you experience fear, anger, or other strong emotions when you think of that experience? If so, consider the possibility that you could benefit from professional counseling.

3. Obtain the name of the agency and the emergency phone number for obtaining help in your community or state for the following situations:

   a. Reporting child abuse

   b. Reporting a rape

   c. Reporting domestic violence

   d. Obtaining emergency shelter for a victim of domestic violence

   e. Filing a complaint about sexual harassment in the workplace (after the employer's established procedures have been followed, without results)

4. Describe normal reactions a person may experience as a result of trauma.

5. Consider the following situations in terms of the trauma experienced by the victim and appropriate action by you as a friend or a health care professional:

   a. A child is brought to the emergency department by both parents, who report that the child fell down the stairs. After determining that the arm is broken, the physician asks you to take the child to the cast room and directs the parents to the waiting room. En route to the cast room, the child whispers to you "I did *not* fall down the stairs." What is an appropriate action for you to take?

   b. Your best friend has been married almost a year. At first you and she continued your custom of having lunch and going to a movie once a week. Then, she began to cancel at the last minute; once, she didn't cancel but failed to meet you. Today, she arrives at the restaurant wearing dark glasses. She says she cannot stay for the movie, as her husband expects her home in an hour. When she adjusts her glasses, you notice bruises on her arm. What are some appropriate statements you could make to her? Or should you just ignore what you have seen?

   c. Your coworker tells you she has a problem and asks if you will meet her after work. She reveals that, as a child, she was sexually abused by her father. She left home as soon as she finished high school and visits her parents (in a nearby city) only on special occasions. She is divorced and has custody of her 10-year-old daughter. Now, her parents are insisting that she allow the daughter to spend one weekend a month with them. The daughter is excited about this, but has told you that Grandpa kissed her on the lips during their last visit. What factors should influence the coworker's decision?

References and Suggested Readings

Centers for Disease Control and Prevention (CDC). (2019). *Leading causes of death: Males. All races and origins; United States, 2016.* https://www.cdc.gov/healthequity/lcod/men/2016/all-races-origins/index.htm#anchor_1571144769

National Coalition against Domestic Violence (NCADV). (2020). *Domestic violence.* https://assets.speakcdn.com/assets/2497/domestic_violence-2020080709350855.pdf?1596811079991

Substance Abuse and Mental Health Services Administration. (2022). Resources for child trauma-informed care. https://www.samhsa.gov/childrens-awareness-day/past-events/2018/child-traumatic-stress-resources

Tomaz T., & Castro-Vale I. (2020, September 14). Trauma-informed care in primary health settings—which is even more needed in times of COVID-19. *Healthcare* (Basel), *8*(3), 340. doi:10.3390/healthcare8030340

U.S. Department of Health and Human Services. (2022). Child maltreatment 2020. https://www.acf.hhs.gov/cb/report/child-maltreatment-2020

U.S. Department of Justice. (2022). Violent victimization by sexual orientation and gender identity, 2017–2020. https://bjs.ojp.gov/library/publications/violent-victimization-sexual-orientation-and-gender-identity-2017-2020

Chapter 11

Defense Mechanisms

Objectives

After completing this chapter, you should be able to:

- State the purpose of defense mechanisms.
- Describe common defense mechanisms.
- Compare substance dependency and defense mechanisms.
- Explain how occasional use of a defense mechanism can contribute to good adjustment.

Key Terms

Abstinence
Addiction
Alcoholism
Alcohol use disorder
Codependency
Dependency
Displacement

Dysfunctional
Enabler
Fetal alcohol syndrome
    (FAS)
Habituation
Hallucinogenic
Hypnosis

Perceptions
Projection
Psychotherapy
Rationalization
Repression
Self-deception
Withdrawal

There are certain mental devices that all of us use at times in order to feel more comfortable and make our behavior seem reasonable to ourselves and others. These devices are known as *defense mechanisms*.

The Purpose of Defense Mechanisms

When we find ourselves in a situation that we cannot handle effectively, feelings of threat are aroused: fear, anxiety, hostility, frustration, or other negative feelings. Inability to handle the situation can threaten self-esteem and possibility expose us to physical or psychological harm. When we feel unable to deal with a situation, we may use a defense mechanism.

Defense mechanisms are attempts to protect our self-esteem. They help us handle feelings of discomfort, make it possible to "save face," provide an *apparently* logical reason for our behavior, and enable us to maintain self-respect in spite of the outcome. Defense mechanisms can be useful—provided that we do not make a habit of using them to avoid reality. Defense mechanisms can help us, or they can become crutches that substitute for more effective ways of dealing with difficult situations.

As a health care professional, being able to recognize common defense mechanisms will help you understand behavior. It is also desirable that you recognize your own use of defense mechanisms in order to develop effective ways of dealing with difficult situations. This chapter explains seven common defense mechanisms: rationalization, projection, displacement, repression, withdrawal, and escape into illness. The remainder of the chapter addresses substance dependency. You will encounter friends, perhaps family members, and patients who have some type of substance dependency.

Common Defense Mechanisms

Rationalization

Rationalization involves offering an apparently reasonable, socially acceptable explanation for behavior, when the true reason would be too painful for the individual. Thus, rationalization helps relieve disappointment, provides a means for avoiding a situation perceived as threatening, and avoids admitting an inadequacy that would be damaging to self-esteem. Unfortunately, rationalization is a form of self-deception; frequent use of rationalization is self-defeating because it displaces efforts to improve one's competence in dealing with life situations. Consider the following example:

Cam has been invited to a party. The other teens know the latest dance moves. Cam does not dance. Although Cam wants to be a part of the group and have a good time, Cam imagines that trying to dance in front of the other teens will feel embarrassing. Missing the party is preferable to being embarrassed. Cam's mother is in poor health, but she is not so sick that Cam needs to stay home with her and miss the party. Nevertheless, Cam's mother's health provides a graceful way to avoid the party.

For Discussion and Reflection

Have you ever used rationalization to avoid an uncomfortable situation? For example, have you ever told someone you could not participate in an event because you had to work, complete an assignment, and so on, when in reality you simply preferred to avoid the event?

FIGURE 11-1 Defense mechanisms are attempts to protect our self-esteem. They help us handle feelings of discomfort.

By rationalizing, Cam has avoided admitting a fear of feeling embarrassed at the party and has given a socially acceptable reason for being absent. When rationalization is used habitually, it becomes an *unconscious* mechanism. Friends of the habitual rationalizer may be unaware of the fears and anxieties that are the basis for hard-to-understand behaviors. They may regard the habitual rationalizer as a person who always makes excuses.

Projection

Projection is blaming our own inadequacies on someone else or on circumstances. Projection is also used to attribute our own unfavorable characteristics and desires to someone else; a person who is often critical of other people may be exhibiting projection. When projection is used to an extreme, the individual develops distorted **perceptions** of life situations and of people.

James is a health occupations student who is not making satisfactory grades. In discussing his academic standing with the counselor, he says that he cannot study at home because his mother wants him to help around the house. When one of the instructors corrects James on his technique in performing a procedure, he complains that the instructor does not like him. When hostility develops between James and a classmate, James explains the situation by saying that his classmate is jealous because James is dating Kim.

Every undesirable situation in James's life is explained as the fault of something or someone other than himself. His use of projection is preventing an honest appraisal of his

FIGURE 11-2 Projection is blaming our own inadequacies on someone else or on circumstances.

problems and how he himself helps create them. Other people may be saying, "Why doesn't James take responsibility for his own actions?" But James is more comfortable projecting blame than looking at himself. He avoids having to admit to himself that he has some shortcomings.

Some people use projection and other defense mechanisms instead of learning to see themselves and situations realistically. Each of us makes mistakes at times. *Being able to recognize how we contribute to an undesirable situation and being able to learn from our mistakes lead to growth as a person.* Frequent use of projection interferes with such growth. Projection is self-deception and a distortion of reality.

Displacement

Displacement is the redirection of strong feelings about one person to someone else. Displacement occurs when there is fear or inability to direct the feeling toward the object or person who aroused the feelings. Usually, displacement involves negative feelings, but it can also occur with positive feelings.

Bryson is a health care professional with hostile feelings toward his supervisor. He is well aware that the supervisor makes out the assignments and the schedule; also, the supervisor must recommend any member of the staff for a raise. It would be unwise for Bryson to be openly hostile to one who has so much control over his daily work and over progress in his career. Bryson recognizes this and is always pleasant to the supervisor. Whenever Bryson has a conference with the supervisor, the next person he sees is likely to become the object of his hostility. Sometimes Bryson carries his hostility home and is irritable and short tempered with his family or the family pet. Bryson is displacing the hostility he feels for the supervisor to others who did nothing to create his negative feelings.

Obviously, displacement creates interpersonal problems. Family and friends may be tolerant for a while, especially if they recognize that the hostility has been aroused by someone else. They may even take sides with the individual and attach unflattering names to the person who aroused the anger. Usually, however, the person who habitually displaces negative feelings is perceived by others as irritable and "hard to get along with."

You have learned that the energy generated by negative feelings needs to be worked off, preferably through physical activity. Displacement is an *unhealthy* method of using negative energy. It is an undesirable pattern of behavior, both because of the self-deception involved and because of its unfavorable effects on relationships.

Repression

Repression is forcing an unpleasant memory into the subconscious mind. Once a memory has been forced into the subconscious mind, it cannot be remembered at will. Although deeply buried, the memory is still a powerful influence on behavior. Repression occurs most often with painful experiences of childhood, but it can also occur with an adult experience. Anyone who has had a traumatic experience may repress the memory because the experience is too painful to keep within conscious awareness. Family members may, at some future time, be surprised to hear that individual say, "I don't remember that," or actually deny that such an experience ever occurred. Repression is less susceptible to conscious control than the defense mechanisms discussed previously.

Repressed memories usually come to light only during **psychotherapy**. Many therapeutic sessions are necessary to bring repressed memories back into the conscious level. **Hypnosis**, possibly with age regression, is sometimes used to identify and/or help a patient "relive" a traumatic experience that has been repressed. This is usually accomplished with only a few hypnosis sessions. These methods require the skills of a psychiatrist or psychologist with specialized training.

You, as a health care professional, should be aware of the influence of repressed memories on behavior. A traumatic experience, especially during childhood, may exert a powerful influence on adult behavior, even though the adult does not recall that experience. As a health care professional in contact with pediatric patients, try to prevent the child's experience with the health care system from being psychologically traumatic.

Withdrawal

Withdrawal as a defense mechanism involves either shutting off communication or removing oneself physically from a situation that feels threatening. Withdrawal makes sense in a situation in which danger is likely, as in a disagreement when the other person becomes physically threatening. Extremes of withdrawal are characteristic of some psychiatric conditions. A less extreme, but quite serious, example of withdrawal is the desertion reaction of some pediatric patients if no member of the family stays with the child. Lying in the fetal position, a tendency of some chronically ill patients and many geriatric patients, is also an example of withdrawal. If your role as a health care professional will involve caring for patients who exhibit these types of withdrawals, you will study these conditions in other courses.

In every health care role and in your personal life, you will see examples of withdrawal used as a coping strategy in difficult situations:

- If a discussion becomes unpleasant and you refuse to participate further, you are using withdrawal.

- If a conference with your supervisor arouses anger and you excuse yourself from the conference, then you are withdrawing physically.

- If you do not do assignments and have made low grades on the tests, then drop the course the week before exams, you are withdrawing to avoid the threat to your self-esteem that a failing grade represents.

Suppose your first position as a health care professional requires that you work with someone you dislike. Every day you have one or more contacts with this person, and each encounter leaves you angry or unhappy. Except for this one person, you like your job very much. Should you resign? Should you keep the job in spite of these daily annoyances? This situation requires a decision between "fight" or "flight." You can stay on and try to cope with your reactions to this person, or you can "flee" to another job.

There are times when it is a better strategy to withdraw physically from a situation than to put up with the problems it involves. There are other times when the satisfactions of a situation can balance the unpleasantness. Decisions about whether to withdraw or remain should be made on a *rational*, rather than an *emotional*, basis; but the probable long-term effects of the alternatives should enter into the decision.

For Discussion and Reflection

After reading the explanation of withdrawal above, describe a time you have used this defense mechanism to avoid an uncomfortable situation. Looking back, was withdrawing a helpful choice, or could you have resolved the situation in a more productive way?

Escape into Illness

Escape into illness involves periodic illnesses that serve a definite purpose, but the individual is not aware of the purpose. Illness as an escape usually has its beginnings in childhood. Parents tend to be especially attentive when a child is sick, even if the illness is a minor one. Sometimes busy parents do not give children much more attention than is necessary for the daily routine until a problem arises involving the child. Then the child becomes the center of attention. When the problem has been taken care of, the busy routine may be resumed, with the child again receiving only necessary attention. Thus, the child learns that illness is rewarded with parental notice and concern.

If illness during childhood is rewarded by special attention, gifts, permissiveness, sweets, or other things desired by children, then illness serves a definite purpose—the reward of being "special" and of having privileges *not usually allowed when well*. If the parents permit a child to use illness to avoid a dreaded situation and/or to gain advantages available only during an illness, then these early learnings can become an unconscious mechanism that will influence behavior throughout life. Once the child has learned that a headache, a cold, or other minor physical complaint can serve a purpose, illness may be used to get special attention or to avoid certain situations. Eventually, the purpose is no longer in the conscious mind and periodic illnesses have become "real."

Many people habitually use escape into illness as a means of avoiding some of their life problems. When the stress of accumulating problems reaches a certain point, or when an anticipated event arouses fear or anxiety, a minor illness can conveniently provide temporary escape. The symptoms experienced are real; the misery the individual feels is real. There may even be great annoyance at the inconvenience caused by this illness, yet the pattern of behavior is based on the individual's inability to face certain situations. Let's look at Janelle, who is enrolled in a program for surgical technicians.

Janelle is 19 years old, a high school graduate. She likes sports and has high ideals about team spirit and fair play. She can hold her own with peers, whether in sports or in standing up for her beliefs.

The surgical technician program proved very interesting to Janelle—until the class went into the operating room. Suddenly Janelle had some feelings she did not understand. Patients on stretchers, containers of body organs, hospital staff members with masks and floppy gowns—it was a frightening and unreal world to Janelle. After several days, Janelle's negative feelings about the operating room were stronger than on the first day. Increasing familiarity did not relieve the intense feelings, whereas most of her classmates had become accustomed to the sights and smells of the operating room suite.

Over the weekend, Janelle could think of nothing but the operating room and its effect on her. She played basketball with friends, but did not play as well as usual. On Monday morning, she could not eat breakfast. When her mother anxiously inquired about her health, she said she must have hurt her back playing basketball. Janelle, with her mother's encouragement, went back to bed and slept all day.

Janelle was not pretending to be sick. Her doubts and fears had mounted to the point that stress was manifested as physical symptoms. Janelle really did feel terrible! Retreating into illness was an unconscious escape.

At this point, Janelle's early learnings will influence the behavior pattern of the next few days. If she has learned to use illness as an escape, her back pain will become worse and she will withdraw from the surgical program because of a "bad back." If Janelle is able to face life realistically, she will eventually recognize that her emotional reactions to the operating room are affecting her unfavorably. An honest and realistic appraisal of the job requirements of a surgical technician should be made. If Janelle is not temperamentally suited to the operating room, she should feel free to withdraw from the program on that basis, without the need to project blame on an "injured back."

Sometimes a person develops insight into tendencies to use escape into illness and, through determination and effort, learns to face problems rather than trying to escape them. Many people, however, have used this device for years and are unable to develop insight into the purposes of the illnesses without professional counseling.

Substance Abuse and Dependency

Defense mechanisms involve mental tricks—the use of the mind to deal with uncomfortable situations. Another approach to dealing with difficult experiences is the use of substances that have physical effects, thereby providing some relief from stress or diminished awareness of discomfort. Like the defense mechanisms, these substances—tobacco, alcohol, and drugs—provide an escape. With repeated use, one may develop **addiction** to one or more of these substances.

Nicotine Addiction

It is now known that nicotine, contained in all tobacco products, is highly addictive. Evidence that tobacco is a major threat to health has been increasing for several decades. As a result, many public buildings and most hospitals have been declared smoke-free environments and smoking is prohibited on airlines. Many smokers refuse to give up their habit until they experience a major health problem, such as a heart attack. Others choose to give up smoking as part of a larger plan for a more healthful lifestyle. But for those smokers who choose to continue their habit, current societal restrictions are sources of frustration and anger.

Why do people smoke? The usual reason is that smoking provides relief from feelings of stress. For an individual whose parents were smokers, the smell of a cigarette, cigar, or pipe may arouse pleasant childhood memories and feelings of comfort and security. Once a person has become addicted to nicotine, smoking is a response to subtle signals from the body that it needs a nicotine "fix." According to the CDC, as of 2020, over 30 million adults in the United States were cigarette smokers. Interestingly, between 14 and 15 percent of adults ages 25 to 65 were smokers, compared to only 7.4 percent of adults ages 18 to 24.

In recent years, the use of electronic cigarettes ("vaping") has increased as an alternative to traditional cigarette smoking, particularly among young people. The CDC reported that as of 2021, over 11 percent of high school students surveyed reported using e-cigarettes regularly. Most e-cigarettes contain nicotine, the same addictive chemical that is found in tobacco. Nicotine use has been shown to impact the brain development and mental health of teens (CDC, 2021). Some e-cigarettes may contain other substances, ranging from herbal formulas, to marijuana or its variants, to various illegal drugs.

The decision to give up tobacco or e-cigarettes may be made voluntarily or under pressure from one's physician, family, or friends. Many smokers are able to give up their habit simply by deciding to do so. When an addictive substance is no longer available to the body, physical symptoms of withdrawal occur. (This meaning of "withdrawal" is different from its meaning as a defense mechanism.) Nicotine withdrawal results in nervous agitation and intense craving for a cigarette (or whatever form of tobacco the individual uses). People who cannot tolerate withdrawal symptoms may use nicotine chewing gum or a skin patch. Psychotherapy also can provide assistance through hypnosis or relaxation with guided imagery.

As a health care professional, you will encounter people who either continue to smoke or are trying to quit. These people may be patients, coworkers, family, or friends. Learn about the dangers of tobacco and the various approaches to giving up tobacco products, so you can be a source of information for anyone who seeks your help.

Alcohol Abuse/Alcoholism

The use of alcohol, like tobacco, may begin as a social activity and a desire for peer approval and acceptance. It is readily available, more affordable than most drugs, and present in many homes, making it accessible to children and adolescents.

Social use of alcohol can provide quick relief from stress, anxiety, guilt, insecurity, and other uncomfortable feelings. These effects may lead to occasional abuse—overindulgence to

FIGURE 11-3 The use of alcohol and other substances provides a temporary escape from stress or unpleasant feelings.

the point of becoming intoxicated. Regular use of alcohol over a period of time can result in psychological **dependency** and, eventually, physiological addiction—**alcohol use disorder**.

Alcohol use disorder has been defined as "an impaired ability to stop or control alcohol use despite adverse social, occupational, or health consequences" (NIAAA 2021). According to the Centers for Disease Control and Prevention, from 2015 to 2019, approximately 140,000 deaths per year were attributed to excessive use of alcohol. In industry, high rates of absenteeism, errors, low productivity, and occupational accidents are attributed to alcohol. Alcohol is involved in a large percentage of crimes, especially murders, and in domestic violence, child abuse, and sex offenses.

Why do people drink? Alcohol provides *escape*. Although classed as a central nervous system depressant, alcohol is considered by many people to be a stimulant, because it lowers inhibitions and releases muscular tension. Unfortunately, these relaxing effects are accompanied by diminished judgment, thinking skills, and memory—effects that make the drinker a danger to themselves and others. The use of alcohol to escape the feelings of despair and hopelessness that characterize clinical depression and the depressive phase of manic depressive illness is common. If such patients have also developed **alcoholism**, their clinical status is "dual diagnosis."

Why do some people progress from social drinking to dependence on alcohol? Many factors have been implicated: physiological, metabolic, nutritional, genetic, emotional, and social. Regardless of causative factors, the condition is treatable, but only when the individual can admit to needing help. This may occur only after numerous arrests, hospitalizations, and various losses (job, spouse, home) have occurred. Medical treatment is required for acute phases, especially during withdrawal, and the ongoing support and encouragement of family and friends is crucial to an alcoholic's long-term recovery.

Effective treatment includes helping the individual learn to face reality and deal with life's problems, instead of trying to escape them. This learning can be facilitated by counseling and participation in group therapy. Alcoholics Anonymous (AA), whose membership consists of recovering alcoholics, has proven to be effective for many people. AA emphasizes total **abstinence** from alcohol; newcomers are encouraged to avoid having a drink and to cope one day at a time. Making it through one day is achievable for many people, but vowing to "never take a drink again" is a promise too easily broken. Researchers have found that no one treatment approach works for everyone, and today a variety of treatment models for alcoholism are available. Treatment may include medication, behavioral therapy, support groups, and treatment of co-occurring physical or mental health conditions.

One consequence of drinking is **fetal alcohol syndrome (FAS)**. This disorder is the result of a woman drinking during the prenatal period. *Drinking even one or two glasses of wine per day during early pregnancy increases the probability that the baby will be born with FAS, since alcohol penetrates the placental barrier and enters the fetal bloodstream.* Serious damage to the brain results, so the baby is born with an *untreatable disability.* The newborn infant is small, has characteristic cranial and facial features, and may have deformities of the limbs. Growth and development will be inhibited; an intellectual disability may be diagnosed when the child is old enough for testing. This condition is so definitely related to drinking during pregnancy that the National Institute on Alcohol Abuse and Alcoholism issued a statement in 1980 that *pregnant women should totally abstain from alcohol consumption.*

Drug Abuse

The use of drugs is so pervasive in modern society that few people are unaffected. Any drug can be abused, but those most likely to be abused are drugs that relieve pain, alter one's mood, have a stimulant effect (provide a "high"), relieve anxiety, or have a **hallucinogenic** effect. Regular use of these types of drugs leads to **habituation**, which is psychological dependence on the drug. If usage continues over a period of time, *tolerance* may develop, meaning that larger and larger doses are required to get the desired effect. *Addiction* exists when there is a physiological need for the drug at regular intervals. *Drug dependency* and *chemical dependency* are now the preferred terms, without concern about whether the patient's condition is habituation or addiction. *Withdrawal*, when used in relation to drug dependency, refers to the symptoms that occur when a drug is withheld. These symptoms range from nervous agitation and anxiety to psychotic behavior and convulsions, depending upon the specific drug being withdrawn.

The Substance Abuse and Mental Health Services Administration (2021) has noted the following trends in the use of illegal drugs in the United States from 2015 to 2020:

- In 2020, there were 59.3 million Americans over the age of 12 who reported using an illegal drug in the past month. This represents 21.4 percent of the population.

- Drug use is highest among 18- to 25-year-olds. Over a third of this age group reported using illegal drugs within the past month.

- The use of marijuana has increased, with 49.6 million Americans reporting using the drug in the past month. As of 2022, marijuana is legal for recreational use in 19 states and legal for medical use in 37 states. While marijuana continues to be illegal under federal law, individuals are rarely prosecuted for its use in states where it has been legalized.

Based on 2020 data, the number of Americans over age 12 who reported using drugs within the past month was as follows:

- 9.3 million Americans reported using prescription medication such as painkillers for nonmedical purposes.
- 5.2 million Americans reported using cocaine.
- 5.1 million Americans reported using prescription stimulants for nonmedical purposes.
- 2.5 million Americans reported using methamphetamine.

While some individuals are able to use illegal drugs recreationally without long-term effects, doing so is a risky proposition. Each year, millions of Americans struggle with addiction and drug dependency. Substance abuse disorder has been defined an "impairment caused by the recurrent use of alcohol or other drugs (or both), including health problems, disability, and failure to meet major responsibilities at work, school, or home" (SAMHSA, 2021, p. 27). In 2020, almost one in four Americans age 18 to 25 met the criteria for substance abuse disorder at some point during the previous year. For individuals 26 and older, 14 percent met the criteria for a substance abuse disorder.

As a health care professional, you are almost certain to encounter individuals whose families, careers, finances, and health have been impacted by drug use. When appropriate, based on your job role and your employer's guidelines, you will have the opportunity to share information about treatment options and recovery support groups in your community.

Codependency

Codependency is a situation in which the **dysfunctional** behavior of an individual with alcohol or substance use disorders meets some need of the spouse or another close family member. The role of rescuer or protector becomes such an important part of the codependent's life that the possibility of giving up that role is quite threatening. Family members may have spent years "rescuing" the individual and pleading for a change in behavior. They cling to the belief that life would be good if and when the individual with an alcohol or substance abuse disorder takes control and gives up the addictive substance. Eventually this interaction becomes an important part of life activities; the rescuer role fulfills an important need. At that point, family members *unconsciously* encourage and support the addiction. If the individual undergoes treatment, family problems increase because family members who are codependent cannot adjust to the individual's new behavior.

A codependent's *conscious* belief is that the family's problems will be resolved when the alcohol or substance abuse disorder has been treated. The reality is that a codependent *unconsciously* functions as an **enabler** by facilitating the addiction. Enabling takes many forms, such as "lending" money that the enabler knows will be used for drugs, even though the individual promises to use the money for food and rent. In the case of alcohol abuse disorder, the enabler may insist on going to parties where alcohol will be served or continue to keep liquor in the home for personal use, knowing that its presence is a temptation for the person with alcohol abuse disorder. In the mental health field, codependency is itself considered a condition that requires therapy.

Where codependency exists, treatment must include treatment of the codependent person also. Ideally, the entire family will be involved in therapy, so that any dysfunctional family dynamics may be corrected. The individual with an alcohol or substance abuse disorder must learn to cope with life problems effectively, without escaping through substance use or relying on the codependent for solving their problems. The codependent must learn to encourage the individual to be self-reliant and must be willing to give up the role of rescuer, protector, and caregiver. *Effective treatment for substance abuse must involve family members.* Otherwise, the "cured" individual will return to a dysfunctional family situation that does not support being drug-free. A difficult adjustment for the recovering individual is giving up old friends and associates who continue to use drugs. New relationships must be developed that include a drug-free lifestyle and ongoing support and encouragement as the recovering individual struggles against the temptation to resume the use of drugs. The desire to experience that drug-induced state of euphoria may remain, even after years of being drug-free.

Defense Mechanisms and Adjustment

All of us need to use adjustment mechanisms at times, including defense mechanisms. At one time or another we all have unhappy experiences, problematic situations to face, and obstacles to overcome. We all experience disappointment and failure at times. We all need to feel good about ourselves, but our self-esteem is always vulnerable to negative experiences. When circumstances threaten self-esteem, we tend to become defensive.

A situation that you perceive as threatening may not bother your best friend. Conversely, you may be puzzled about your friend's defensive reaction to a situation you consider to be ordinary. Some of us become defensive whenever we are criticized. Some of us become apprehensive when we are expected to show achievement. Some of us become uncomfortable in the presence of an authority figure. Some of us distrust others, always expecting a

FIGURE 11-4 When circumstances threaten self-esteem, we tend to become defensive.

put-down or criticism. Threat, then, is quite personal. It is based on our own specific areas of sensitivity, the psychological scars that are the result of hurtful experiences in our past.

The Patient

As a health care professional, keep in mind that illness and medical treatment represent a threat to many people. Therefore, you are likely to see many examples of defense mechanisms as you work with patients. If you work with psychiatric patients, you will need to learn about other mechanisms and about behavior deviations that psychiatric patients manifest. In the meantime, observe behavior and learn to recognize defense mechanisms.

When you become aware that someone is using a defense mechanism, realize that the person feels threatened by a situation. It is *not your role to point out the defense mechanism.* Your role is to *reduce the degree of threat the individual feels.* Through reassurance, acceptance, and sincere interest in the patient's well-being, you can usually reduce a patient's need for defensive behavior.

The Health Care Professional

How can you use knowledge about defense mechanisms to improve your own adjustment? First, keep in mind that defense mechanisms can be useful in relieving discomfort or negative feelings. Suppose a friend drops in just as you are about to leave home for a movie. At first, you feel quite irritated, but then you tell yourself, "I didn't really want to see that movie anyway." Having thus rationalized, you disposed of the angry feelings toward your friend and are free to enjoy the unexpected visit.

The key to healthful use of a defense mechanism is awareness. If you are aware of using a defense mechanism and of your reason for using it, then you are probably using it healthfully.

Suppose, on the other hand, your supervisor criticizes your performance frequently, but each time you place the blame on someone else or on circumstances. For example, the supervisor comments that you should have explained a procedure to your patient before carrying it out, but your reaction is, "I didn't have time." For every criticism you have an excuse. Then your use of projection is an obstacle to improving your performance as a health care professional. *Self-deception and distorted perception of situations interfere with learning and improved performance.*

In striving to improve your own adjustment, be aware of the frequency and purposes of the defense mechanisms you use. As you learn to recognize your use of each defense mechanism, you will be able to identify the types of situations that are threatening to you. Then you can seek ways of effectively dealing with such situations. If you have a habit of projecting blame, you may have to force yourself to admit a shortcoming now and then. Eventually, you will find it easier to admit being wrong or having made an error. By discarding the defense mechanism, you open the way to learn from experience.

As you become more aware of your tendencies to use defense mechanisms, you will begin to recognize those you have previously been using unconsciously. With increased understanding of yourself and your use of defense mechanisms, you will be ready to eliminate **self-deception**, learn to face reality, and use appropriate behavior in a variety of situations. Through practice in dealing with problems rather than "fleeing" from them, you will improve your skill in solving problems—even those that involve some unpleasantness. At that point, you will have less need for defense mechanisms.

Activities

1. Reflect on your own behavior, and rate each of the following defense mechanisms as follows:

   0 = I never or almost never do this.

   1 = I sometimes do this.

   2 = I often do this.

   a. I tend to use rationalization when I must choose between responsibility and fun. *Example:* This is often true for me. When I want to watch a show, I convince myself that I have studied enough. The next day, I wish I had studied. I will rate this item 2.

   b. I do not like to be criticized, even when I know the criticism is true.

   c. I am easily hurt by other people's remarks. It seems to me that people are too ready to be critical or to say unkind things.

   d. I have a lot of trouble with teachers (parents, supervisors, etc.) because of things other people did. I also have a lot of bad luck.

   e. Other people often make me angry (or unhappy), but I usually do not let them know it. I wait until I am home and then "let off steam."

   f. Sometimes my daydreams are more pleasant than what is going on around me. Then I have trouble keeping my mind on my work.

   g. I don't believe in getting upset. When the going gets rough, I leave.

   h. Some people irritate me, so I don't talk to them unless I have to.

2. Review the description of escape into illness in the chapter. Have you or someone you know ever used illness as a way to escape from an unwelcome situation?

3. Search online to find the following sources of help in your community. Note the phone number and types of services available for each:

   a. Alcoholics Anonymous

   b. Alcohol abuse 24-hour helpline

   c. Drug abuse 24-hour helpline

   d. Your local community agency for alcohol and drug abuse

4. Participate in a class discussion on the topic "Watching television/social media/the Internet serves as an escape for many people." Identify how to determine whether escape or any of the other defense mechanisms discussed in the chapter are being used in ways that support good adjustment or which interfere with good adjustment.

References and Suggested Readings

Centers for Disease Control and Prevention. (2022). Current cigarette smoking among U.S. adults aged 18 years and older. https://www.cdc.gov/tobacco/campaign/tips/resources/data/cigarette-smoking-in-united-states.html

Centers for Disease Control and Prevention. (2022). Deaths from excessive alcohol use in the United States. https://www.cdc.gov/alcohol/features/excessive-alcohol-deaths.html

Centers for Disease Control and Prevention. (2021). Quick facts on the risks of e-cigarettes for kids, teens, and young adults. https://www.cdc.gov/tobacco/basic_information/e-cigarettes/Quick-Facts-on-the-Risks-of-E-cigarettes-for-Kids-Teens-and-Young-Adults.html

National Institute on Alcohol Abuse and Alcoholism (NIAAA). (2021). Understanding alcohol use disorder. https://www.niaaa.nih.gov/publications/brochures-and-fact-sheets/understanding-alcohol-use-disorder

Substance Abuse and Mental Health Services Administration. (2021). *Key substance use and mental health indicators in the United States: Results from the 2020 national survey on drug use and health*. U.S. Department of Health and Human Services. Publication Number PEP21-07-01-003.

Sources of Additional Information

Alcoholics Anonymous, http://www.aa.org
For over 50 years, AA has offered community support for alcoholic individuals.
Narcotics Anonymous, http://www.na.org
Narcotics Anonymous offers community support for individuals recovering from drug addiction.

Chapter

12

Frustration and Inner Conflict

Objectives

After completing this chapter, you should be able to:

- Name internal and environmental factors that could be sources of frustration.
- Discuss emotional and behavioral reactions to frustration.
- Describe strategies for dealing with frustration and resolving inner conflict.
- Explain the importance of understanding frustration and inner conflict for yourself and in your role as a health care professional.

Key Terms

Alternative
Analgesic
Aspirations
Attitude
Debilitating

Digital
Frustration
Incompatible
Manipulative
Narcotic

Perfectionism
Proficient
Prognosis
Prosthesis

You now know that everyone experiences threats to adjustment at intervals and reacts to such threats according to learned patterns of behavior. **Frustration** is a threat that can arouse negative emotions and evoke aggressive or defensive behavior. The effects of frustration can seriously interfere with interpersonal relationships and adjustment.

Frustration exists when progress toward a desired goal is blocked. Everyone feels frustrated at times, but how we react to frustration determines to a large extent whether or not we reach the desired goal.

Understanding Frustration

Frustration may evoke irritation or a major emotional reaction. Minor frustrations occur almost daily: The car won't start when we are in a hurry; a pencil point breaks just as we begin a test; we miss the bus; someone keeps us waiting; a button pops off when we do not have time to sew it back on. Such experiences arouse feelings that range from annoyance to intense anger—these feelings are due to frustration.

Major frustrations involve larger aspects of living. A person whose job is not satisfying—who has many job-related problems or has been passed by repeatedly for promotion—has frustrations in the workplace. Individuals who experience discrimination due to race, national origin, sexual preference, gender identity, or other factors will face numerous frustrations in the community or workplace.

Minor frustrations cause annoyance for a relatively short period of time, though a frustration encountered in the morning often sets the pattern of the day. On such days we might comment, "I should have stayed in bed today." Major frustrations, however, may affect the individual's total personality—behavior patterns, values, beliefs, moods, attitudes, and general outlook on life. Major long-term frustrations can negatively impact an individual's adjustment.

Cumulative Effects of Frustration

Minor frustrations are significant if they lead to a buildup of negative feelings, with sudden release over a seemingly minor incident. A series of frustrations during the day may be the underlying cause of a parent's explosion when their teen asks for twenty dollars. Or the parent may show annoyance on Friday after giving the teen five dollars every morning. Unknown to the teen, the requests for money are frustrating the parent's efforts to make their money hold out until payday.

People differ in their tolerance for frustration. Some react emotionally whenever their goals are blocked, and others show the effects of frustration only when it is major. Most people react to minor or moderate frustration by taking action to resolve the problem; but when frustration is overwhelming, deciding the best action to take becomes challenging.

Occasionally the news media report an incident of bizarre or violent behavior. A tobacco farmer who believed his livelihood was being taken away from him by government intervention in the tobacco industry drove his tractor to Washington, DC, and threatened to set off explosives. Workers have gone to their workplace and shot colleagues, supervisors, and innocent bystanders. Although each case of such behavior would require detailed study for a full understanding of the individual's behavior, it is likely that cumulative frustration and a sense of powerlessness for dealing with the sources of frustration were major factors.

Sources of Frustration

Blocking of progress toward a goal can arise from many sources: personal characteristics, the environment, other people, illness, or prejudice.

Self When we set goals, we do well to consider many factors: our own interests and abilities, the opportunities available to us, and the resources (financial or otherwise) at our disposal. Setting an ambitious goal, "dreaming big," can be a powerful motivation, but doing so should be accompanied by a realistic assessment of the steps needed to reach the goal. When we set goals without considering "what it will take" to reach them, we increase the chances of experiencing frustration.

As high school seniors, Kendi and Riley shared an interest in the health field. Both students discussed their futures with the school counselor, taking into consideration many types of information, including high school records, achievement and aptitude test scores, vocational interest surveys, personal interests, family finances, and other factors.

Kendi's record indicated a good chance of success in college. Family finances were strained, and Kendi did not like to think of four or more years of school. Deciding to become a laboratory assistant, Kendi enrolled in the nearby technical institute. After completing the course with honors, Kendi accepted a position in the local hospital. Soon, Kendi asked the laboratory supervisor how to do some of the complex procedures but was told that only the registered medical technologists were allowed to do these tests. Kendi felt resentful and became increasingly hostile toward coworkers. By setting objectives

FIGURE 12-1 Setting an ambitious goal can be a powerful motivator, but doing so should be accompanied by a realistic assessment of the steps needed to reach the goal.

For Discussion and Reflection

Consider your own experience in selecting career goals, as well as the experience of close friends or family. In your opinion, how can the advice "You can do anything you set your mind to" be balanced with a realistic assessment of abilities, interests, opportunities, and resources?

that were not challenging enough, Kendi became frustrated at work by not being allowed to function like the more highly trained technologists.

On the other hand, Riley applied to a college despite having had difficulty with high school classes. The school counselor had encouraged Riley to plan vocational goals rather than academic ones. Riley's parents always wanted their child to be a doctor, so Riley had grown up with the idea of attending medical school. Refusing to recognize evidence that succeeding in college courses was unlikely, Riley failed three out of four courses at the university and came home confused and upset. By setting objectives that were too high, in spite of guidance that could have helped with planning more realistically, Riley created a situation that ended in frustration.

Frustration, then, can result either from trying to reach what is unreachable or from achieving unchallenging goals. A career goal should be carefully selected on the basis of all information available about the individual and occupations in which the person is interested. Career goals are important to achievement, development of one's potential, job satisfaction, and, ultimately, to adjustment and happiness.

Goals are also involved in short-term aspects of living. To some students, failure to make the school sports team is a shattering experience. Athletic ability is, to a great extent, based on physical characteristics and motor skills. If one's goal is to make the football team in spite of small physical build and limited stamina, then frustration is almost certain to occur. If one enjoys singing, the short-term goal of being accepted into the school chorus is probably realistic. On the other hand, the goal of becoming a pop star is realistic only for those few who have rare talent, the resources to develop the talent, and the determination and perseverance to strive many years for that goal.

Goals are more realistic when related to what we enjoy and learn readily. Satisfaction is greater if goals continue to offer challenge. In measuring goal progress, it is better to compare yourself today with yourself in the past, rather than with other people. Aspiring to be "the best" in anything is more likely to lead to frustration than aspiring to "continue to improve."

The Environment Environment—either physical or social—can be a source of frustration. The environment is less subject to control than one's goals and **aspirations**. As adults, we learn to accept some frustrations, such as rain on the day of a picnic or lack of snow for skiing.

The opportunities an environment offers should be considered in making long-range plans. If you decide to follow a career for which there is no locally available opportunity, frustration will occur unless resources can be made available or a move to another community can be arranged.

Sometimes the customs and practices of a community are the source of frustration. The health care professional who wants to improve health habits in a community must give careful consideration to the established beliefs, values, and customs of that community. Cultural aspects of the social environment may block efforts to change established practices.

Discrimination In some communities, discrimination based on race, nationality, sexual preference, gender identity, or other factors may create additional obstacles toward meeting personal goals. While federal laws prohibit discrimination in hiring, housing, and education, local attitudes and practices in many places remain unfairly biased against members of certain groups. Taking legal action against a potential employer or institution can be time-consuming and costly. When facing discrimination, individuals have a difficult choice: to confront discrimination directly and advocate for fair treatment, or to look for opportunities in another location where there are fewer barriers. Some professional groups and consumer advocate organizations provide legal assistance to people whose rights to equal opportunity have been violated.

If you have personally experienced discrimination, you are already aware of the tremendous frustration and sense of injustice it causes. If you have not experienced discrimination directly, as a health care professional committed to helping all clients, you can now begin noticing opportunities to speak out against or refuse to participate in discriminatory practices whenever possible.

Other People Many obstacles can be overcome through persistence, problem-solving techniques, or an approach that removes the obstacle or allows one to get around it. When the obstacle is a person, however, overcoming the obstacle is more difficult.

Kendi's laboratory supervisor was an obstacle to Kendi's learning advanced techniques, even though the supervisor was basing the decision on hospital policy, role differentiation, and Kendi's lack of educational preparation to perform advanced procedures. Suppose Riley had been refused admission to college. Then the admissions committee would constitute an obstacle to Riley's attending college.

In some cases, people are obstacles because of their beliefs, prejudices, attitudes, superior ability, dependency, and many other factors. When achieving a goal requires changing an **attitude** or belief of the person who is an obstacle, then the frustration is not likely to be overcome easily; people do not readily change their values and beliefs. In competition, the abilities of other people determine whether or not an individual makes the team, wins a gold medal, or gets a promotion. When the obstacle is a competitor's superior ability, then personal effort to surpass such ability is necessary to reach the goal.

Illness Illness may cause either minor or major frustration, depending upon the duration of illness and the patient's life situation. A minor illness that lasts a few days may simply be an inconvenience, or possibly a welcome relief from the daily routine—a chance to stay home and take it easy. But even a minor illness can create intense frustration if it interferes with some important event.

If the illness is serious or life-threatening, the patient experiences numerous frustrations. Individuals may feel that they are losing control of their life. Suddenly someone else (a doctor) is telling the patient what to do. Often these mandates include major life changes: stop smoking; change jobs to minimize stress (or physical exertion or exposure to hazardous situations); stop playing tennis; eat fresh vegetables; do not eat red meat; stop drinking

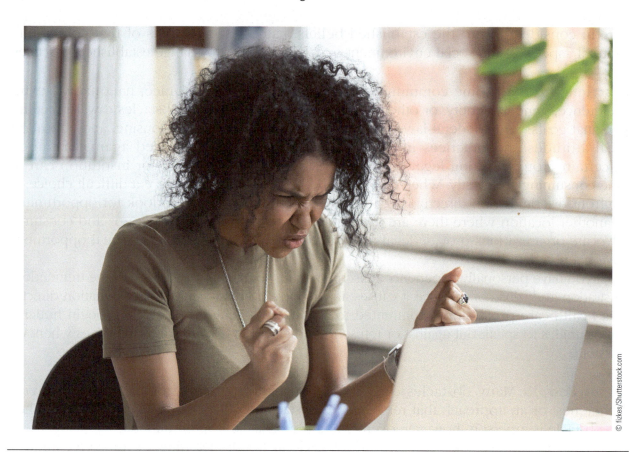

FIGURE 12-2 **Frustration is usually experienced as anger.**

alcoholic beverages; stop drinking sodas; exercise at least 20 minutes every day; have at least two rest periods; stay out of the sun between 11 A.M. and 3 P.M.; agree to a course of chemotherapy (or radiation); go to a medical center for special tests or treatment. Whatever the mandate includes, it will impact the patient's lifestyle. The significance of each thing that must be given up determines the degree of frustration. The specific treatment may also be a source of frustration, especially if there are side effects.

Frustration is usually experienced as anger. When you, as a health care professional, realize that a patient's behavior seems to be an expression of anger, consider what impact the illness is having on the patient's life. Show interest in the patient's life situation with an expression of caring and concern, such as, "I imagine this illness is really changing your life." If the patient is willing to talk about the effects, it will help defuse the anger. As you carry out your responsibilities for health care, be aware that the recipient of your services is a person who may be angry and/or sad about the losses involved as his or her life is disrupted by illness.

For Discussion and Reflection

Consider a situation within the last month that frustrated you. Was the frustration major or minor? What frustrated you about the situation?

Effects of Frustration

Each of us reacts to frustration according to patterns we have learned throughout life. These reactions, therefore, vary from one person to another, but they often involve either hostile behavior or withdrawal. Frustration arouses negative emotions: fear, anger, disappointment, anxiety, resentment, or a combination of these. Both behavior and emotional reactions to frustration are influenced by the importance attached to the goal as well as the individual's adjustment. A person who is insecure and inclined to perceive frustration as a threat is likely to feel a mixture of fear and anger. A person who is self-confident is likely to feel some degree of anger, with little fear. The person who is easily discouraged is likely to give up when there is an obstacle to success. Quitting, remember, is a form of withdrawal. The person who is stimulated to try harder in the face of difficulty is likely to react to an obstacle by increased effort or a change in strategy.

Frustration and Behavior Patterns

Everyone who has cared for a baby or young child has seen examples of behavioral responses to frustration. The pattern of response is learned behavior, largely based on how others react to the child's frustration. Ideally, an adult would recognize that the child is frustrated and take action to assist the child or remove the source of frustration. Frequently, however, the child's need is not recognized and the frustration is viewed as misbehavior. Thus, patterns become established based on whether or not the child's behavior led to satisfaction of a need.

Early Learning Experience with frustration may begin almost with birth. The infant who is fed according to a rigid schedule, rather than when hungry, experiences frustration as well as the physical discomfort of hunger. Each developmental task (such as turning over, sitting, and standing) requires many efforts before success is realized. Early efforts to perform such activities are frustrating, but the infant persists until bodily control has been mastered. Many infants show distress when these early efforts result in failure.

Toddlers know what they want long before they can state their needs verbally. When a toddler is unable to make wants known, the reaction may involve falling to the floor, kicking, or crying. The child's frustration is due to inability to communicate verbally—a lack of competence for the task attempted. The parent who does not understand frustration may punish the child. Then the child feels anger as the result of frustration and fear as the result of punishment. Such experiences affect the child's learning about frustration and also about the "right" to express feelings. The parent, without realizing it, is teaching the child that it is "wrong" to express negative feelings. This can be the beginning of ineffective patterns for dealing with frustration. It can also be the beginning of a pattern that you have already learned is undesirable—suppression of emotions.

Childhood During childhood, many frustrations result from the child's lack of competence for tasks being attempted, parental restraints, and rules at school, in clubs, and other organizations. Adults should make a conscious effort to help children understand the necessity for placing limits on behavior, especially where there are groups of children.

Yet, even when the need for rules is understood, the child is frustrated when these limits interfere with a desired activity. If the frustration is great, the child may feel resentment toward the source of the rule—a parent, teacher, club sponsor, or whatever authority figure seems to be preventing a desired activity. If punishment is also involved, fear and distrust of authority figures may develop. Rebelliousness or hostility toward authority, beginning with such childhood experiences, may later interfere in relationships with authority figures, such as supervisors in the job setting.

Adulthood Adults experience frustration in many forms and in every aspect of living. For the majority of people, probably the most common frustration is lack of enough money to have the material possessions desired. The major adaptations required by marriage, parenthood, and a job all involve numerous frustrations. Even after one has learned to function within the various roles of adulthood, frustrations periodically occur in each role.

As a health care professional, you are likely to have patients who are experiencing frustration. Illness and injury interfere with one's life. Loss of income due to inability to work and difficulty in performing self-care tasks, such as buttoning a shirt, are common problems for patients. Some patients, however, have long-term frustrations. The person with an amputation who must learn to use a **prosthesis** and the patient who survived a stroke and has lost the use of one side of the body are examples of patients who live with frustration. Be aware that some of your patients are experiencing intense frustration; try to anticipate their needs and be sensitive to the feelings they are experiencing.

Perfectionism and Frustration

A personal trait that leads to frequent frustration is **perfectionism**. This trait probably has its roots in childhood, with the child seeking parental approval through performance of assigned tasks, school work, or athletics. Parents' efforts to motivate a child to improve performance may result in the child learning that no performance is ever good enough ("Well, it's good that you passed the audition for chorus. Now, I expect you to be a soloist by the end of the year."). In this situation, one child may give up hope of winning unqualified approval; another may become determined to please, to turn in the perfect performance that is sure to win approval.

The perfectionist may expect perfection from themself or from others, especially a spouse, one's children, or coworkers. When perfectionism is focused inward, the individual views any less-than-perfect performance as unacceptable, even humiliating ("You may make mistakes, but not me!"). This person may agonize over a mistake or social blunder that others hardly notice. Self-forgiveness is not even considered.

The person whose perfectionism is directed outward is repeatedly disappointed in the performance of other people. Being intolerant of mistakes or poor performance by others, the perfectionist tends to be critical and irritable, leading to poor relationships within the family and on the job. These high expectations of self and others inevitably result in frustration for a perfectionist.

Coping with Frustration and Inner Conflict

You will experience frustration at intervals throughout life. This is a good time to evaluate your behavior patterns and decide whether you need to find new ways of dealing with frustration. By learning to handle frustration effectively, you can spare yourself much unhappiness and increase the proportion of satisfying experiences in your living.

There are numerous ways of dealing with frustration. The most desirable method of handling one particular frustration may be inappropriate for handling another. The general approach requires three steps:

1. Expect a certain amount of frustration in living and avoid overreacting emotionally or using defense mechanisms to avoid dealing with the problem.

2. Recognize frustration when it occurs.

3. When experiencing frustration, evaluate the situation and use the systematic procedure described next to select an approach for dealing with the obstacle.

Overcoming the Obstacle

There is no guaranteed way to overcome any and all obstacles. Recognize that the negative feelings of the moment are due to frustration, and then use a rational approach to solve the problem at hand. If dealing with the frustrating situation can be delayed, it is helpful to put it out of your mind for a while; take time to "sleep on it." You may then be able to return to the problem with a fresh viewpoint and with less emotional influence on your thinking. The following questions can help in planning to overcome the obstacle:

- Exactly what goal am I trying to reach?
- What is preventing my reaching that goal? (Identify the obstacle.)
- How can I overcome or get around this obstacle? List *all* possible ways to deal with the obstacle.
- What additional information do I need to make an informed decision?
- Who could I ask for additional information about my options? (In other words, who is knowledgeable or experienced in this area?)
- How is each possible solution likely to affect my achieving the goal?
- How is each possible solution likely to affect the way I feel about myself?
- How is each possible solution likely to affect other people?
- Is this *my* goal, or did someone else set this goal for me?
- Which solution is most likely to help me reach my goal?
- Is the goal important enough to me to justify the expenditures (time, effort, energy, money) required for reaching the goal?
- What other benefits (such as new competencies, widened experience, and future opportunities) am I likely to gain from continued efforts to achieve the goal?
- Shall I persist in striving for this goal? Or shall I substitute another goal?

For Discussion and Reflection

What is one of your career or personal goals? When you honestly assess your abilities and resources, is this a realistic goal? If yes, what are some short-term goals or steps that can help you move toward your long-term goal? If your original goal is not realistic, what are other options you could explore?

- Make a decision:

  a. If you decide to continue to pursue that goal, select a method for dealing with the obstacle and follow through.
  b. If your first effort does not remove the obstacle, try another approach.
  c. If you decide not to continue to pursue that goal, modify the goal or substitute a different goal.

Preventing Frustration

It is also desirable to use a preventive approach to frustration. As illustrated by the cases of Kendi and Riley, unrealistic goals can be the source of much frustration. Long-term goals, such as preparing for a career, usually include numerous short-term goals. There may be many frustrating experiences before the long-term goal is reached. If the short-term goals provide stepping-stones to be reached one by one, then frustration is offset by achievement of these intermediate goals.

Inner Conflict

Another common cause of poor adjustment is inner conflict. Perhaps you are accustomed to thinking of conflict as a fight or argument. Such conflicts involve two or more people and are *interpersonal* conflicts. Inner conflict, on the other hand, exists *within one person*. Other people may contribute to a person's inner conflict and others may be affected by the behavior resulting from inner conflict, but it is the individual with the conflict who is most affected.

Inner conflict exists when an individual has two **incompatible** needs or goals, or when the individual must choose between two or more **alternative** means for meeting a need or achieving a goal. The conflict arises because of the incompatibility of these needs, goals, or means, but other behavior influences may also be involved. One's value system, standards of behavior, beliefs, interests, personality traits, character traits, and self-concept may all contribute to inner conflict.

The person who has an inner conflict is usually aware of the need to choose between two goals or two courses of action. However, the individual may be unaware of the basic needs, values, interests, beliefs, and other factors that contribute to the conflict.

Conflict between Needs Adolescents are often faced with a conflict between the need for acceptance by the peer group and the need for maintaining their beliefs about "right" and "wrong" behavior. Suppose someone in Bri's crowd proposes a risky adventure involving behavior Bri believes to be wrong. Bri must choose between participating in the adventure or refusing to participate. The need to belong, feel accepted, and be approved by members of the peer group is in conflict with the need to maintain Bri's standard of behavior, beliefs, and self-concept— "I am a person who does not do things that are wrong." Going along with the adventure requires lowered standards of behavior, which is a threat to Bri's beliefs, values, and self-concept. Opposing the proposed adventure

FIGURE 12-3 Inner conflict exists when an individual has two incompatible needs or goals.

involves risking status with the group, which is a threat to Bri's need to belong. Bri is in a situation that requires a decision between two alternative actions, both of which threaten something Bri values.

Conflict between Means Conflict also exists when a goal can be reached in two or more ways. Mrs. P. has a chronic condition that causes her much discomfort. She usually relies on **analgesic** drugs, but more and more often she must have a **narcotic** to obtain full relief from pain. Her physician now warns her that continued use of drugs will have undesirable effects. He recommends surgery to correct her problem.

Mrs. P.'s goal of restored health requires choosing between habitual use of drugs and surgery. To be free of pain, she must use one means or the other. When Mrs. P. was a child, her oldest brother died during surgery. Since then, she has heard numerous stories about unsatisfactory surgical results, each one adding to her fear of surgery. Now, the thought of going to the operating room terrifies her, yet she desperately wants to be free of pain. To Mrs. P., with her deep-seated fear of the operating room, this conflict between two remedies for her health problem may be far more distressing than the physical discomfort associated with surgery.

Types of Inner Conflict

Regardless of whether a conflict is between needs, goals, or the means for achieving them, the individual must choose between alternatives. These alternatives may be positive (desirable) or negative (undesirable). Even in a choice between two positives, unhappiness may result from giving up one alternative. The degree of difficulty in making a decision is often influenced by whether the alternatives are both positive, both negative, or positive accompanied by a negative outcome.

Approach-Approach Conflict—Two Desirable Goals

Approach-approach conflict involves two needs or goals that are incompatible. Ali is working in the local hospital as a nursing assistant. Ali enjoys the work and is especially good with older adults. The supervisor recommends Ali to the director of the practical nursing program. The supervisor points out the advantages of being a licensed nurse and indicates belief in Ali's potential for succeeding in the program. Ali is proud of receiving the supervisor's recommendation and is suddenly fired with ambition to undertake the educational preparation for a promising career.

At the same time, Ali and Ali's partner have been saving money to buy a home together. Enrolling in the nursing program would reduce Ali's income for a year or more. Ali has two goals: saving money to buy a home and completing educational preparation for a promising job. Ali has a conflict between two strong but incompatible needs—they cannot be met at the same time.

Approach-Avoidance Conflict—Desirable Goal with a Negative Effect

Ryan is enrolled in a dental laboratory technology course. He is having difficulty developing some of the **manipulative** skills necessary for constructing dental prostheses. His teacher discusses the problem with him, emphasizing that he must spend more time on laboratory practice to develop the necessary **digital** skills. The only time Ryan has for this extra practice is the period the basketball team practices. Ryan is top scorer for the team.

Ryan wants to pass his lab course, but to do so he has to miss basketball practice. To achieve his goal of becoming **proficient** as a dental laboratory technician, Ryan has to accept the negative aspects of giving up his prized position on the team: feeling disloyal to the team and relinquishing an activity that gives him much satisfaction. Regardless of which choice he makes, Ryan will lose something that he values.

Approach-avoidance conflict is a special type of conflict involving a desirable goal with undesirable effects. The individual alternates between trying to reach a certain goal and abandoning the goal. The decision to abandon a goal usually occurs as the individual approaches achievement of the goal or when the time for a desired event approaches. Jordan is a high school student who has been offered a full scholarship to attend a nursing program at a prestigious university in another state. Despite the advantages of the program, Jordan is reluctant to move many hours away from friends and family. Jordan struggles to decide whether to accept the scholarship or to attend the local community college.

Avoidance-Avoidance Conflict—Two Negative Alternatives

Avoidance-avoidance conflict exists when an individual must choose between two alternatives, both of which will have a negative outcome. Carolyn is a student in a medical assistant program. Last week her best friend in the class broke an expensive piece of equipment and returned it to its storage case without reporting the breakage. Carolyn was present at the time, and her friend insisted that Carolyn promise not to tell anyone. Today, Carolyn learns that another student in the class has been blamed for the broken equipment and told to pay for it.

Carolyn has strong feelings about loyalty to friends. She also has strong feelings about keeping promises, honesty, truthfulness, and fair play. Carolyn knows who actually broke the equipment, but the guilty person refuses to report herself. Carolyn can break her promise to this friend and report the incident, or she can keep silent and permit an innocent person to take the blame. Carolyn's values are involved, yet either course of action will violate personal traits on which she places a high value. Carolyn's self-concept is also involved: she does not want to be a person who breaks promises, nor does she want to be a person who permits an injustice when she could prevent it. She has to choose between loyalty to her friend and her sense of fairness. She has to choose between telling the truth and breaking a promise.

How Carolyn handles this situation will probably be determined by her values. She must place a higher value on one set of traits than the other in order to select an alternative. If she reports the breakage, then honesty and fair play assume a higher place in her value system than loyalty to friends and keeping promises.

Carolyn's behavior patterns will affect how she works through this conflict. She may put off a decision and, by her inaction, allow the wrong person to be blamed. She may project blame by saying to herself that it is her friend's responsibility to tell the truth. She may rationalize by telling herself it is not really her business. Which choice she makes and how she justifies that choice to herself will result from many years of forming behavior patterns to deal with unpleasant situations.

For Discussion and Reflection

Consider a time when you felt torn between two possible courses of action. After reading about types of inner conflict, would you describe your experience as approach-approach conflict, approach-avoidance conflict, or avoidance-avoidance conflict?

How to Deal with Inner Conflict

Inner conflict may be handled effectively *only by making a decision between alternatives.* Obviously, the choice will be better if the individual recognizes that a conflict exists and identifies the competing needs or goals. Insofar as possible, the feelings and values related to the conflict should also be examined.

Thinking through a Conflict Situation The following steps provide a rational approach to resolving a conflict:

1. Recognize that there is a conflict.
2. Identify the two incompatible needs (or goals).
3. Examine the situation in terms of interests, values, immediate needs, long-term needs, and other relevant factors.
4. Decide how each need could be met (or each goal achieved).
5. Think through the probable effects of each possible action: what will be gained, what will be lost, and whether or not the action would be in accord with your beliefs, value system, interests, goals, and needs.

6. After thorough consideration of the probable effects of each possible choice, make a decision.

7. *Fully accept your decision.* One alternative has been selected; the other has been discarded. Do not flounder in doubt about whether the right choice was made. Set out to prove that you made a good decision. Do not develop feelings of guilt or failure about the alternative that was discarded. Remember: *A choice had to be made.*

Identifying Opportunity Cost In business, a concept known as "opportunity cost" may be used to assist in making decisions. This concept, when applied to inner conflict, can help the individual focus on facts rather than vague fears in order to make a *rational*, rather than an *emotional*, decision. Opportunity cost refers to what one must give up (an opportunity) when choosing one course of action over another.

In resolving inner conflict, opportunity cost consists of what will be given up if action 1 is pursued, and what will be given up if action 2 is pursued. Opportunity cost may be the basis for anxiety about choosing either action. The cost of a specific decision, then, includes not only the obvious consequences of that decision, but also the opportunity cost involved in not following the other course of action.

In the examples described above, Ali must choose between continuing to work full time in order to save money to buy a home or enroll in a practical nursing program that promises, in the long run, to provide greater career opportunities. If Ali chooses to continue working full time, the opportunity to pursue a more advanced career is lost, at least for now. If Ali chooses to enroll in the educational program, the opportunity to buy a home is lost or delayed.

For Jordan, the cost of accepting the scholarship and attending college out of state will be time lost with friends and family. On the other hand, the cost of remaining close to home to attend college will be losing a full scholarship and the chance to attend a prestigious university.

Inner Conflict and Adjustment

The approach just described illustrates the familiar saying "You can't have your cake and eat it too." Even minor conflicts cause a certain amount of inner discomfort until they are resolved. If you put off doing an assignment in favor of more pleasant activities, you eventually reach the point of having to resolve the conflict. You must either decide to do the assignment instead of some preferred activity, or decide not to do the assignment and accept the consequences. You are probably a little uncomfortable as long as you continue to put off the decision.

Many people react to conflict with indecision, either procrastinating as long as possible or making one choice and then changing to another. Only a firm decision truly resolves a conflict. Sometimes the decision is necessarily accompanied by an unfavorable effect, either on oneself or on others. *The ideal result in handling conflict is to gain the desired goal with the least possible undesirable effect. In many situations, a new solution to the conflict can be discovered by talking the situation over with a trusted friend, relative, or coworker.*

Frustration, Inner Conflict, and the Health Care Professional

As a health care professional, you can make good use of your understanding of frustration, conflict, and their effects on behavior and emotions. Health care professionals frequently have inner conflict. Health care professionals often possess confidential information. People tend to put health care professionals into conflict situations by asking about patients or seeking health advice. The necessity for providing many health services on a 24-hour basis requires that some health care professionals have a schedule different from that of their families. Staffing problems give rise to occasional changes in time off, sometimes on short notice. Urgent situations require working overtime, being "on call," or returning to work unexpectedly after putting in a full day's work.

The health care professional who is dedicated to serving others and has a strong sense of duty is likely to experience conflict between loyalty to the job and loyalty to the family. There may be occasions when there is a conflict between job responsibilities and "rights" as a person.

Medical ethics and the policies of your place of employment can help you with some of these conflicts. For example, when a close friend asks about a patient, your *ethical responsibility* to hold in confidence what you learn about patients in the course of your job helps you resolve the conflict between responsibility and desire to have your friend's approval. At times, you may have to justify your *sense of duty* when job requirements interfere with plans involving family or friends. Thinking about such possible conflicts in advance can help you resolve them if they actually occur.

Inner Conflict and the Patient

Many patients have inner conflict related to their illness. Mr. B. has orders for strict bedrest, yet he feels capable of returning to work. He has a conflict between his need for self-interest (perhaps self-preservation) and his need to fulfill his job responsibilities. Ms. J., who is having diagnostic studies, may have a conflict between the need for relief from distressing symptoms and the fear of learning something unfavorable as a result of the studies.

Family members, too, have inner conflict when decisions must be made. It is difficult to agree to painful procedures on someone you love, yet refusing permission for the procedure may contribute to continued illness or the loved one's death. The decision on whether or not to consent to surgery involves many emotions, including the possibility of guilty feelings if the outcome is unfavorable. An emotionally wrenching conflict for family members is a decision to discontinue life support. Even if the patient's status fits the conditions specified in an advance directive, an inner conflict exists for each person involved in the decision. Some physicians try to protect families from decisions that may lead to guilty feelings. However, it is desirable that the family be involved in decisions about painful or **debilitating** treatments and the use of life-support systems for persons whose illness involves a hopeless **prognosis**.

Using Knowledge About Inner Conflict

As a health care professional, be aware that some of the distress you see in patients and their families is due to inner conflict. With such understanding, you are better able to accept behavior that appears unreasonable and accept emotional reactions that seem out

© smolaw/Shutterstock.com

FIGURE 12-4 Family members often experience inner conflict when making difficult treatment decisions for a loved one.

of proportion to the seriousness of the illness. Be aware, too, that sometimes the physician has given the family or patient information that you do not have, such as an unfavorable prognosis.

Applying knowledge about inner conflict to your personal life can help you resolve conflict situations rationally to achieve the best possible outcome for you and your family. Applying your knowledge of inner conflict to relations with patients can help you be more understanding and more accepting of your patients and their families.

Activities

1. Review the sources of frustration discussed in this chapter. Which of these have caused frustration for you personally? Are there other sources of frustration in your life not mentioned in the chapter?

2. How do you typically respond to frustration at home? At school? At work? Does your reaction to frustration differ based on where you are and whom you are with?

3. Consider one conflict you have had during the past month.

   a. Describe the conflict: What incompatible goals, beliefs, or values were involved?

   b. Describe how you handled of this conflict and how you felt afterward.

   c. Identify the results of your actions for yourself and for others involved.

   d. Looking back on the situation, what have you learned? In the future, would you solve a similar situation in the same way? If not, what might you do differently?

4. You have a 2-year-old male patient who is to be hospitalized for about a month. During the first days in the hospital, the child tries to talk to those caring for him, but no one can understand him. He frequently throws himself down in bed and kicks violently; sometimes he bangs his head on the crib.

   a. Explain the child's behavior.

   b. How should you as a health care professional react to this behavior?

   c. How could those in frequent contact with this child best help him?

   d. Describe this child's primary need.

   e. List some possible long-term effects on the child if health care professionals:

      (1) Label the child "spoiled" and avoid the child whenever possible.

      (2) Make a sincere effort to understand what the child is trying to say.

References and Suggested Readings

Duke, A. (2020). *How to decide: Simple tools for making better choices*. New York: Portfolio.
Heath, D. (2020). *Upstream: The quest to solve problems before they happen*. New York: Avid.
Johnson, E. (2021). *The elements of choice*. New York: Penguin Random House.

Effective Human Relations and Communication

The technological advances of the health field tempt the health care professional to become absorbed in complex equipment and the details of technique. To the patient, however, the *social climate* that health care professionals create has great importance. Each contact with a member of the health team affects the patient's peace of mind, emotional state, and outlook. *Scientific breakthroughs and sophisticated procedures cannot replace the human element in patient care.*

Section IV is designed to help you learn ways to promote a favorable outlook for the patient. Remember to relate to each patient as a human being and develop your own personal technique for identifying patient needs. As you learn to select the behaviors that promote favorable reactions in others, you will also enrich your personal life. Thus, you can grow not only as a health care professional, but also as a thoughtful, self-directing person, gaining increased satisfaction in living and at the same time enriching the lives of others.

Chapter 13

Effects of Illness on Behavior

Objectives

After completing this chapter, you should be able to:

- State possible physical effects of illness.
- Discuss common emotional effects of illness.
- Describe factors that influence how individuals respond to illness.
- Explain strategies you can use as a health care professional to better serve clients facing illness.

Key Terms

Desertion reaction
Disguised behavior
Incapacitated

Lethargy
Mindset

Separation anxiety
Verbalize

Illness is always a threat to one's sense of security. Even a minor illness or injury poses a challenge to an individual's physical and emotional well-being. Illness disrupts everyday routines, causing discomfort and inconvenience and often arousing feelings of fear, anger, or grief. These feelings are often manifested through the patient's behavior, but are not verbalized.

In other courses you are learning about specific illnesses: symptoms, diagnostic procedures, therapeutic techniques. Such knowledge is essential to safe and efficient performance as you provide patient care. Your *effectiveness* as a health care professional, however, is dependent upon your skill in applying knowledge about human behavior to relationships with patients. An effective health care professional/patient relationship promotes the patient's well-being. For one patient, reassurance in large amounts is needed to counteract fear and anxiety. For another patient, you may need to build confidence in the health team in order to gain the patient's cooperation in following the therapeutic plan.

Trying to provide a therapeutic atmosphere that is favorable for each patient is an ongoing challenge. Human variability is so great that no one method will work for all patients. By applying your knowledge about human behavior and the effects of illness, you can become sensitive to patient behaviors and their possible significance in terms of mental and emotional needs.

Physical Effects of Illness

Patients not only experience the signs and symptoms of a specific illness, but also various physical effects related to emotional reactions, change in daily routine, drugs, and numerous other factors. Examples of such general physical effects are fever, pain, nausea, lack of appetite, urinary problems, and difficulty with elimination. The overall effect may range from extreme **lethargy** to extreme restlessness. These general effects may be just as distressing to the patient as the symptoms of a specific illness. *The patient's complaints about general or vague effects should be noted.* These general symptoms may indicate either physical or emotional needs. Since interpretation may be beyond the scope of your role, report such complaints to your team leader or supervisor.

Emotional Effects of Illness

Most people react to illness with negative emotions that vary in type and intensity:

- Some patients are mildly annoyed at being sick; others are quite angry.
- Some patients are apprehensive; others are almost in a state of panic.
- Some feel sorry for themselves, while others react with pronounced self-pity.
- Some people feel bitter about their misfortune; bitterness is a combination of anger and self-pity.
- Some patients readily **verbalize** their feelings. The patient who says, "Why me?" is probably expressing anger.

Obviously, the words alone do not carry the full message. Be alert for additional evidence about the patient's emotional reaction to illness: facial expression, tone of voice, body posture, choice of words, and emphasis given to certain words.

Negative feelings may also be expressed through **disguised behavior**. The patient who is very talkative may be covering up fear. The patient who is eager to please may be covering up fear, hostility, or other negative feelings. Such patients are just as much in need of understanding and interest from health care professionals as those who verbalize their feelings. Do not make the mistake of thinking that the patient who is pleasant does not have fears and anxieties; for these patients, too, illness is a threat. *Each patient reacts to threat in a very individual way.*

Effects of Serious Illness on Behavior

During serious illness, an individual's mental and emotional functioning may decline. The individual's energy resources are used to cope with the physical stress of illness. A person with a serious illness may be less aware of their surroundings and less concerned about life problems. A calm, interested, and caring manner on the part of health care professionals is essential to provide these patients with emotional support, reassurance, and, hopefully, some relief from fear.

Sometimes a patient who has been very cooperative during the serious stage of illness shows a marked change in behavior as convalescence begins. Energy resources are no longer fully required for coping with physical demands. The patient is now more aware of discomfort and has energy for emotional reactions and for conscious attention to symptoms and life problems. You may find it difficult to cope with this change in behavior, because you probably believe the patient should now exhibit positive emotions. Accept a patient's behavior as indicative of needs and problems, rather than condemning their behavior because it is different from what you think it should be.

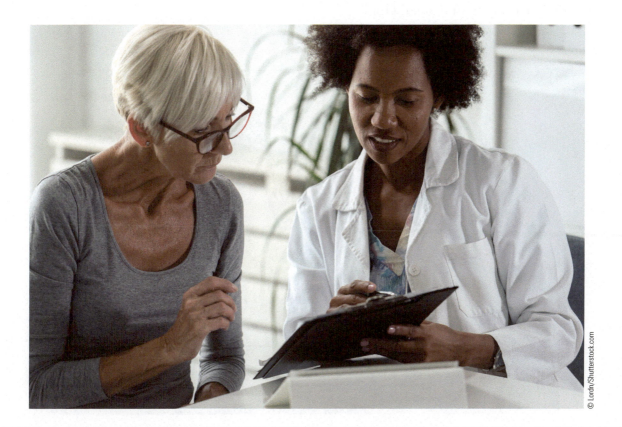

FIGURE 13-1 Patients will benefit from your taking time to explain a procedure and to answer questions.

Influences on Patients' Reactions to Illness

As a health care professional, you will see situations involving pain, discomfort, disability, and even death. The atmosphere of the health agency is your work environment, but to a patient, it may seem unfamiliar and uncomfortable. The equipment you use daily and the clinical sights, smells, and sounds that are so familiar to you may be frightening to other people. Most patients will benefit from your taking time to explain a procedure and to answer questions, no matter how routine that procedure has become for you. By dealing with the strangeness of a situation and by helping the patient understand, you can have a positive influence on patient behavior.

Childhood Age influences patient reactions to illness, especially if the patient is at either extreme of the life span. The young child reacts to illness with all the characteristics of the stage of development, in addition to the child's fear of strange places, the discomfort of illness, and expectations developed from past experiences with health care professionals.

Hospitalization may result in a desertion reaction or separation anxiety, unless some member of the family stays with the child. **Desertion reaction** is a form of withdrawal in which the child retreats to a corner of the crib or curls up into the fetal position. The child is unresponsive when caregivers try to communicate. **Separation anxiety** is a type of panic reaction when the child realizes the parent is going to leave them in a strange place. Young children cannot understand the need for hospitalization; nor do small children understand that they are not being abandoned and the family will return later. Because of these two common reactions of small children, most hospitals now allow, or even encourage, a member of the family to stay with a small child.

© fizkes/Shutterstock.com

FIGURE 13-2 Accept each child according to their current stage of development.

How to work effectively with sick children of various ages is a full course of study. By observing some general rules, however, you will improve your effectiveness with young patients. Accept each child according to his or her current stage of development:

- Allow the young patient to express feelings—do not suggest that a 3-year-old "be brave" and not cry when something hurts.

- Do not expect cooperation from those who are too young to understand. Be aware that the child does not understand what is happening.

- Accept that the child is afraid.

- Remember that children often sense the feelings of adults. If you have negative feelings, the child is likely to sense your true feelings. Some child behavior is actually a reaction to the feelings of an adult.

As a health care professional, it is your task to win the child's confidence. *When a treatment or diagnostic procedure must be done, indicate that you accept the child's feelings and are sorry that the child is having pain.* Be aware that any traumatic experience will influence the child's behavior throughout this illness, create negative feelings toward health care professionals in general, and influence behavior in future illnesses.

Senescence Many older adults fear becoming bedridden or otherwise losing their independence. For the senescent patient, any illness is especially threatening. An older adult may have greater anxiety than you think is justified by the particular illness. Such patients need your sincere interest and concern as they cope with the threat their illness represents.

In caring for an older adult, encourage independence insofar as it is reasonable. The need for help with buttoning a shirt may be due to arthritic hands—very different from a child who needs help with buttons! Consider the following guidelines:

- Do not assume that the older adult's need for help with some aspects of daily living also means that the patient is to be treated like a child.

- Allow the patient to make decisions whenever appropriate, rather than insisting that the patient conform to every routine of the facility.

- Keep in mind that some routines are for the convenience of the staff and may not be in the best interest of every patient.

Above all, remember that this older adult, now somewhat dependent on you, was at one time independent and self-reliant. The loss of one's independence is a difficult loss to accept.

For Discussion and Reflection

Have you or a close relative ever experienced a serious illness? How did the illness affect daily routines for the person who was ill? For others in the family?

Life Role One's life role assumes great importance during illness. A parent with small children has anxiety about their care while **incapacitated**. Possibly, there is also anxiety about the ability to fulfill parenting responsibilities. The parent's reaction to illness may be quite different from that of an individual with the same illness whose family is less dependent on them.

Occupational role also influences the degree of threat. Illness can seriously threaten job security; even if one's job is secure, there may be loss of income. Sick leave, salary continuation plans, whether or not one works on commission, whether or not insurance will help with the costs of illness—all influence the amount of anxiety the patient feels. If there is permanent disability, a change of occupation may be necessary. For most of your patients, you will not know the details of their life situation; hence, you cannot know what their worries are. You can, however, be sensitive to manifestations of anxiety, and you can listen when a patient indicates a need to talk.

Financial Concerns In addition to worry about losing income from missed work during an illness, many patients worry about the cost of treatment itself. Cost of care and access to care pose a challenge for those without health insurance as well as to those who do have insurance. According to a 2021 study, the United States is the only high-income nation that does not offer universal health coverage, leaving almost 30 million people uninsured. Despite spending significantly more money on health care as a nation than other high-income nations, the access to care in the United States is lower than in any other high-income country (Schneider et al., 2021, p. 11). Even when patients do have insurance, deductibles, copayments, and noncovered treatments can mean that patients incur significant out-of-pocket medical costs.

Adjustment The usual adjustment of a patient has much influence on reactions to illness. The patient who has a sense of security and usually copes with life problems effectively is very likely to cope with illness effectively also, even though adjustment will not be as good as usual. *Even for the well-adjusted person, illness is accompanied by inconvenience and discomfort, which alters the degree of adjustment.*

Those same personality traits and patterns of behavior that influence adjustment also influence how one reacts to illness. A person who tends to use defense mechanisms will continue this pattern during illness. The person who often finds escape from unpleasantness will try to avoid facing the reality of illness. Sometimes the defense mechanisms fail the individual during illness; then the patient may be unable to cope with the situation. When the usual patterns of coping fail, the individual may become fearful and may even panic. Patients who seem overly anxious may not know how to cope with illness.

Dependency Some people are quite independent, in the sense of being self-reliant. Others are inclined to lean on someone else whenever possible. This trait is known as dependency. People who are extremely dependent may react to illness in a way that reflects this characteristic. It is expected that the sick be dependent on others; therefore, illness justifies dependency. During illness, *dependent persons* escape the self-reliance normally expected of adults. Therefore, *unconsciously* wishing to prolong an illness, they find it difficult to admit they are improving. New complaints may be offered as evidence that they are still sick.

It is easy to be critical of such patients. Yet if you had that patient's life problems, background, and patterns of behavior, then you would probably be using the same behavior pattern the patient is using. Instead of being critical, the health team should plan ways for such a patient to resume self-care progressively during convalescence.

Cultural Background and Language Barriers Another influence on patient reactions to illness is cultural background. According to the Migration Policy Institute, as of 2019, the population of the United States included over 44 million people born in other countries. Over a fourth of U.S. residents are members of immigrant families (immigrants and their U.S.-born children) (Esterline, 2022). You have likely met people from many parts of the world living in your own community. Being aware of your own culture and learning about the culture of your clients will help you better serve clients who come from diverse backgrounds.

Each culture has certain beliefs about sickness, death, and dying. In some cultures, members of the family and the community care for the sick. Hospitals and doctors may be viewed with suspicion and are consulted only if the situation becomes desperate. When a person moves from that type of culture to one where medical care is a common occurrence, admission to the hospital may be perceived as meaning the patient's illness is hopeless. These patients present an opportunity for the health care professional to learn about the patient's culture, perceptions of illness, and lifestyle.

The patient with a limited understanding of English presents a special challenge to health care professionals. The patient may have difficulty describing symptoms or conveying needs—frustrating for both patient and health care professional. Such patients should be given careful explanations of procedures and routines to alleviate fear and prevent misunderstandings. Many health care agencies provide access to interpreters to assist clients who speak languages other than English. Clients may need assistance in learning about how to access these services.

Cultural differences also include religion, dietary practices, and other lifestyle choices. The patient whose religious or personal beliefs influence diet and other practices needs assurance that the practices will be respected. Your philosophy of individual worth should guide you in providing quality care for each patient, regardless of cultural background.

Past Experience Experience creates in each of us a mindset toward certain types of experience. **Mindset** influences how we perceive a situation. How we perceive the situation influences how we react. The patient who has had unfavorable experiences with sickness, health care professionals, or health agencies is likely to perceive greater threat than a person who has not had such unfavorable experiences. The patient who expects health care professionals to be cold and impersonal may perceive coldness even in a friendly care professional. If the patient expects inefficient care, then examples of inefficiency will be found. Evidence of defensiveness, distrust, hostility, or fear toward health care professionals may indicate traumatic past experiences.

You cannot undo past damage quickly. Mindset is a fixed expectation that is not easily modified; it creates readiness to behave according to the *expectation*, rather than according to the specific situation. When you encounter a patient who seems to have had unfavorable experiences with health care professionals, do not expect to establish rapport immediately. However, your efforts may be more effective than you realize and pave the way for new and more favorable attitudes in the future.

The Challenge for Health Care Professionals

As a health care professional, you will sometimes be extremely busy performing all the procedures required to complete your assignment. Both time pressure and workload can be quite stressful. At such times you may tend to focus on task completion, rather than identifying patients' needs, being aware of patients' emotional reactions to their illnesses, and understanding that certain behaviors are reactions to illness. Actually, *giving your attention to human relations as you perform various procedures* will help you manage your own stress. You will be able to enjoy interacting with each patient and be less aware of job pressures.

Relating to the Patient

Practicing effective human relations is not time-consuming; it is a matter of *where you focus your attention*. Familiar procedures do not require a lot of concentration, so you can focus on relating to the patient while you carry out a procedure. If you do need to concentrate on the task, you can simply state to the patient, "I really need to focus on what I'm doing; we'll talk some more when I have finished."

Relating to your patients effectively requires certain attitudes: genuine concern for others, the belief that other people are important, and willingness to see a situation from the patient's point of view. In fact, these three attitudes are essential to feel empathy for another person. The caregiver who truly feels empathy for a patient is likely to be perceived by the patient as warm and caring.

Certain personal traits also contribute to effective relationships, especially sincerity, truthfulness, and honesty. In addition, behavior patterns affect relationships. Attentiveness, giving one's full attention to the patient, is absolutely necessary to convey caring and concern. Two health care professionals who carry on a conversation with each other while performing a procedure on a patient are sending the message: "We are not really interested in you as a human being. We are just here to do this task." Making eye contact at frequent intervals also conveys attentiveness. Have you ever tried to have a conversation with someone who looked over your shoulder or kept glancing around the room while you were talking? If so, you probably felt that the other person was not really interested in you or what you had to say. Probably the most important of all caring behaviors involves just "being there" when someone needs comfort and emotional support. Being there may or may not include conversation. It may involve simply taking the patient's hand in yours for a moment, or simply asking, "Do you need anything?"

Communicating with the Patient

Your purpose in communicating with a patient affects your communication style. Interviewing a patient to obtain information, instructing the patient in self-care, explaining a procedure or the patient's care plan, or conveying empathy are examples of different purposes that would require somewhat different approaches. Regardless of purpose, however, it is important to convey caring and concern for the patient. Communication includes both verbal and nonverbal messages, so you should become aware of your own communication style, especially your use of body language as you communicate verbally. Chapter 15 discusses verbal and nonverbal communication in greater detail.

FIGURE 13-3 Being there for a patient may or may not include conversation. It may involve simply taking the patient's hand in yours for a moment, or simply asking, "Do you need anything?"

Activities

1. Give three examples of how illness can affect an individual's physical functioning.

2. Consider some past illness you have experienced. Describe your reactions to this illness in terms of the following:

   a. Perception of threat

   b. Emotional effects

   c. Your behavior when you were uncomfortable

   d. Inconvenience of the illness

   e. Effects on your daily habits

   f. Effects on your state of adjustment

   g. Influence of one or more personality traits on how you reacted to illness

   h. Expectations or mindset that affected your relationship with those caring for you

> **Note**
>
> Reactions to illness occur even if the illness is a minor one. If you have never had any illness that could provide a basis for this activity, interview a friend or member of your family who has had a recent illness.

3. Describe how each of the following factors can affect an individual's response to illness: life roles, cultural background, language barriers, previous experience with the health care system.

4. Describe how you would respond to each of the scenarios below in your role as a health care professional:

   a. Your neighbor comes to you to talk about her recent experiences with diagnostic studies. She states, "The doctor says there is nothing physically wrong. He says I should stop being so nervous. I don't know what he means." How could you help this neighbor understand what the doctor means, without exceeding your role as a health care professional?

   b. A member of your family has a disorder that can only be treated by extensive lifestyle changes. List specific suggestions for helping this relative make the necessary changes.

   c. A friend informs you that her husband has a malignancy and describes some changes in his behavior. How could you help her understand her husband's behavior?

   d. You are assigned to a patient whose treatment includes bedrest. As you prepare to give a bed bath, you put on gloves. The patient says angrily, "Am I so dirty that you can't touch me with your bare hands?" How will you respond?

References and Suggested Readings

AARP. (n.d.). Family caregiving. https://www.aarp.org/caregiving/

Esterline, C., & Batalova, J. (2022). *Frequently requested statistics on immigrants and immigration in the United States.* Migration Policy Institute. https://www.migrationpolicy.org/article/frequently-requested-statistics-immigrants-and-immigration-united-states

National Cancer Institute. (n.d.). *Resources for caregivers.* https://www.cancer.gov/resources-for/caregivers

Schneider, E., Shah, A., Doty, M., Tikkanen, R., Fields, K., & Williams, R. (2021). *Mirror, mirror: Reflecting poorly. Health care in the US compared to other high-income countries.* The Commonwealth Fund. https://www.researchgate.net/profile/Roosa-Tikkanen/publication/358397629

Chapter 14

Human Relations and Coping with Patient Behavior

Objectives

After completing this chapter, you should be able to:

- Describe strategies for positive interactions with patients.
- Discuss common emotional reactions patients may have to illness and how health care providers can help them adjust.
- Apply guidelines for interacting with patients to a variety of situations.
- Explain common patterns of patient behavior and appropriate ways health care professionals can respond.

Key Terms

Covert
Egocentric

I-statements
Overt

Passive aggression
Regression

Behavior is highly individualized. Each person has typical patterns of behavior for various situations, including reacting to the stress of illness. Do not expect to know exactly why each person behaves in a certain way. You can, however, be aware of *possible* reasons for behavior and thus be more accepting of whatever behavior the patient does exhibit. If you demonstrate an accepting attitude rather than a judgmental attitude, you will be able to develop more effective relationships with patients and coworkers.

Practicing Effective Patient Relations

To become an effective health care professional, you will be expected to:

- Know your job
- Perform well all tasks within the scope of your responsibilities
- Understand and apply the concepts and facts relevant to each task
- Observe safety precautions

Most of the courses you are now studying prepare you to fulfill these requirements. But to be truly effective, you must also focus on developing human relations skills. As you improve your skills in interacting with coworkers and patients, you will find your work more satisfying, and you will gain confidence in handling a variety of challenging situations.

Helping Patients Adjust to Illness

Your patients come to the health agency with the effects of illness added to their usual problems. There are some—perhaps many—stressors in their life situations; illness is an additional stressor. To some people, the health care facility is a strange place. For some, it is so threatening that the patient enters only as a desperate effort to get help. Patients may also be worried about how they will cope with the high costs of health care. In a stressful situation such as the hospital, the patient uses patterns of behavior that have proven useful in past threatening situations.

Identifying a Patient's Needs

You are learning about influences on patient behavior. Use this knowledge to understand and accept each patient as a person. You do not serve a patient's needs when you tell your coworkers, "They just act like that because they have a conflict." You may or may not be right about the cause of the behavior. Your role is to be aware of *possible* meanings of behavior in terms of patient needs. Recognizing some of the possible influences on behavior is the key to identifying patient needs, not the source of conversational topics.

If you think a patient's behavior indicates unmet needs, discuss the patient's behavior with your supervisor. Sometimes, the health team needs to study a patient situation in an effort to identify needs. The need driving a particular behavior may not be obvious at first. For example, children may cry because they are tired, hungry, afraid, or missing a parent. Similarly, an adult may display aggressive, hostile, or uncooperative behavior for a variety of reasons—they are worried about finances, in pain, angry with family members for "not being there for them," and so on.

FIGURE 14-1 If you think a patient's behavior indicates unmet needs, discuss the patient's behavior with your supervisor.

Striving to understand the behavior of your patients should be approached in a *thoroughly ethical and responsible way*.

Each person's behavior is highly individual. We each have typical patterns of behavior for various situations:

- Reacting to stress
- Feeling out of control
- Feeling afraid or anxious
- Expressing anger
- Expressing worry

You may never know exactly why each person behaves in a certain way. However, you can be more accepting of patients' behavior by considering *possible* reasons for the behavior. By choosing to have a nonjudgmental attitude toward your patients rather than a judgmental one, you will be better able to form effective relationships. *Keep in mind that skill in interpersonal relations comes through applying your knowledge and understanding to every relationship with another person—at work, at home, and in all activities involving other people.*

Being Sensitive to Feelings

Unpleasant behavior is usually due to a negative emotional state, ignorance, or an unfavorable attitude. When patients behave in undesirable ways, it is almost always the result of inner feelings; these feelings affect the patient's well-being. *When you encourage a patient to adopt a positive, realistic outlook, you contribute to that patient's well-being.* Negative feelings indicate a need; try to identify the need and respond appropriately.

Guidelines for Interacting with Patients and Clients

Practicing the strategies that follow will improve your ability to interact effectively with patients or clients. As you read the description of each strategy, consider how you could use each approach not only with patients but also with friends, family, or coworkers:

- Set aside your own personal problems.
- Accept the patient.
- Show interest and concern.
- Listen and observe.
- Recognize significant behavior.
- Adapt your behavior.
- Maintain confidentiality.

Practice applying these strategies to your verbal and nonverbal behavior both. For example, you can show interest and concern verbally by asking, "How are you feeling today?" You can show interest and concern nonverbally by smiling, turning to face the patient as he or she speaks with you, and taking time to listen.

Putting Personal Matters Aside

Do you have the right to inflict your personal problems on this troubled patient? Your role is to provide health care. To do so effectively, you must handle your own problems of living well enough to give your full attention to your patients. When you report for work each day, the problems of your personal life, as well as your personal interests and plans, must be set aside until you have completed that day's work. *You cannot deal with job problems and home problems at the same time.* Put personal matters aside while you are on the job, so you can give your full attention to your patients. With practice over time, the ability to rise above your own problems will increase your effectiveness as a health care professional. The following strategies can help you focus on work, saving personal matters for later:

- Put your mobile phone away during work hours, and silence message alerts. If you need to check for messages from friends and family, do so only on your breaks.
- Let friends and family know that you will not respond to texts or emails during work hours. Provide the appropriate number they can call to contact your workplace if a true emergency arises.
- If your situation makes it imperative that you do check your mobile device regularly, for example, if you are the parent of a young child in daycare or have a sick family member, you will need to be disciplined about quickly checking for the relevant information and letting other nonessential messages wait until later.
- When talking with coworkers during work hours, keep the conversation focused on work matters as much as possible. Occasional light topics (such as weekend plans or a new restaurant) may sometimes be appropriate to discuss with coworkers, but discussion of personal relationships, finances, or other serious matters should not be conducted during work hours. If your coworker is also your friend, ask if they have a few minutes after work to talk, or if they would like to meet after work for coffee.

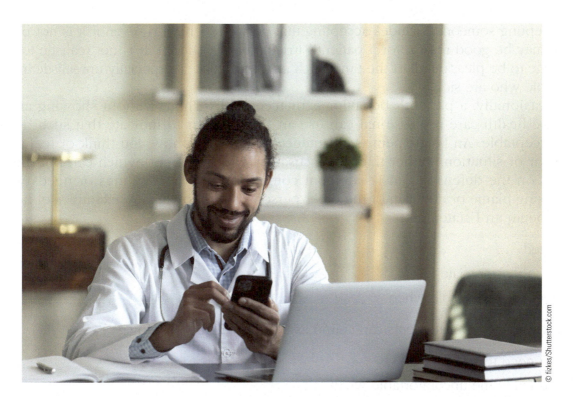

FIGURE 14-2 **Put personal matters aside while you are on the job.**

- Have a plan for when and how you can "get things off your chest" outside of work hours, such as by talking to friends, calling a relative, or writing in a journal. Allowing personal worries to accumulate makes it difficult to concentrate at work.

- Before you begin your shift each day, take a few moments to clear your mind and visualize setting personal matters aside for later. If needed, write yourself a note or set a reminder on your device about something you need to take care of later.

- As much as possible, avoid expressing strong personal opinions in the workplace on matters which are not work related. This does not mean that you should not stand up for what you believe to be right in a situation in which someone is facing unfair treatment. However, strongly stated opinions about controversial topics can make coworkers and clients uncomfortable and can interfere with establishing caring, trusting relationships.

Accepting the Patient

Each patient needs to feel accepted by health care professionals. Many patients are sensitive to any evidence of irritation, impatience, indifference, or hostility on the part of a health care professional. Accepting every patient may require effort, because each of us has some prejudice or lack of understanding toward those who are different from ourselves. Through increased experience with a variety of people, you can grow in understanding of others—provided you avoid a critical or judgmental attitude. This is the key to learning to accept others—*recognize that other people are like you in many ways, even though different in other ways.*

Accepting someone includes accepting that person's behavior—even if it is not pleasant. There may be good reason for a patient's irritability or criticism. It is not realistic to expect everyone to be pleasant all of the time; such an expectation is especially unrealistic in regard to people who are sick.

Occasionally, a patient's behavior *is* unacceptable. Then, without showing anger or fear, the health care professional can use an **I-statement** to indicate that such behavior is unacceptable. An I-statement is a sentence which states how you think or feel about a behavior or situation. Rather than an accusatory you-statement, which can put the other person on the defensive, an I-statement communicates your feelings or needs without expressing blame or criticism of the other person. The following are examples of how you could begin an I-statement:

- I need . . .
- I would appreciate . . .
- I feel uncomfortable when . . .

In contrast, you-statements can sound as though you are blaming:

- You need to . . .
- You made me uncomfortable when . . .

With practice, using I-statements can help you communicate concerns clearly and directly without blaming the other person.

Showing Interest and Concern

While you are caring for a patient, give that patient your full attention. Address the patient by name, listen, respond appropriately, and show willingness to act on any requests. In many situations, hospital routine requires that things be done at a certain time; usually, an explanation will gain the patient's cooperation. In other situations, health care professionals unnecessarily force patients into a routine. If a patient customarily bathes at bedtime, why insist upon a morning bath while in the hospital? Some patients deeply resent unnecessary interruptions or changes in their daily routine. Before insisting that such patients conform to the usual hospital routine, be sure that such conformity is really necessary.

For Discussion and Reflection

Consider a time when a friend, family member, or coworker behaved in a way that you found unacceptable. How did you respond? If this situation were to occur again, how might you use an I-statement to respond to the other person?

Listening and Observing

The patient who has fears and anxieties can benefit from talking out these feelings. Most patients, however, do not readily "open up." Be sensitive to subtle indications that something is bothering the patient. Linger in the patient's unit to chat casually and respond to any hint of anxiety by showing interest in how the patient feels. Be available as an interested listener. A patient's readiness to express feelings to you is, in a sense, a test of the effectiveness of your relationship with that patient. Usually acceptance, demonstrated interest, and concern pave the way for a patient to express fears, anxieties, and uncertainties.

Recognizing Significant Behavior

Nonverbal behavior often provides a clue to the patient's feelings. Consider the following examples of patient behavior:

- Nervous movements, restlessness
- Unwillingness to participate in conversation
- Not making eye contact when speaking
- Sleeping excessively
- Watching television when you are speaking to them

The patient who states, "My doctor says I should have surgery," is probably signaling a need to talk about it. You can shut off conversation, or you can encourage it by your response. Saying, "I know that. I took your preoperative orders from the doctor" may be interpreted by the patient to mean, "This health care professional doesn't care how scared I am." On the other hand, if you respond, "How do you feel about having surgery?" the patient is more likely to verbalize feelings about the impending surgery.

When you encourage patients to express feelings, you are providing a valuable service. A patient may gain more from verbalizing anxieties than from taking a tranquilizer. Asking open-ended questions can encourage patients to open up about their concerns. Several ways to ask open-ended questions and to respond to patient feelings are discussed below.

Using Appropriate Responses

When patients make "loaded statements," it is usually effective to repeat what the patient has said, using essentially the same words but with a questioning inflection. This type of response, known as *echoing*, is a safe response; it does not give information, and it does not show your reaction to what the patient said. It merely says to the patient that you heard; the rising inflection in your voice implies, "Please continue. I am listening." Some patients will not understand the meaning of the rising inflection and simply be annoyed by your use of echoing.

It is good to have a range of communication techniques so you can use the most appropriate one for a particular situation. Some other useful techniques are: reflecting, clarifying, validating, questioning, and confronting. *Reflecting* is similar to echoing, but requires that you restate what the patient said, indicating that you have heard the message and are aware of the patient's feelings. Your response may begin with a phrase such as, "It sounds like. . ." or "It seems like you. . ." This type of response is also called *mirroring*. When you use reflecting, you are essentially providing a mirror for the patient to view what he or she just said. The patient then has an opportunity to confirm, deny, or modify the meaning of the comment.

Clarifying is a technique used to test your interpretation of what has been said. After stating something like, "Let me see if I understand what you mean," you state the message, as you understand it, in your own words. The speaker can then confirm or deny that you understand the intended meaning. This may require several repetitions before the speaker will agree that you understand the message.

Validating is a technique used to check the meaning of certain nonverbal behaviors of the speaker. Often, the spoken message conveys one meaning, but certain nonverbal clues indicate a different meaning or indicate that the speaker's emotional state is different from what the verbal message implies. The technique for validating involves such statements as, "I sense that. . ." followed by a description of a feeling or "I notice that. . ." followed by an observation of some behavior, posture, or facial expression. This technique invites the patient to express feelings, doubts, anxieties, worries, annoyances, and frustrations.

Questioning is often required in the performance of patient care, usually to obtain specific information. Questioning can also be used as a therapeutic tool and as a means of avoiding a misunderstanding. Questioning should be done with a caring attitude. It is better to ask only one question, allow time for the patient to answer, then converse briefly before asking another question. It is especially important that you listen while the patient responds and allow the patient to finish before you speak again.

Adapting Your Behavior

Accept each patient as a worthy person. Remember that the patient's behavior is an effort to deal with the present situation. If it becomes apparent that you are having an adverse effect on the patient, change your behavior. Some patients enjoy a cheerful, talkative health care professional; others find cheerfulness annoying. As you become more sensitive to the feelings of others, you will be able to adapt your behavior to each patient.

Maintaining Confidentiality

Legally and ethically, health care professionals are required to protect patients' privacy and to hold patients' health information in confidence. In 2003, the Health Insurance and Portability and Accountability Act (HIPAA) Privacy Rule took effect. This federal legislation protects the privacy of individuals' medical information. Clients are generally given information about their privacy rights on their first visit to a particular health care office or facility. HIPAA stipulates that consumers have the right to request copies of their medical records, and to correct any errors they may contain. Consumers also have the right to decide who can receive their medical information and for what purposes. Violations of the HIPAA Privacy Rule may be reported to the Department of Health and Human Services Office of Civil Rights.

An exception to confidentiality is information *relevant to the patient's well-being.* For this reason, it is unwise to commit yourself to promises. If a patient offers to tell you something that requires a promise "not to tell," do not be flattered that the patient wants to share a secret. Even more important, do not make such a promise. Simply state, "Whatever I learn about a patient is kept in confidence, unless the patient's well-being requires that I share the information with the health care team." Then indicate that you are listening if the patient wishes to talk.

Common Behavior Patterns of Patients

Egocentrism

Most people become **egocentric** during illness. This means that the patient becomes self-centered—the primary concern is with self. Much of the demanding behavior that health care professionals (and families) resent in patients is actually a manifestation of the egocentric reaction to illness. This behavior can test your acceptance of the patient, yet egocentrism is just as much a reaction to illness as physical symptoms. If you accept egocentrism as a reaction to illness, you will find it easier to tolerate a patient's self-centered behavior.

Regression

Regression involves reverting to behaviors that are appropriate to an earlier level of development. The most extreme form of regression is lying in the fetal position and not responding to one's surroundings. This is often seen in older adults who have been bedridden for a long period of time.

In the home, a young child may regress when a new baby arrives. For example, a toddler who has mastered drinking from a cup may ask for a bottle. Regression can be seen with patients of all ages. Dependence on others for personal care, when one is capable of self-care, is an example of regression.

Unfriendly Behavior

Place yourself in the following situation. Today you are assigned to Mr. A., who is totally indifferent to all your efforts to be pleasant. You feel annoyed and wonder why you are wasting good cheer on this cold, unfriendly person.

Then you tell yourself that there may be reasons for Mr. A.'s behavior. Your thoughts run through some of the possible reasons. "Maybe Mr. A. fears his illness, but he does not want me to know he is frightened. Perhaps he does not admit to himself that he is frightened. He may have had unfavorable experiences with health care professionals and is transferring hostility from his previous experiences to me."

There is no one way to cope with an unfriendly patient. Every person reacts as an individual and may or may not be aware of the reaction or its effects on other people. Do not take unfriendliness personally. Accept it for what it is: a manifestation of how the patient feels at the moment. Maintain your own pleasant manner. Continue to show interest and concern. Visit the patient's room at intervals, but not so frequently that you are an annoyance. Sometimes your efforts will pay off without your knowing; your sincerity and interest lead to trust and the patient begins to respond to you.

Aggressive Behavior

Aggression may be physical or verbal. Physical aggression is most likely to occur if the patient is a child, is facing emotional or mental challenges, is inebriated, or is in an irresponsible state. A simple aggressive act such as pushing your hand away may indicate fear, anger, or other negative emotional reactions to you or to what you are planning to do. It may be an effort at self-defense. If the aggression is more serious—an actual attack on you, for example—you must handle the situation as best you can to avoid being hurt and then summon help from a professional worker. Because there are legal and ethical implications in handling aggression, avoid any action that could result in your being accused of assault on the patient. Protect yourself from injury, but secure the assistance of your supervisor as quickly as possible.

A child is likely to use physical aggression defensively, due to the expectation of pain. The child's age, condition, and other factors determine the best way to handle aggressive behavior. If you are in doubt about how to work with a particular child, discuss the problem with the pediatric supervisor and obtain specific instructions. Your general approach, however, must include an accepting attitude. Never say to a child, "You are bad." Instead, tell the child you cannot accept kicking, biting, or whatever form the aggression is taking. Set limits to the behaviors you will accept. Even if the child does not respect these limits (example: no kicking), they will understand why you are using restraints during a procedure. When you have finished working with the child, demonstrate acceptance with friendly behavior. Keep in mind that the child who fights you is manifesting an intense emotional state.

With adults, aggressive behavior is usually in the form of verbal attack or resistance. Verbal aggression may involve criticism, loud talking, profanity, or arguing. If the patient is critical, listen to the complaint and how it is described. If there is a valid complaint, corrective steps should be taken immediately. If the complaint does not seem to be valid, consider the complaint to be an expression of feelings. Arguing may be a disguised request for an explanation: the patient is challenging you to justify some aspect of the therapeutic plan, some policy of the health agency, or some procedure.

Passive aggression, on the other hand, is likely to consist of overt or covert non-cooperation. In **overt** noncooperation, the patient resists by refusing to take medicine, accept a treatment, undergo a diagnostic procedure, or carry out some self-help routine. **Covert** noncooperation involves deceit. The patient wants the health team to think they are cooperating, but actually are not. Patients who ask that their medication be left on the bedside table ("I'll take it later") may intend to flush it down the toilet. If you discover that a patient has been covertly noncooperative, you will probably feel anger. It is hard to accept that someone has deceived you. But consider for a moment: Why would a patient not cooperate with the therapeutic plan?

Perhaps the patient fears drug reactions and believes that quietly disposing of the drug is easier than trying to explain to health care professionals "who do not understand how I feel about drugs." Perhaps the patient's religion discourages the use of drugs. Perhaps the patient knows (or thinks) that this is a terminal illness and does not want to prolong life, if the cost is pain and helplessness or depleting the family's financial resources. Whatever the reason for this noncooperation, you may be sure it makes sense to the patient. It is your responsibility to (1) refer this problem to the professional staff, (2) remain nonjudgmental toward this patient, (3) accept that you may never understand the reasons for the patient's behavior, and (4) remember that noncooperation serves a purpose for the patient.

Hostility

Dealing with verbal or passive aggression is largely a problem of dealing with hostility. Team planning is more likely to be effective than isolated efforts by one or two members of the team. In general, each health care professional should give undivided attention to the hostile patient, listen without defensiveness or argument, indicate respect for the patient's feelings, show concern, and encourage expression of thoughts and feelings. Sometimes, it is effective to reflect what the patient has just said: "You think the food is terrible." At other times it may be more appropriate to question, using the patient's ideas but adding your own interpretation followed by "Is that what you mean?" It may be more appropriate to test your guess about the feelings behind the patient's comments: "Are you unhappy about this?" or "You seem to be quite angry about this." Use a pleasant tone and phrases that help the patient feel free to express feelings. Your responses should convey acceptance, caring, and willingness to listen. Sometimes such an approach has unexpectedly good results. The patient, after expressing feelings, may say something such as, "I guess that's a pretty small thing to be fussing about."

The worst thing you can do with a hostile patient is to return hostility. This simply confirms the patient's belief that you do not care or understand—your hostility has justified the patient's hostility. To avoid hostile behavior toward the patient, you *must* avoid hostile feelings. Accept the patient's hostility as indicative of a need, perhaps a need to develop trust in the health care team. If you develop negative feelings toward a patient, avoid defensiveness, criticism, arguing, short answers, or otherwise showing your negative feelings. If the patient detects your negative feelings, someone else should be assigned to care for that patient.

Crying

Crying can result from any degree of anger, fear, or grief. Some people cry whenever they experience sentimental feelings. Crying is an emotional release and should not be stifled.

When you find a patient crying, avoid such comments as "Let's stop crying now," or "You are much better, so there is nothing to cry about." These remarks may make you feel better, but they indicate to the patient that you are not trying to understand the patient's feelings.

Sometimes it is appropriate to ask the reason for the crying. At other times, it is better just to show acceptance, encourage freedom to express feelings through crying, and wait for the patient to volunteer information. It is not difficult to find out if the patient is crying because of pain and discomfort, fear, or sadness. If the crying seems to be due to personal problems, avoid prying questions, which could be an invasion of the patient's privacy.

With the crying patient, always indicate that you approve of crying as a means of relieving feelings. Sometimes holding the patient's hand or placing your hand over the patient's hand provides reassurance and conveys your interest and concern. Offer to stay, but if the patient shows a preference for being left alone, then say you are available if anything is needed, and leave. But return after 15 to 20 minutes and use appropriate behavior to respond to the patient's status at that time.

Each situation with a crying patient must be handled according to your best judgment and knowledge about the patient. Exactly what to say and do is dependent on the patient's situation. In every case, however:

• Do not offer false hope. (For example, "Everything's going to be OK.")
• Do not make promises you cannot keep.
• Do not minimize the patient's cause for crying.
• Do not express disapproval of crying.

Noncooperation

When an adult patient is uncooperative, there is usually a reason. Most adults recognize that cooperation with the health team is in their interest. Some possible reasons for noncooperation are lack of understanding, misinformation, suspicion or distrust, preference for one's own way of doing things, or negative feelings.

To understand a patient's failure to cooperate, inquire in an interested but uncritical manner about the reason for the patient's behavior. You may find that an explanation is needed, the patient needs to be taught a health principle, a false belief needs to be corrected, a misunderstanding needs to be cleared up, or feelings of fear or distrust need to be relieved.

Patients cannot be forced to cooperate. Cooperation must be gained by eliminating the cause of noncooperation. If you are unable to learn why the patient is not cooperating, discuss the situation with your supervisor. Sometimes the problem must be referred to the patient's physician. If cooperation is essential to recovery, then it must be secured in some way. If the patient is objecting to a procedure that is not essential to recovery or well-being, then the physician may discontinue it rather than antagonize the patient.

The Overly Friendly Patient

Occasionally, you may have a patient who is overly friendly. Such behavior may consist of personal questions or physical contact. The person who begins to ask personal questions may be trying innocently to make conversation or may be attempting to establish an overly familiar relationship. It is better to avoid discussing your personal life and your own experiences with patients. Instead, direct the conversation to the patient or to impersonal topics. One health care supervisor tells staff, "We are *friendly* to our patients, but it is not our role to be their *friends*."

Situations involving familiarity should be discussed with your supervisor. Be sure to report facts—what actually happened. Do not color your report with what you would have liked the situation to be, with judgmental statements, or with opinions. The supervisor can best assess the situation if you give an accurate account of what the patient said or did and what you said or did. The supervisor's professional judgment can provide guidelines for members of the health team who are caring for the patient.

Inappropriate Sexual Behavior

Occasionally a patient may display inappropriate sexual behavior. The behavior may include sexual remarks, inappropriate touching, or self-exposure. If inappropriate sexual behavior occurs, you can use the techniques described below to let the patient know that the behavior is unacceptable and to set limits. However, if the behavior persists or if you feel unsafe, you should seek assistance from other staff immediately and notify your supervisor. You should also be familiar with your employer's policies and procedures regarding sexual harassment.

Responding to Inappropriate Behavior

The following techniques can be used to set limits in response to inappropriate patient behavior: "I think, I feel, I want" and the positive/negative warning.

The "I think, I feel, I want" technique involves a series of I-statements:

- The first sentence describes or assesses the situation.
- The second sentence includes a statement of how the inappropriate behavior makes you feel.
- The third sentence states the appropriate behavior you expect from the patient.

For example, if a patient has made a sexually suggestive remark to you, you might reply as follows: "I think you meant that as a joke. However, I feel uncomfortable with your remark. I want our conversation to remain professional if I am going to continue your treatment."

The *positive/negative warning technique* sets limits by stating the positive outcome if the patient behaves appropriately as well as the negative outcome if the patient persists in inappropriate behavior. To use this technique, follow these steps:

1. State the appropriate behavior you would like the patient to exhibit.
2. State the positive outcome if the patient behaves appropriately.
3. State the negative outcome that will occur if the inappropriate behavior continues.
4. Follow through with either the positive or negative outcome based on the patient's continued behavior.

If a patient intentionally exposes themselves during treatment, you might reply as follows: "If you stop lifting your gown, I will stay with you and help you get stronger. However, if you continue, I will leave and cancel the rest of this treatment."

Following an incident of inappropriate behavior, follow your employer's policies and procedures regarding documentation of the behavior. If you are unsure about your employer's policies and procedures, ask your supervisor.

For Discussion and Reflection

Think of a time someone's behavior has made you feel uncomfortable, whether in a health care setting or another setting. How did you respond? Was your response effective in stopping the behavior?

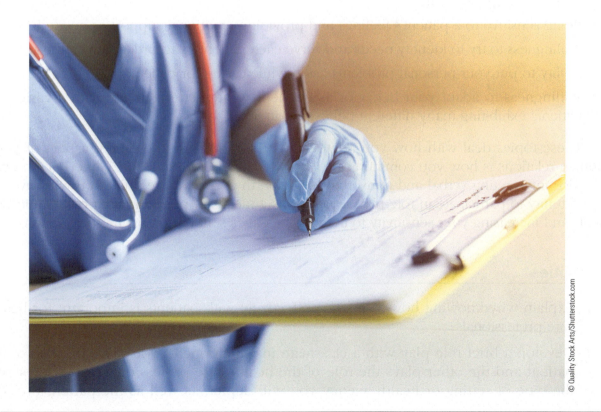

© Quality Stock Arts/Shutterstock.com

FIGURE 14-3 Following an incident of inappropriate behavior, follow your employer's policies and procedures regarding documentation of the behavior.

Conclusion

In this section, you have studied several topics that will help you be sensitive to the needs of a patient and understand common behaviors of patients:

- Physical and emotional effects of illness
- General effects of serious illness
- Influences on a patient's reaction to illness (age, life role, usual state of adjustment, dependency, cultural background, past experience)
- Common behavior patterns
- Strategies for coping with certain problem behaviors

You have also studied several topics that are relevant to you as a health care professional—*the beliefs and attitudes that you personally bring to the role*—and are important aspects of your personal effectiveness:

- Acceptance of each patient as a worthwhile human being (including tolerance for those who are different from you)
- Interest in and concern for each patient
- Willingness to listen
- Accuracy in observing
- Ability to recognize significant behaviors
- Respect for confidentiality
- Being sensitive to a patient's feelings and providing emotional support as needed
- Willingness to try to identify needs and serve each patient in accordance with those needs
- Ability to put your personal problems aside while caring for patients
- Willingness to adapt your behavior as needed to interact effectively with a variety of patients exhibiting many different behavior patterns

These topics deal with how you relate to your patients. Another major aspect of good human relations is how you communicate, verbally and nonverbally. In Chapter 15, you will practice interpreting verbal and nonverbal behavior. In each of these units, you will have the opportunity to participate in role-play situations as a means of polishing your communication skills and increasing your sensitivity to the real messages sent to you by another person.

Activities

1. Explain why knowing how to interact effectively with patients is important for health care professionals.

2. Develop a brief role play with a classmate in which one of you plays the role of the patient and the other plays the role of the health care professional. Briefly describe the type of setting or health agency you will depict, as well as the patient's reason

for seeking health care. As the "patient," select one of the following behaviors to demonstrate (the classmate playing the role of health care professional should select an appropriate response to the behavior demonstrated):

Option 1: Demonstrate the role play to the class or a small group of classmates. The observers can identify the patient behavior that was demonstrated and discuss additional options for responding appropriately.

Option 2: Practice this activity in groups of three, with the third classmate taking the role of observer. Rotate roles until all three have practiced each role. The observer can identify the patient behavior demonstrated and provide feedback about the response of the health care professional.

List of patient behaviors to demonstrate:

Egocentrism

Regression

Hostility

Crying

Aggression

Asking staff to "keep a secret"

3. For each of the following guidelines, give an example of an action you could take or a statement you could make to put the guideline into practice in your work as a health care professional:

Putting personal matters aside

Accepting the patient

Showing interest and concern

Listening and observing

Maintaining confidentiality

4. Conduct an informal interview with a friend, relative, or acquaintance currently working in health care. What types of patient behavior have they encountered? What responses have they found to be most helpful?

References and Suggested Readings

Hsueh, L., Hirsh, A. T., Maupomé, G., & Stewart, J. C. (2021). Patient–provider language concordance and health outcomes: A systematic review, evidence map, and research agenda. *Medical Care Research and Review, 78*(1), 3–23. https://doi.org/10.1177/1077558719860708

Mento, C., et al. (2020). Workplace violence against healthcare professionals: A systematic review. *Aggression and Violent Behavior, 51*. https://doi.org/10.1016/j.avb.2020.101381

Notaro, E., Pascoe, V., Shinohara, M. M., & DeNiro, K. (2019). Sexual harassment from patient to provider. *International Journal of Women's Dermatology, 6*(1), 30–31. doi: 10.1016/j.ijwd.2019.09.001 .PMID: 32042881; PMCID: PMC6997839.

Practicing Effective Communication

Objectives

After completing this chapter, you should be able to:

- List examples of nonverbal behavior and interpret the message of nonverbal behavior.
- List ways to make verbal communication as clear as possible.
- Describe how paraverbal communication can influence the way spoken communication is received by the listener.
- Practice skills for effective listening.
- Practice strategies for improving your communication skills.

Key Terms

Ambiguity
Assumptions
Clarification
Enunciation

Expectation
Inconsistency
Paraphrase
Paraverbal

Selective observing
Stance

You have heard much about "good human relations" since you began your preparation for a career in the health field. Skill in interpersonal relationships may be thought of as *controlled* interaction with others. It means control over what happens by *consciously deciding* what to say or do to bring about the response you desire from another person.

When your behavior arouses positive feelings in others, then it is likely that the behavior of the other person toward you will be favorable. On the other hand, your behavior can arouse negative feelings in others: anxiety, anger, a sense of threat, self-pity, feelings of being "put down," or just plain irritation. When your behavior arouses negative feelings, then the behavior of the other person toward you may be unpleasant: noncooperation, complaints, withdrawal, or disagreement with whatever you say.

Any interaction with another person involves three types of communication—verbal, paraverbal, and nonverbal:

- *Verbal* communication uses words and language to convey a message.
- **Paraverbal** communication refers to *how* a verbal message is spoken—the tone of voice, volume, and rate of speech.
- *Nonverbal* communication refers to body language and facial expressions.

Many experts have stated that nonverbal communication accounts for half or more of the messages we send to other people. By learning to observe others' nonverbal behavior more closely, you can make a more informed decision about how you will communicate with them. By becoming more conscious of your own nonverbal behavior, you can increase the chances that the other person will receive your message in the way you intend.

Observing and Interpreting Nonverbal Behavior

Most of us think we are observant and that our observations are reasonably accurate. **Selective observing** means that we notice some details of a situation, while completely missing many other details. Left to chance, observations are likely to be made according to one's interests or curiosity. To become skillful in observing nonverbal behavior, make it a habit to consciously observe others' nonverbal behavior.

Most people communicate feelings through nonverbal behavior, often unconsciously. But regardless of whether or not the nonverbal behavior is conscious, it signals that the person is responding to something—perhaps to you as a person, something you said or did, your tone of voice, the expression on your face, and the other person's interpretation of what it means. It is also possible that the behavior indicates the individual's response to the total situation: the stress of a job interview, anger at being ill, fear of surgery, or the expectation of an unfavorable diagnosis. Nonverbal communication, then, provides a clue to a person's inner feelings. In some cases, it is also a signal that more specific behavior, such as an angry outburst, is about to occur.

The message of nonverbal behavior is lost unless you note it and interpret the meaning correctly. To improve your use of nonverbal communication, consciously practice observing the nonverbal behavior of others. Next, practice interpreting that behavior and check your interpretation against further evidence. When you interact with another person, note any changes in facial expression, slight movements of facial muscles, position of the lips, direction of gaze, position of the eyelids, body movements, **stance** (how a person stands), general posture, and the hands—position and movements. Experts use the ability to read people to help them select members for a jury or screen job applicants.

FIGURE 15-1 **Most people communicate feelings through nonverbal behavior.**

After noting the nonverbal clues, try to interpret that behavior. Does a twitching facial muscle indicate stress? Or repressed anger? If stress, why does the individual feel stressed in this situation? Do the restless movements of the hands indicate nervousness? If so, why does the person feel nervous in this situation? What is the person's emotional state? What expectations does the person have? Are you sending nonverbal messages to which that individual is responding? By associating the nonverbal behavior of a specific person with additional evidence as it becomes available, you can learn to "read" that person with a reasonable degree of accuracy.

Interpretation of nonverbal behavior carries the risk of misinterpretation. This is a serious risk, for *misinterpretation can lead to more misunderstanding than simply ignoring the nonverbal communication.* The risk of misinterpretation can be decreased by following six steps:

1. Note the nonverbal behavior.
2. Make a *tentative* interpretation.
3. Continue to observe for more evidence, especially evidence that is easily interpreted—a display of anger, statements of disapproval, objections, or complaints.
4. Revise your interpretation if there is evidence that the first interpretation was not accurate.
5. Watch for *consistency*, that is, occurrence of a specific nonverbal behavior every time that individual is in a particular situation, such as making a decision, doing something new, speaking before a group, or coping with conflict.
6. Use verbal communication to clarify the meaning of the nonverbal behavior. For example, if it is appropriate in a given situation, you could say, "Pat, you seem upset. What's going on?"

Once you have detected the pattern and determined that certain nonverbal behaviors consistently indicate a specific feeling state of that person, you have learned to "read" that person's nonverbal behavior.

For Discussion and Reflection

Think about someone you know well, such as a close friend or family member. What nonverbal behaviors provide a clue to this person's mood? How do you know, even without speaking, what kind of day this person has had?

With friends and coworkers, you may become quite accurate at reading their feelings without any words being exchanged. Accuracy in interpretation is achieved only over a period of time and through frequent opportunities to observe an individual in a variety of situations.

With people you see less frequently, you will not be able to learn the meaning of their nonverbal clues as readily. And with people you see only occasionally or for brief periods of time, you must make your best judgment of the probable meaning of nonverbal behavior and try to confirm that interpretation as the relationship proceeds.

In relating to patients and their families, look for nonverbal behavior that may mean a buildup of feelings, especially fear, anxiety, confusion, and anger. When you detect such signals, it is likely that the patient would benefit from extra attention in the form of sincere interest, concern, consideration, and emotional support while adapting to strange surroundings and illness.

The special attention you provide may encourage the patient to talk. You might invite questions with, "Is there something you would like me to explain? I will try to answer any questions you have." You may be able to answer some questions but find it necessary to refer others to appropriate persons—the patient's physician, the supervisor, or another department of the health facility. You will be safe in giving information about routines and the facility itself. Questions about the patient's condition should be handled by others, usually the physician. Your role is to provide emotional support for the patient when you listen to questions, show sincere concern, and state that you will pass any questions you cannot answer on to the person who can provide answers.

A *full exploration of feelings* is best left to professionals with counseling skills. However, you can encourage *expression of feelings* and still remain within your role as a health care professional. Be aware that your patient is a human being going through a stressful experience, indicate your willingness to listen, and give your full attention to the patient. But, in order to recognize those who need an understanding listener, you must receive the message. A *message of need is most likely to be sent nonverbally.*

The following exercises are designed to help you practice recognizing and interpreting nonverbal communication.

Exercise 15–1: Observing Nonverbal Behavior

Purpose

In this exercise, you will discuss the messages conveyed by a series of nonverbal behaviors.

Instructions

1. Work in groups of two. One partner will be the actor and the other the observer. In round 2, you will reverse roles.

2. Without speaking, the actor will demonstrate each of the nonverbal behaviors listed. After each behavior, the observer will comment briefly on the message he believes the behavior is sending. (There are a number of possible explanations for each behavior.)

Nonverbal Behaviors: Round 1

1. Cross your arms.
2. Roll your eyes.
3. Look at the floor.
4. Jiggle your leg for several seconds.
5. Fiddle with your pencil or pen.
6. Sit up very straight in your chair.

Nonverbal Behaviors: Round 2

1. Clench your fists.
2. Sigh loudly.
3. Smile.
4. Tap your fingers on the table repeatedly.
5. Look at your phone or a wall clock.
6. Make direct eye contact with your partner.

Exercise 15–2: Observing and Interpreting Nonverbal Behavior

Purpose

In this exercise, you will observe and interpret nonverbal communication and test your interpretation against the person's explanation of the thoughts and feelings that accompanied the nonverbal behavior.

Instructions

1. Divide into groups of four. Two people will be actors and two will be observers. In round 2, you will reverse roles.
2. Select one of the situations below to role-play. The actors may take a few minutes to plan their performance.
3. Actors role-play the situation for three minutes. During this time, observers list the nonverbal behaviors they see and note what was happening in the role-play when the behavior occurred. One of the observers should call time after three minutes.
4. Observers describe the nonverbal behaviors they witnessed and offer a possible interpretation for each behavior. Actors confirm whether each interpretation matches what they were thinking or feeling at the time.
5. Reverse roles so that the actors are now observers and the observers are now actors. Repeat the exercise using a different situation.

Role-Plays for Exercise 15–2

1. Kori often arrives late to work and asks to leave early. The supervisor decides to discuss the matter with Kori.

2. Ravi, an experienced lab technician, notices a new technician using sloppy procedures and taking shortcuts. Concerned about accuracy and a reprimand from the supervisor, Ravi confronts the coworker.

3. Arturo has recently immigrated to the United States and must get a physical for his new job. He has never been examined by a doctor before, and his English is limited. A nurse sits down to help him fill out paperwork and to get a medical history.

4. An older adult who is hard of hearing takes several prescription medications. The patient asks a staff person to explain how much of each medication to take and when.

5. Fifteen-year-old Lisa has come to the clinic for a pregnancy test, which is positive. A clinic worker gives her the test results and discusses her options with her.

Verbal Communication

Workers in the health field spend much time communicating with others: patients and their families, visitors to the health agency, other members of the health team, and supervisors. As a health care professional, you need a high level of communication skill. Whenever and wherever people talk to one another, communication problems may occur.

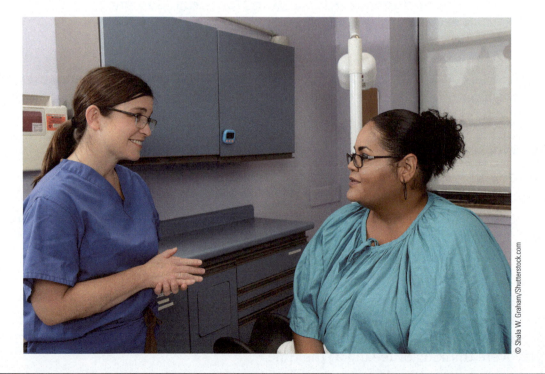

FIGURE 15-2 Health care professionals spend much time communicating with others.

We often assume that whatever we say to another person is understood—that the listener gets the meaning we intend to convey. In reality, there are numerous sources of communication breakdown:

- Our language permits different meanings for many words.
- Speech and hearing factors may distort what is heard.
- Nonverbal messages may differ from the spoken message.

Many examples of misunderstanding, noncooperation, criticism, and other forms of conflict between people can be traced to a communication problem. Your preparation for working in the health field includes practice in improving your communication skills so you will have a minimum of communication problems.

Ambiguity

Ambiguity is the state of being *ambiguous*, or vague and unclear. The opposite of ambiguity is clarity. The word *unambiguous* is sometimes used to mean completely clear or free of ambiguity.

It is difficult to avoid ambiguity in verbal communication for a number of reasons:

- A word may have several different meanings.
- The word used by the speaker may not be the best word for expressing the desired meaning.
- A pronoun may not clearly indicate whom or what it represents.

For example, the word *smart* is used by some people to mean very intelligent; another person uses *smart* to mean sassy or disrespectful. Can you think of other meanings for this one word?

Some words or phrases have double meanings. They can be interpreted literally, or they may be used to mean something entirely different. The following joke illustrates this type of ambiguity:

A: *"This cat is really good for mice."*
B: *"How can you say that? He is afraid of mice. He even runs from them."*
C: *"That's just what I mean. He is very good for the mice."*

In attempting to avoid ambiguous statements, you should:

- Use words that have a single, precise meaning whenever possible.
- Use the best word for what you want to say.
- Use a noun to indicate who or what; if you use a pronoun (he, she, it, they), it should clearly refer to *one specific noun* used in the same sentence.

Discrepancies in a Message

Most of us are careless about verbal communication, especially when we are trying to attend to many things at once. In haste, we say *approximately* what we mean, then *assume* that

For Discussion and Reflection

Consider a situation in which you experienced a communication breakdown with another person. Were you the sender or the receiver of the message? What might have caused the breakdown? How was the situation resolved?

the message received by the listener is the same as the message we intended to send. Also, we sometimes send one message nonverbally and state a different message verbally. Which message is the listener to believe?

Message discrepancy means that the message sent and the message received differ in meaning. The difficulty may be with the sender of the message or the receiver. When the problem is with the sender, it may be caused by:

- Ambiguity in the message.
- **Inconsistency** in the verbal and nonverbal messages.
- Poor **enunciation**, causing some words to sound like other words with a different meaning.
- Use of language the listener does not understand. (This is likely to occur if the listener is a child, a person from a different culture, or an older adult who may not be familiar with newer meanings of a word.)

If the problem of message discrepancy lies with the receiver, it may be caused by:

- Poor hearing.
- Selective listening (the individual listens only to certain parts of a statement).
- Inability to understand the words used by the speaker, such as medical terminology.
- Acceptance of the wrong message when there is inconsistency in the sender's verbal and nonverbal communication.

An example of inconsistency in verbal and nonverbal messages is the crying patient who says, "I'm all right. I feel fine." Sometimes the health care professional who is alert to nonverbal messages can pick up the true situation, as when a patient says, "There is nothing really wrong with me. The doctor says these are just routine tests." At the same time, the patient's countenance reflects a high level of anxiety. Whenever there is inconsistency in verbal and nonverbal messages, the listener must decide which message to believe.

In your endeavors to convey messages that are received (interpreted) as you intend:

- Avoid ambiguous statements.
- Select words and phrases the listener will understand.
- Speak clearly.
- Control your nonverbal signals to avoid sending a message that is different from your verbal message.
- Face the person to whom you are speaking.

Paraverbal Communication

Tone of voice is a key aspect of paraverbal communication, or *how* you say a message apart from the actual words used. You have probably heard a parent or teacher scold a child, "Don't take that tone with me!" Tone of voice can be as important as the choice of words in conveying a message to a listener. Responding to someone who is angry in a calm tone of voice often helps defuse the person's anger. On the other hand, an impatient or harsh tone of voice may hurt or anger the listener. Becoming conscious of your tone of voice helps your listener take your words in the spirit you intend them. Tone is particularly important when talking on the telephone because the listener does not have the benefit of seeing your facial expressions and other nonverbal behavior.

Two other components of paraverbal communication are volume and rate of speech. You have likely experienced listening to someone who spoke so quietly that you strained to hear each word. Very quiet speech may send a message that the speaker is shy, anxious, or afraid. Likely, you have also heard someone speaking too loudly, which can give the impression that the person is angry or upset. When someone speaks at a very slow rate, the listener may become impatient, question the intelligence of the speaker, or feel that the speaker is being condescending. On the other hand, a very fast rate of speech may send the message that the speaker is in a hurry, and the listener may have difficulty catching all the information in the message.

As you communicate with others, notice both their use of paraverbal communication and your own. You may have heard the phrase, "It's not what you say, it's how you say it." By consciously choosing a tone of voice, volume level, and rate of speech which fits the message you want to send, you can increase the chance that your message will be received accurately.

FIGURE 15-3 Tone is particularly important when talking on the telephone because the listener cannot see your facial expressions and other nonverbal behavior.

Effective Listening

In addition to expressing ideas clearly, a good communicator takes care to "hear" others accurately. The following techniques will help you become an effective listener:

- Give your full attention to anyone who is speaking to you.
- Listen to the words and observe nonverbal behavior in an effort to get the "real message."
- **Paraphrase** or restate what the person says to make sure you have understood correctly.
- Use questions to clarify the speaker's intended meaning, especially (1) if the speaker uses ambiguous or unfamiliar words and (2) if the verbal and nonverbal messages are inconsistent.

Assumptions and Expectations

Underlying many communication problems are **assumptions** and expectations held by the speaker or by the listener. An assumption is *acceptance of something as fact without any evidence or proof.* Sometimes we assume that another person "knows" how we feel or what we are thinking, even though we did not verbally express our thoughts or feelings. In fact, the person to whom we are speaking may be completely unaware of how we feel or what we are thinking. Or the other person may make assumptions about how we think or feel and the assumptions are completely wrong! Making assumptions is certain to create misunderstandings and communication breakdowns.

Another frequent cause of communication problems is the expectation of a person, either the sender or receiver of the message. An **expectation** means thinking that something will occur. An expectation can cause the receiver to "read into" a message something that the sender did not intend. For example, suppose your supervisor walks in while you are taking a shortcut on a task, then later the supervisor sends for you. Having been "caught" taking an unauthorized shortcut, your expectation is that the supervisor is going to correct you. You are probably set to defend yourself or to accept blame and say you will not do it again. But perhaps, instead of reprimanding you, the supervisor says, "I noticed you were not following procedure. Let's take a close look at the method you were using. It may be more efficient than our present procedure." Let us hope you did not misinterpret the supervisor's opening statement before you found out that your expectation was wrong! Sometimes an expectation can even lead the listener to "hear" a message that is quite different from the words spoken. This takes the speaker by surprise because the speaker is unaware of the other person's expectations.

Being careful to avoid assumptions and expectations is important in all your communications, but especially when working with clients who come from another culture or who have cognitive disabilities. These clients may or may not fully grasp the meaning of the words and nonverbal communication you use. When possible, check for understanding when providing information and provide a written or visual copy of the information if possible. Encourage clients to ask questions, and be aware of other resources that can support these clients, such as translation services, transportation, or community agencies.

Improving Communication Skills

Improving your communication skills requires that you test your habits as both a sender and a receiver of messages. Fortunately, the same practice that helps you become more precise in your sending can also contribute to your skill in listening. As you become sensitive to ambiguities, inconsistencies, assumptions, and expectations, you will ask for **clarification** rather than risk a misunderstanding.

The following exercises are structured to provide practice in speaking, listening, and interpreting messages. In Exercise 15–3, you will increase your awareness of how the tone of a message can alter the meaning you convey to your listener. In Exercise 15–4, you will practice expressing your ideas clearly and listening effectively to the ideas of others.

When you have made progress on each of these skills, the probability of your having a communication breakdown is less. As an effective communicator, you will also be more effective in establishing good relationships.

Exercise 15–3: Using Tone to Alter the Meaning of a Statement

Purpose
In this exercise, you will practice using and listening to different tones of voice.

Instructions
1. Work in groups of two. One partner will be the speaker and the other the listener. In round 2, you will reverse roles. Note that although the statements are the same in both rounds, the tones of voice used are not.
2. Role-play the following situations, using the tone of voice indicated. After the speaker has made the statement, the listener comments on how the tone affects the message they "hear."

Role-Plays: Round 1
In this exercise, you will practice making statements that convey your intended meaning to another person, with minimal chance of misinterpretation by the listener.
1. A nurse says to a patient, "Are you ready for your treatment, Mr. Jones?"
   Tone: impatient
2. A supervisor says to an employee, "I expected you at work an hour ago. What happened?"
   Tone: concerned
3. A patient says to a health care professional, "There was a mistake on the last bill I received from your office."
   Tone: hesitant
4. A lab supervisor asks a lab technician, "Are those test results ready yet?"
   Tone: curious
5. A health care professional comments to a coworker, "Here we are, working the late shift again."
   Tone: resentful

Role-Plays: Round 2

1. A nurse says to a patient, "Are you ready for your treatment, Mr. Jones?"

   Tone: kind

2. A supervisor says to an employee, "I expected you at work an hour ago. What happened?"

   Tone: irritated

3. A patient says to a health care professional, "There was a mistake on the last bill I received from your office."

   Tone: demanding

4. A lab supervisor asks a lab technician, "Are those test results ready yet?"

   Tone: hurried

5. A health care professional comments to a coworker, "Here we are, working the late shift again."

   Tone: joking

Exercise 15–4: Expressing Ideas and Listening Effectively

Purpose

In this exercise, you will express your opinion on a topic as clearly as possible. You will also use the listening techniques described earlier to check your understanding and to gain more information about another person's opinion.

Instructions

1. Organize into groups of three. Each person should get a turn to play the role of the speaker, the observer, and the listener. The roles are described below.

2. The opinion statements that follow will serve as the basis for your discussion. Select a different opinion statement for each of the three rounds.

3. The speaker will discuss an opinion (agree or disagree) about one of the statements. The listener will use the listening skills described in this unit to check for understanding and to gain more information. After three minutes, the observer will call time and will provide feedback about the communication skills and listening skills observed.

Speaker Your objective is to communicate your opinion clearly to the listener. Select for discussion one of the opinion statements listed following this exercise. Explain why you agree or disagree with the statement. Feel free to use your personal knowledge and experiences to support your opinion.

Listener Your objective is to use effective listening techniques to gain a full understanding of the speaker's opinion. You are not to express your own opinion while playing the role of listener.

Observer Your objective is to provide feedback for the speaker and listener according to these guidelines:

- How clear was the speaker's first statement of opinion?
- How did the listener show that they were listening?
- Which listening skills did you observe?
- What additional information did the speaker share as a result of the listener's responses?

Opinion Statements to Serve as a Basis for Discussion

1. Health care professionals should be allowed to go to classes during duty hours if they want to work on a higher certification.
2. Most people entering a health career want to help the sick.
3. Patients should not expect health care professionals to listen to their personal problems.
4. The government should provide universal health care coverage for all Americans.
5. An individual who is pregnant has the right to decide whether or not to continue the pregnancy.
6. Sex education should not be allowed in the public schools.
7. Managed care is the best system for providing health services.
8. Select a health-care related topic of your own based on current events or information you are studying in your health occupations program.

Communication and the Health Care Professional

So far we have explored three types of communication: nonverbal, verbal, and paraverbal. In everyday situations, all three types of communication occur simultaneously, working together to create an overall message. As you practice your communication skills in the workplace and elsewhere, the following guidelines can help:

- When someone is upset, angry, or afraid, often the most helpful approach is to listen to their concerns. Most individuals will calm down once they feel that their concerns are being heard.
- An anxious or upset individual is unlikely to "process" information from you at that time, so keep your own statements as clear and brief as possible.
- Pay attention to both verbal and nonverbal messages.
- If you are unsure what another person means, follow up with clarifying questions or by restating the message to check for understanding.
- If you can remain calm and professional in your communication, others are more likely to do the same. By remaining calm, you can avoid escalating a negative situation.

Activities

1. The next time you watch a movie or show, select one or more of the following exercises to increase your awareness of nonverbal communication:

   a. Concentrate your attention on one of the lead actors and note examples of nonverbal communication. Did any specific example lead to a misunderstanding or conflict between two of the characters?

   b. The next time you watch a comedian who does imitations, note the various mannerisms and facial expressions the comedian portrays. Comedians are keen observers of human behavior, and imitators are especially observant of small bits of behavior that characterize an individual. Note the specific mannerisms portrayed in the actor's imitation of a certain person.

   c. Do you notice an actor who has a frozen countenance (facial expression does not change) most of the time. What nonverbal behaviors does this actor use to communicate?

   d. Do you see an actor who uses subtle changes in facial expression. What "body language" does this actor use to supplement facial expression?

   e. Look for an actor who conveys feelings primarily through facial expression. Does this actor also make use of body language to communicate feelings and/or reactions to the action occurring?

   f. Turn down the volume for at least five minutes during a show and observe the characters' facial expressions and body language without sound. Can you follow the plot, based on the actors' nonverbal communication?

2. What factors can cause misunderstanding in verbal communication? What strategies can reduce the chance of a misunderstanding?

3. Describe how tone of voice, volume, and rate of speech can influence the way a spoken message is received by the listener.

4. Has someone ever misunderstood your meaning because they expected or assumed that you would behave in a certain way? What happened, and how did you react?

5. List three strategies you can use as health care professional to improve your communication with clients.

References and Suggested Readings

Schiavo, R., Van Wye, G., & Manoncourt, E. (2022). COVID-19 and health inequities: The case for embracing complexity and investing in equity- and community-driven approaches to communication. *Journal of Communication in Healthcare, 15*(1), 1–6, doi: 10.1080/17538068.2022.2037349

Schlögl, M., & A Jones, C. (2020). Maintaining our humanity through the mask: Mindful communication during COVID-19. *Journal of the American Geriatrics Society, 68*(5), E12–E13. https://doi.org/10.1111/jgs.16488

Section V

Death and Loss

You have now learned about human behavior, ways people react to threat, and how to communicate effectively. This knowledge will be especially valuable as you work with people who are struggling to cope with loss. The ultimate losses are death (loss of one's own life) and bereavement (loss of a loved one).

In order to provide effective care to a terminally ill patient or to help those who are facing the loss of a loved one, the health care professional must have arrived at full acceptance of their own mortality and must have resolved any "unfinished business" related to past losses.

The purpose of Section V is to help you acknowledge your own mortality, clarify your beliefs about death, and become sensitive to the needs of terminally ill patients and their families.

16

Chapter

Grief and Loss Throughout Life

Objectives

After completing this chapter, you should be able to:

- Discuss strategies for coping with loss, sadness, and depression.
- Explain why loss is a natural part of everyone's life.
- Explain how the circumstances of a loved one's death can affect surviving friends and family.
- Describe the grief process and how it can affect behavior.
- Discuss strategies for assisting the family of a dying patient.

Key Terms

Anticipatory grief
Bereavement
Condolences

Displacement
Grief work
Mortality

Survivor guilt
Transference

Life involves a continuous series of changes that require us to adjust and readjust. Some of these changes represent a gain of some type—new home, new member of the family, graduation, new job, or a promotion. Some changes represent a loss—being fired, losing an important object, losing a spouse through divorce, or losing a loved one through death.

Many events involve both gains and losses. Moving to a new home is exciting, but it involves losing the familiarity of the old home and relationships in the old neighborhood. Graduation is usually a happy event—it symbolizes moving on to bigger and better things. But graduation also means giving up a favorite teacher, no longer spending much of the school day with your classmates, and giving up a familiar role for a new role and new responsibilities. You expect the big events of life to have a happy effect, so it is confusing to find that, instead of being happy, you are sad or even depressed. These negative feelings are due to awareness (perhaps at the unconscious level) of losses that will result from an otherwise happy event.

Most people do not need to learn how to be happy about a gain, but many people do not know how to cope with loss. Loss definitely is one of life's most important lessons because unexpressed grief is a powerful influence on behavior and on emotional/mental health.

Coping with Change and Loss

If we learn early in life to deal effectively with the small losses that are part of living, then we are better prepared to deal with those losses that cause a radical change in our life situation. If we do not learn to "let go" of whatever was lost and to grieve appropriately for each loss, then there is an accumulation of suppressed emotions—grief, anger, guilt, and fear. Suppressed emotions are eventually expressed in some form, such as uncontrolled outbursts, depression, or inability to cope with daily life problems. Failure to express such feelings is characteristic of people who develop phobias, commit suicide, or develop alcohol/drug dependency.

Actually, we have a choice. We can learn to accept the inevitable losses of life and express our grief appropriately, thereby maintaining control and emotional well-being. Or we can go through life without learning how to deal with loss—reacting with anger about the "unfairness" of life or suppressing our grief, thereby risking loss of control when these feelings eventually erupt.

Dr. Elisabeth Kübler-Ross (1926–2004) was a psychiatrist who worked with dying patients for many years. According to Dr. Kübler-Ross, the loss process extends throughout life, and each of us goes through the stages of this process repeatedly as we experience specific life changes, especially those that involve some type of loss. The best preparation for dealing with death, according to Dr. Kübler-Ross, is to learn to grieve appropriately for the small losses that accompany any major life change. Once we have learned to grieve, we are able to cope better with the big losses that will, inevitably, occur in each of our lives. Learning to cope with loss involves several specific steps:

1. Recognize the losses involved in a life event.

2. Grant yourself the right to grieve for each loss—no matter how small.

3. Recognize and accept the various emotions involved in your reaction to a specific loss.

4. Allow yourself time to grieve.

5. Accept that grief is a *process* that extends over a period of time.

FIGURE 16-1 The significance of a loss is very personal.

Significance of Loss

Losses are of many types: objects, people, relationships, jobs, money, body image (e.g., amputation, radical mastectomy), or intangibles such as beliefs, faith, one's sense of security, or self-esteem. The significance of a loss is very personal. A person's reaction to a loss *reflects its meaning to that person*, rather than its value as perceived by others.

Some types of loss may be experienced at any time throughout life: moving, personal relationships, death of a loved one, personal property, health. Reactions to such losses are influenced by the period of life in which they occur. Children often do not understand the reasons for a loss, and adults may fail to note or accept the child's emotional reaction. Adults have the advantage of being involved in some decisions that result in a loss, such as moving, so their emotional reaction is tempered by an understanding of the reasons for the decision. For older adults, a great loss is losing control over decisions that affect the remainder of their lives. Moving into a child's home or into a nursing home results in partial loss of control over one's daily activities. The reaction to such a change often includes hopelessness and resignation. The most devastating loss is the loss of life—one's own or that of a loved one.

Losses Throughout Life

Preparation for coping with a significant loss comes from experiencing a variety of losses throughout life. The individual who learns during childhood to grieve for small losses is better prepared to cope with a major loss than someone who has not learned to recognize and grieve for a loss. Learning to cope with loss begins in infancy; the types of loss and their significance vary according to the period of life.

Losses of Infancy and Early Childhood

The prenatal period is a very special time for both mother and fetus. If there are no complications or difficult circumstances, the pregnant individual experiences positive feelings during most of the pregnancy. For the fetus, life in the womb is the ultimate in security and safety. At the time of delivery, the family gains a new member—one of life's happiest events. But birth is the end of pregnancy—the loss of a once-only relationship between mother and infant. If the baby is breast-fed, the mother and infant establish another very special relationship. Weaning is a small loss because it requires both mother and infant to "let go" of this special relationship.

During infancy and early childhood, any separation from the parents (or other caregivers) is perceived as loss. The child, not knowing that the parents will return, feels deserted. Sadness is a natural reaction to separation; but separation from those who represent security can also arouse fear, anger, and even guilt. When a young child is hospitalized and no member of the family remains with the child, the child's emotional reaction may be manifested as withdrawal. Early separation experiences may be the source of fears and anxieties in later life about the loss of a relationship.

The importance of parental attachments, especially during infancy and childhood, should be understood by parents who must leave their children at frequent intervals. Special efforts should be made to establish a loving relationship and minimize the child's distress at being left in day care or with a babysitter. A good day care center offers a loving and supportive atmosphere for the child, in recognition of the distress felt by an infant/child as a normal reaction to separation from parents.

Health care providers need to understand separation anxiety, spend as much time as possible with a child whose parents have left, and provide emotional support as needed. Honest, age-appropriate explanations will help the child understand what has happened. Above all, do not subscribe to the value judgment that a crying child is "just spoiled." Be aware that the crying child may feel abandoned.

Many changes in relationships occur during early childhood. The child achieves more independence (and less dependence) as growth and development occur. Dependency is another type of special relationship, so the child's achievements also involve changes in relationships. Entering kindergarten or school is an exciting, sometimes frightening, experience. The child loses the comfort, safety, and security of home, but gains new experiences, a peer group, and new adult contacts. The parent loses their dependent "baby" and gains a schoolchild who is increasingly independent.

Losses of Middle Childhood

Throughout the school-age years a child repeatedly experiences losses and gains. Each promotion means leaving a familiar teacher and gaining a new one. There may be a loss of some classmates, although new children may come into the class at intervals. Friendships may break up, with any grief over the loss obscured by anger or guilt about the cause of the break-up. A change of school during this period includes numerous losses, which may or may not be offset by gains available in the new school. Completion of the elementary grades includes the loss of some relationships and also the loss of a familiar role. Promotion to middle school or high school usually means giving up childhood activities and entering the world of adolescence.

Losses During Adolescence

Gains and losses related to growth and development, dependence versus independence, and promotion from one grade to another continue through adolescence. For the most part, the emotional effects of these types of losses or gains are manageable. A person with adequate adjustment copes with these changes reasonably well. But some events of adolescence have the potential for arousing very strong emotional reactions: establishing a romantic relationship, becoming sexually active, experiencing peer pressure (to smoke, to use drugs, to consume alcoholic beverages), getting a job, and graduating. During this period romantic relationships are established. When such a relationship ends, one or both parties may experience intense emotional reactions to the loss.

Adolescence is also the time when many young people obtain their first job, which requires learning a new role and includes a significant gain—one's own income. If the job is terminated, both role and income are lost; the circumstances may include loss of self-esteem.

Graduation from high school is perceived by students and their families as a happy event. The losses involved are seldom talked about. A high school graduation results in the end of many friendships. It also represents the beginning of passage into adulthood and many new responsibilities. Although some students maintain their dependence on parents through additional years of education, for many the relatively carefree life of childhood and adolescence ends forever with graduation from high school.

Losses of the Young Adult Years

The adult period of life is characterized by vocational choices, the struggle for financial independence, establishing adult coping strategies, affirming one's sexuality through marriage or a relationship, starting a family, setting up a home, and developing a satisfying lifestyle. Each of these activities may provide much satisfaction and happiness. Each also includes the possibility of loss: getting fired from a job; ending a marriage through divorce; losing property through theft, fire, or natural disaster; losing friends or family members through death; moving, which often includes loss of a support network of friends and family.

The adult period of life involves a continuous sequence of gains and losses, both large and small. Accepting the joy that life may bring and also learning to cope with the pain of loss leads to continued growth and a full life. Trying to escape pain by avoiding life experiences that include the risk of loss, such as marriage or a loving relationship, does not lead to growth and precludes living a full life. *Part of the adult life experience is accepting the risk of losing some of what we have gained.*

Losses of Middle Age

Ideally, middle adulthood is a period for enjoying the rewards of one's labors during the early adult years. For many, however, this is a period of continued struggle for financial survival. The expenses of a family peak as children reach high school and college. If the family's income has increased through the years, these expenses are manageable. Otherwise, adolescent members of the family may have to become wage earners.

The struggle for financial security involves relatively frequent gains and losses. For example, a promotion may mean additional salary and prestige, but result in the loss of free time if new responsibilities require longer hours or taking work home at night. Any unexpected expense may result in loss. For example, a long-awaited vacation at the beach may be lost because the car needs a new transmission.

Parents usually welcome the growing independence of their children. There may also be some sadness at the loss of the child/parent-dependent relationship. As children leave home to attend school, set up their own apartments, or marry, parents experience a sense of loss. Departure of the youngest child is especially difficult. "Empty nest syndrome" is a well-known depressive reaction to this event.

During the middle adult years, many people begin to realize that they will not be able to achieve some of their career or financial goals. As this realization reaches full consciousness, the individual may experience a profound sense of loss. Attitudes toward the job may change, the quality of work may be lower, and there may be expressions of hopelessness.

Recognition of a significant loss—namely, the loss of one's youth—occurs sometime during the middle years. This may occur on a 40th or 50th birthday, or it may develop gradually as physical stamina diminishes, physical proportions change, baldness develops, wrinkles appear, or once-firm tissues become flabby. Many people accept the effects of time and adapt their lifestyles to accommodate physical changes. Some people, however, experience a "midlife crisis" and set out to prove to the world (and to themselves) that they are still young. A long-term relationship may break up during this period, as one partner seeks younger companions to bolster the belief, "I am still young and attractive." Loss of youth is very painful to those who subscribe to the current emphasis on youth and sex appeal in the media. Menopause represents a very significant change for a biological woman—namely, loss of the ability to reproduce. For a biological man, occasional periods of impotence threaten self-esteem.

Middle age is also the time of life when potentially serious health problems may develop. As life span has increased during the past 50 years, the incidence of chronic diseases has risen markedly. Loss of health is so unacceptable that many people, upon being told that they have a particular disease, react with, "I don't believe it."

Denying a newly diagnosed disorder is not limited to serious illness. An adult who is told that recurrent sore throats are due to allergy may refuse to have allergy studies performed. This person's self-concept may not include "I am a person with an intolerance for certain foods and other substances in my life situation." A person who is diagnosed as having early arthritis may think immediately of people with deformed hands or those who complain constantly of their joint pain. The initial reaction is, "I will not become deformed, and I will not accept continuous pain in my life." Denial eventually gives way to acceptance of the diagnosis, after the individual has had time to adjust to symptoms and changes in body function.

Losses During Senescence

The fastest-growing population segment in the United States is 65 and older group. Because of this increased life span, we are seeing a relatively new phenomenon—older adults caring for their parents. For these caregivers, death of a parent is a loss that is experienced during old age.

The senescent period of life includes more losses than gains. Physical losses eventually include diminished vision, hearing, taste, mobility, and memory. These losses usually develop gradually, but may be accelerated by any serious illness. Any chronic condition, such as arthritis, increases awareness of losses. When buttoning a shirt or tying a shoe becomes difficult, the individual is reminded daily of lost mobility and dexterity.

Psychological losses are also numerous during senescence. Retirement is a serious threat to mental health. For people who have not developed interests and activities outside of their work, there is no longer a daily routine of meaningful activity. One's work-related identity is lost. Daily interaction with coworkers is lost. Because retirement benefits seldom equal work-related income, financial loss may be significant. All of these losses are a serious threat to self-esteem, so serious that a period of depression following retirement is relatively common. This emphasizes the importance of having a purpose in life and being actively involved in meaningful activities other than work.

Social losses affect older adults more than other age groups. Friends and close family members move or die. The loss of a specific friend may also mean the loss of a social activity shared with that person. The loss of a partner may mean being left out of social activities in which the couple has participated for years. A son or daughter moving to another town means the loss of daily contact with immediate family, especially grandchildren. For many older adults, social life gradually diminishes. Loneliness and aloneness may characterize the daily life of an older person.

The loss that is feared by most older adults is loss of independence. When an older person is deemed unable to live alone, the result is loss of one's home, loss of a familiar bed, and loss of choices in what to eat and when. This loss of independence is accompanied by a loss of self-esteem. Moving to a retirement home or nursing home involves so many losses for the individual that there is often an immediate decline in health. All too often the emotional reactions of older adults to these radical changes in lifestyle are not recognized or acknowledged by caregivers or by family members.

FIGURE 16-2 Following the death of a loved one, survivors may feel sadness, depression, or guilt.

Losses due to Death

The impact of a death on each survivor is influenced by numerous factors, including age of the survivor, relationship to the deceased, the survivor's past experience in coping with significant losses, age of the deceased, and circumstances surrounding the death. For example:

- Was the death expected? Did it follow a lengthy terminal illness?
- Does the death represent a release from pain and suffering?
- Was the death sudden and unexpected? In this situation, the survivors must cope with shock initially, then with loss.
- What was the age of the deceased? If the deceased was older and the survivors believe that they had "lived a good life," the loss is easier to accept. If the deceased was young, grief is likely to be accompanied by anger and a sense of injustice.

Certain circumstances surrounding a death have an especially powerful impact on survivors:

- **The death was accidental.** Was the accident due to someone's negligence or carelessness? If so, anger and blame may delay the beginning of a healthful grieving process. If a survivor was involved in the accident, that person may feel that they were responsible for the death. Or that person may experience **survivor guilt**, wondering "What right did I have to survive?" or believing "I should have been the one who died." Anyone who is experiencing survivor guilt needs professional counseling.

- **The death was related to violence or criminal activity (e.g., mugging, burglary, shooting).** Survivors of this type of death must deal with anger and perhaps a desire for revenge, as well as grief.

- **The death was a murder or homicide.** Survivors must deal with shock initially, then questions of "Why?" and "Who?" If the killer was a member of the family, survivors may divide into two groups. Some will refuse to believe the perpetrator's guilt and will loyally support their defense. Others will direct anger at the accused and seek "justice" for the deceased. In both cases, these emotions interfere with the grief process.

- **The deceased was on life support.** Who made the decision to discontinue it? Even when a living will and advance directives exist, the decision to discontinue life support is difficult for family members. If some family members disagree with the decision, then the decision-maker has to cope with their criticism in addition to personal feelings about making that fateful decision.

- **The death was due to self-inflicted injury—suicide.** This type of death is especially difficult for survivors. Because suicide is widely misunderstood, it is important that health care professionals understand this type of death.

For Discussion and Reflection

Think back to your childhood. At what age did you first experience death, whether the death of a pet, a friend, or a relative? What was your family's attitude toward death?

Suicide

Any suicide attempt is a medical emergency. Although suicide is viewed as a mental health problem, it can be understood only within the context of the person's life situation: social isolation, abuse, pain, disfigurement, disability, loss of a body part, severe mood swings, the "voices" heard by someone with schizophrenia, or any life circumstance that has become intolerable. For a desperate individual, death may seem to be the only way to escape. Members of certain groups are at high risk for suicide: teenagers, older adults, and anyone who is seriously depressed.

Any death by suicide places family members and associates of the deceased in a soul-searching position:

Why did I not recognize the signs that they were in such distress?

Why was I not more sensitive to their unhappiness?

What did I do that caused this terrible act?

Why did I not express my love?

Why was I so critical?

Why did I not insist that they seek help?

What could I have done to prevent this act?

For parents there may be many questions, most pertaining to "How could I have been a better parent?" For siblings, the entire range of emotions is possible, depending upon the relationship with the deceased. For surviving spouses, the emotional impact may range from relief to a devastating sense of loss, depending upon the quality of the marital relationship. Friends and associates may be affected differently by suicide than by a death due to accident or illness. Some of the questions just listed may haunt those who associated with the deceased on a daily basis, especially the question "What could I have done to help?"

Following a suicide, survivors have to deal not only with their loss, but also with psychological trauma: guilt, anger, remorse, confusion, helplessness, or feelings of failure for not having been a better parent, sibling, or friend. Suicide by a child or teenager may affect an entire school, setting off an epidemic of suicides or suicide attempts within the school population.

Suicide is considered an honorable death in some cultures. In certain Asian societies, someone who has lost honor, for whatever reason, is *expected* to commit suicide. Today there is a resurgence of belief in *honorable suicide* among fundamentalist groups throughout the world. The role of suicide bomber is willingly assumed, usually by an adolescent or a young adult, in order to destroy members of a group perceived as the enemy. This activity occurs with disturbing frequency in the Middle East. The mother of a young male suicide bomber was quoted in the news media as declaring proudly that her son had died an honorable death. If the suicide bomber acted on the instructions of a terrorist organization, that organization may pay the surviving family a large sum of money for this sacrifice of their family member. In the United States, suicide is regarded by many people as a dishonorable act. Some life insurance companies do not pay if a death is due to suicide or may exclude suicide for a specific period of time.

One who completes a suicide is found dead, and therefore will not come under your care. Most people who complete a suicide have a history of suicide attempts. Who is to know when a person who survived one suicide attempt will make another attempt that becomes a completed suicide? As a health care professional, avoid thinking that any suicide attempt is "just trying to get attention." The attempt may be a call for help, but "attention" is not the motive.

Why would anyone ingest a poison or take a lethal dose of a drug? Why do some people cut themselves? Why put a bullet through one's head? The only logical answer is that the individual is desperately trying to escape an intolerable life situation, a painful or debilitating physical condition, or the hopelessness that accompanies deep depression.

The greatest danger of suicide is when the person is coming out of a depressed state. Many people who are depressed do not have the energy to carry out a suicide. As they recover from depression, they not only have the energy, but also know that sooner or later they will again experience the hopelessness of depression. One journalist spoke of her depressed periods as a "bottomless hole" or a "black abyss" of hopelessness and despair. After two attempts, she completed a suicide just when her physician and family believed she was recovering from her latest bout of depression. The suicide of a person who is depressed is a desperate effort to escape the effects of depression.

It is likely that you will encounter a hospitalized patient who has attempted suicide. It is especially important for caregivers to keep in mind that they do not know the circumstances of that patient's life situation. Any one of us may at some time in our lives experience emotionally overwhelming circumstances. Without having experienced such conditions, we do not know how we would react. Only those who have experienced hopelessness, depression, or mood swings over a period of time can understand the distress of a person who attempts suicide.

The implications for you as a health care professional are clear. Do not judge the patient who has attempted suicide. Know that this person needs emotional support and respect. Keep in mind your philosophy of individual worth, be a compassionate caregiver, demonstrate caring, and *listen*. Anyone who has attempted suicide should be evaluated by a psychiatrist and, according to the diagnosis, given appropriate treatment. Long-term counseling is needed by most survivors of a suicide attempt, to learn effective ways of coping with depression, mood swings, and life problems.

Death of a Parent

The death of one's parent is a unique type of loss, regardless of one's age and the age of the parent. For each of us, parents provide a link to our ancestry, our own life history, and most of what we learned as children. For a child, the immediate reaction may be anger: "How could Mommy or Daddy leave me?" There may also be feelings of guilt:

> *When she (he) sent me to my room I wished they were dead. It's all my fault.*
>
> *If I had been a better child, my parent would not have died.*
>
> *If only I had said, "I love you" more often.*

A young child is likely to perceive the parent's death as abandonment. Loss of a parent during childhood also means the loss of parental guidance through current and future developmental tasks. The deceased parent will be missing from important life events: graduations, recitals, athletic performances, weddings, the birth of one's own children.

The death of a same-gender parent means the loss of a parental role model. This loss is especially significant during adolescence, a time of struggling to establish one's own

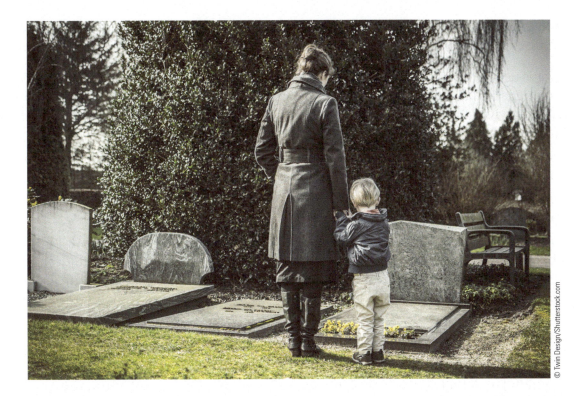

FIGURE 16-3 When a death occurs, a child needs honest explanations, but only enough detail to help the child understand the situation.

identity. Although adolescence is characterized by some degree of rebellion, this period of life involves developmental tasks that are best accomplished under parental guidance. Sometimes the death of a parent forces a child into an adult role, such as caring for younger siblings, managing the household, or working to help support the family.

After a parent dies, surviving children may be profoundly affected psychologically, especially if they do not grieve appropriately for their loss. **Displacement** may occur if feelings were not fully expressed during the mourning period; they may emerge, greatly magnified, later in life when some other loss occurs. **Transference** is manifested by seeking fulfillment from others, placing them in the position of parental substitute.

Understanding Grief

Grief is a normal and natural reaction to loss that ranges from mild disappointment through various degrees of sadness, up to the intense and painful state that we call grief. **Anticipatory grief** occurs prior to the actual loss, usually during a terminal illness. **Bereavement** is separation from or loss of someone who is significant in one's life. Grief is the predominant emotional response to bereavement, although anger and fear may also be experienced. **Grief work** is a process of working through the emotional reaction to loss, reorganizing one's life patterns, and achieving some degree of adjustment. Grief work is important to future emotional and mental health. Uncompleted grief work will eventually manifest as physical illness, poor adjustment, or tendencies to avoid or overreact to situations involving loss, dying, or bereavement.

Some grief reactions include not only sadness, but also some degree of anger, hate, guilt, anxiety, or even panic:

- *Anger* is usually a major component in grief when the age of the deceased is "inappropriate" for dying, such as infancy and childhood, adolescence, young adulthood, or "the prime of life." A survivor may actually feel anger toward the deceased for "going away and leaving me." This reaction is especially likely in a child whose parent has died.

- *Anxiety* is related to the future: "How can I live without . . . (that which was lost)?" or "How can I make certain this never happens to me again?"

- *Panic* is related to the recognition that one does not have the power to control the loss of a loved one.

- *Guilt* may be concerned with control: "Could I have prevented this from happening?" or blame: "If I had been more loving, this wouldn't have happened." Children who are not old enough to understand terminal illness or death are especially prone to guilt, because a child's anger toward a family member or playmate is sometimes expressed as an explosive "I hate you!" or possibly, "I wish you were dead!" A child may recall past actions, words, or thoughts and perceive that behavior and the death or illness as having a cause/effect relationship.

Grief is painful. Grief related to loss of a loved one through death usually results in a profound grief reaction. The remainder of this unit limits discussion of grief to this type of loss.

Effects of Grief

The death of a loved one has both physical and psychological effects on the survivor. Shock is the immediate reaction. Profound shock is likely if a death is sudden or unexpected, the result of an accident or act of violence, or a suicide. In contrast to sudden bereavement, a lengthy illness provides time for anticipatory grieving prior to the actual death. Intensity of the immediate grief reaction, then, is determined by whether the death was expected or unexpected, a sudden or slow process, violent or nonviolent. If shock is severe, the survivor cannot begin grief work until the physical effects of shock have subsided.

In the absence of severe shock, a grief reaction can range from little or no visible reaction to uncontrolled, destructive behavior. The immediate physical effects include tightness in the throat, a choking sensation, shortness of breath, weakness, a feeling of emptiness or a knot in the stomach, and nausea. These effects may subside within a few hours, to be replaced by loss of appetite and/or digestive problems, disturbed sleep patterns, restlessness, frequent sighing, and crying that may continue intermittently for days, weeks, or months.

The mental/emotional effects of bereavement include preoccupation with thoughts of the deceased, lack of interest in other people, irritability, difficulty in organizing thoughts or making decisions, difficulty in concentrating or remembering, feelings of hopelessness, feelings of guilt, and possibly a tendency toward blaming self or others for the loss. Some behavioral effects of grief are lack of interest in grooming, refusal to participate in previous activities or hobbies, poor performance at home or on the job, reminiscing about the deceased, idealizing the deceased (forgetting negative aspects of the deceased), and clinging to personal reminders.

These effects of grief vary in intensity and duration according to a survivor's relationship to the deceased, personal ways of dealing with strong emotion, and patterns of behavior learned in previous life crises. *How a survivor deals with grief influences future adjustment.*

Importance of the Grief Process

Grief is a period of pain from which one recovers over time. It may also be a growth experience in which one learns to accept certain realities:

- We are vulnerable to certain life experiences, including losses.
- We are not all-powerful. We only have control over *some* aspects of our lives.
- We are mortal, not immortal.
- There will be a time for each of us when life comes to an end.
- Loss requires saying "good-bye" to some aspect of life, but loss can also mean a new beginning.
- "Letting go" does not diminish the importance of what was lost, but it does free the survivor to make the necessary adjustments for living without the deceased.

Influences on the Grief Process

Any person who has experienced a significant loss has the right to grieve. A person's grieving tends to be consistent with the personality and usual coping styles. The intensity and duration of grieving are influenced by the relationship to the deceased and past experiences with loss. Friends and family should grant each survivor the right to grieve in their own way.

Working through the stages of denial, anger, and bargaining prior to the actual death seems to facilitate grief work during the bereavement period. Spending quality time with the dying person—sharing memories, expressing feelings, touching and holding—facilitates anticipatory grieving and also eases the dying process. Grieving is facilitated if family members share their feelings and if relatives and friends are supportive throughout the process.

Acceptance of Loss Grief work begins with acceptance of the loss—the finality of death. Sometimes there is intellectual acceptance without emotional acceptance. Only when the finality of the loss is accepted at the emotional level can grief work begin. The survivor needs encouragement to "be with" their feelings by expressing the sadness and pain, rather than denying the feelings or hiding them from others.

Making Final Arrangements Participating in the tasks related to death seems to facilitate acceptance. Before or immediately after the death, someone must notify relatives, friends, coworkers, the minister, and the family lawyer; prepare an obituary; care for and remove the body; plan for the disposal of the body (burial, cremation); plan a service (funeral, memorial); purchase a cemetery lot (or decide how to dispose of the ashes if cremation is chosen); complete paperwork (death certificate, notices to insurance and annuity companies, government agencies, banks). Insofar as possible, the tasks that involve decision making should be completed prior to the actual death, because one who is experiencing powerful emotions may not be able to make important decisions.

Some people want to be involved in the final stages of the dying process, and some want to assist with final care of the body. Being present at the final moments of life is beneficial to survivors and also to the patient. Many dying patients state that dying alone is their greatest fear. For survivors, being with the patient in those last moments is preparation for emotional release. Bathing, dressing, and grooming the body provides an opportunity for saying "good-bye" in the most loving and caring way possible. This is especially appropriate if the deceased is a child. Sometimes the survivors participate in closing the grave with handfuls of dirt. This, too, is a way of saying "good-bye" and moving toward emotional acceptance of the loss.

The body of the deceased and the final service both play a role in acceptance of death. The funeral service and interment provide opportunities to express the intense feelings that immediately follow the death and help prepare the survivors for grief work. Alternatives to a traditional funeral, such as a memorial service, can also facilitate the grief process.

Cultural Differences in How Grief is Expressed Each person's experience of grief will be influenced by their past experiences, their own beliefs and values, and their culture. Culture and environment influence both the resources available to support those who are grieving and the ways in which it is customary to express feelings of grief. For example, mental health support for parents who have lost a child is limited in middle- and low-income countries (McNeil et al. 2020). Clients whose home countries offer little support for grieving family members may not be aware that such support is available or may be reluctant to access it. Culture also affects the language individuals use to express grief, the ways in which emotions are commonly expressed, and the extent and manner in which surviving friends maintain a sense of connection with the deceased (Klass & Chow 2021).

Grief Inhibitors In the belief that people need to be protected, someone may try to keep those closest to the deceased from participating in these tasks. Friends or relatives may encourage survivors-to-be to withdraw from the death scene and to delegate final tasks to others. The survivors may even be deprived of time with the loved one, either during the final moments or immediately after death, in the mistaken belief that witnessing the death or being with the body would be traumatic. No matter how good their intentions, people who influence the family to withdraw from the death scene deprive family members of an experience that facilitates "letting go" and beginning the grief process.

Children, especially, are likely to be excluded. As they observe atypical adult behavior and disruption of the family's normal routine, they may be confused, frightened, or angry. They need explanations about what is happening, much comforting, and a chance to say "good-bye" to the dying person *if they wish to do so.*

Numerous other conditions can inhibit the grief process: a sudden death, an untimely death, the mode of death (accident, suicide, violence), unresolved grief from past losses, past tendency to suppress anger and grief, ambivalent feelings toward the deceased, the use of drugs or alcohol to suppress feelings, resuming normal activities too early, isolation from a death (war in a foreign country), or uncertainty about a death (a plane crash or fire in which the remains are difficult or impossible to identify). The uncertainty created when the body cannot be viewed makes it especially difficult for survivors to accept the death. There is, instead, a tendency to cling to the belief that the victim will come back home some day.

Condolences Most people find it difficult to express **condolences** to the bereaved. All too often, statements that are offered as words of comfort or as reassurance actually deny the importance of grief or imply that the person has no right to grieve. The following are examples of such statements:

- "You must be strong" implies that showing one's grief is a sign of weakness.
- "It's time to get on with your life" is a way of saying, "I do not grant you any more time for grieving."

Often, the most effective form of condolence is simply silence, accompanied by a hug or kiss if appropriate. Friends and relatives who take time to "be there" for a bereaved person are helpful. Staying in touch, either in person or by phone or mail, keeps the bereaved person believing that you care. Over time, having friends and family who are willing to listen facilitates the grieving process for a bereaved person.

If a year has passed, the person may need professional counseling to facilitate the completion of grief work. But a statement such as, "It's time to get on with your life" is totally inappropriate a month, or even several months, after the death of a loved one. An inappropriate statement may indicate that the speaker does not understand the grief process or its importance to a survivor's future adjustment.

Uncompleted Grief Work Some survivors fail to complete the grief process, either because feelings are suppressed or because certain conditions inhibit the grief process. Grief that is not resolved may be indicated by hyperactivity, inappropriate feelings, physical illness (possibly with the symptoms of the deceased, if he or she dies of an illness), changes in relationships with others, hostility, depression, or a lack of feeling.

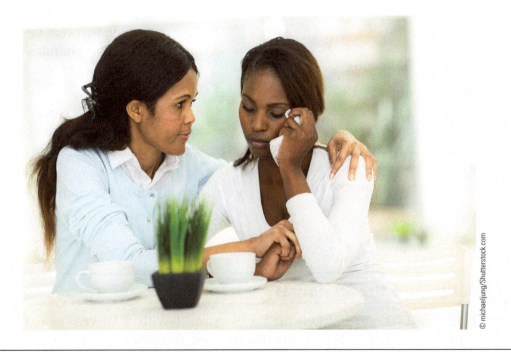

© michaeljung/Shutterstock.com

FIGURE 16-4 Supportive friends and relatives can contribute greatly to successful grief work.

Sometimes the grief reaction becomes chronic; that is, the bereaved becomes locked into the early stages of the process and does not progress toward readjustment. Denial of grief at the time of the loss may result in a delayed grief reaction after weeks, months, or even years, usually at the time of another death or when a close friend is grieving.

Supportive friends and relatives can contribute greatly to successful grief work. Professional counseling is needed, however, when a survivor manifests denial or evidence of uncompleted grief work after one year.

Guidelines for Using Loss and Grief as a Growth Experience

Loss involves pain. The intensity of the pain depends upon the degree of commitment to what was lost. *Coping with the pain of loss is a life skill that is essential to mental and emotional health.* There are many opportunities in health care agencies for a sensitive caregiver to recognize someone's need for emotional support when dealing with significant loss.

The following guidelines may appear simple. They are relatively easy to accept—intellectually. Accepting them at the *emotional level*, however, requires dealing honestly with one's feelings and beliefs. The result should be an increase in readiness to cope with the reality of loss and to help others who have experienced a significant loss:

1. Learn to recognize the small losses that occur in your life.
2. Accept anger, fear, and guilt feelings as part of many grief reactions.
3. Allow time for grieving.
4. Acknowledge your own vulnerability to losses and pain.
5. Acknowledge your lack of total control. You may control some aspects of your life, but some events are beyond your control.
6. Acknowledge your own **mortality**—the fact that your life will end at some time.
7. Accept that life involves change, including losses. Some changes require that we modify our belief systems to fit the new reality.
8. Following a loss, work through the feelings. When you are ready, "let go" of the past (which includes the loss).
9. Believe that you can cope with whatever loss you may experience.
10. Be supportive of those who have suffered a loss.

> **For Discussion and Reflection**
>
> Identify a loss, large or small, that you have experienced in the past three years. Which of the steps above do you feel that you have accomplished in regard to "letting go" of the loss? Are there ways in which you have not finished the grief process?

Role of Health Care Professionals

The health care professional is likely to be in contact with relatives of a dying patient before the patient's death, rather than throughout the bereavement period. Because the physician has primary responsibility for providing information about a patient's condition, health care professionals must know what the patient, as well as the family, has been told. This can be determined by carefully worded questions and by observation of nonverbal behavior. Active listening is effective for learning what the physician has told the patient and family and identifying where the other person is emotionally.

The health care professional's goal is to help the family, not by giving information or expressing personal opinions, but by helping the other to express feelings and work toward acceptance of the loss at their own pace. Various health care professionals are prepared to provide skilled counseling for patients and their families. Large hospitals have chaplains and social workers, some of whom have special preparation for helping others cope with a life crisis. Smaller hospitals and most nursing homes rely on community resources to provide this specialized service.

Each death/bereavement situation is unique, so there cannot be a single procedure to guide the health care professional. But there are guidelines that may help the caregiver adapt to each situation.

Assisting the Family of a Dying Patient

1. Be available to the family as much as possible. (Do not use the nurses' station as a refuge to avoid interacting with the family.)

2. Use active listening to encourage the expression of feelings.

3. Interact with the patient as you provide physical care. Model for family members the expression of caring, even if the patient is not responsive.

4. Be tolerant of what you see and hear. Various members of the family are at different stages of grieving, and each is reacting to a life crisis in their own way.

5. Encourage close family members to stay with the patient, to talk and touch as much as possible throughout the dying process. This is important, even if the patient is comatose.

6. As appropriate, offer to call the family minister, priest, or rabbi. If you observe that a family seems to need assistance in dealing with their grief, contact the hospital chaplain or social worker.

7. Know the available sources of help in your community and share this information with a family as appropriate. For example, *Compassionate Friends* is a support group for parents who have lost a child.

8. Work on your own "unfinished business" related to past losses and on your own fears related to death. Until you have accepted your own mortality and completed your own grief work, you cannot be fully effective in helping others to cope with death and dying.

Activities

1. List significant changes that have occurred in your life, starting with your earliest memories and continuing to the present.

2. Compare the items below with your list of significant life changes (developed in Activity 1). Add any of these events that have occurred in your life.

   a. Death of a grandparent, parent, brother, or sister

   b. Death of a partner, son, or daughter

   c. Death of any other relative who was important to you

d. Death of a friend or classmate when you were a child

e. Separation, divorce, or end of a long-term sexual relationship

f. Marriage or establishment of a romantic relationship

g. Any move—from one neighborhood to another, one city to another, or one state to another

h. Change of school

i. Major purchase—house, car, other

j. Loss of personal possession—theft, foreclosure, fire, other

k. New family member

l. Pregnancy

m. Serious illness of a family member

n. Diagnosis of a serious or chronic illness (yours)

o. Obtaining a new job; being fired from a job

p. Change in job responsibilities or work schedule

q. Radical change in financial situation

r. Moving out of parents' home

s. Your child moves out of your home

t. Loss of freedom—confined to your room, not allowed to date or use the car, jail time

u. Radical change in lifestyle

v. Entered military service, college, other educational program

3. What would your behavior be like following the death of your best friend? Write a description of your feelings, how you would express these feelings, and the people with whom you would share your feelings.

4. Discuss strategies you can use to support someone working through grief (a) as a friend and (b) as a health care professional.

5. Participate in a class discussion about a health care professional's responsibilities when caring for (a) a patient who attempted suicide and (b) a patient who is dying.

References and Suggested Readings

*Indicates a classic reference that introduced new ideas.

Klass, D. & Chow, A. (2021). Culture and ethnicity in experiencing, policing, and handling grief. In *Grief and bereavement in contemporary society.* Routledge.
*Kübler-Ross, Elisabeth. (1969). *On death and dying.* Scribner.
*Kübler-Ross, Elisabeth. (1974). *Death: The final stage of growth.* Simon & Schuster.
McNeil, M. J., Namisango, E., Hunt, J., Powell, R. A., & Baker, J. N. (2020). Grief and bereavement in parents after the death of a child in low-and middle-income countries. *Children, 7*(5), 39.

Chapter 17

Death: Attitudes and Practices

Objectives

After completing this chapter, you should be able to:

- Contrast past and current practices related to death and dying.
- Explain how beliefs and attitudes about death influence individuals with terminal illnesses and their families.
- Define the concept of "death with dignity."
- Discuss definitions of death, the difference between quality of life and quantity of life, and the rights of patients and their families.
- Describe the purpose of the following: the living will, medical durable power of attorney, and advance medical directive.
- Develop a personal philosophy about death and end-of-life care and explain how your philosophy impacts your role as a health care professional.

Key Terms

Advance medical
  directive (AMD)
Assisted suicide
Bereavement
Conservator

Do not resuscitate (DNR)
  order
Durable power of
  attorney (DPA)
Euthanasia

Living wills
Patient Self-Determination
  Act (PSDA)
Proxy
Thanatology

Many people view death as an enemy to be feared and avoided at all costs. A different view is reflected in the writings of Dr. Elisabeth Kübler-Ross, who titled one of her books *Death: The Final Stage of Growth*. As a result of her many years of attending dying patients, Dr. Kübler-Ross proposed that the dying process involves a series of emotional/spiritual changes that, ideally, terminate with feelings of peace and tranquility prior to death. The dying process, then, can be an opportunity for emotional and spiritual growth. Some dying people need help to move through this process. Others seem to undergo this growth through their own beliefs, values, and inner resources.

Between these two opposite views of death, there is a wide range of beliefs. These differences are due in part to cultural attitudes and practices in care of the dying, which have undergone a marked change during the past half-century. This chapter reviews those historical changes, examines some influences on beliefs about death, and discusses attitudes and practices related to death and dying.

Changing Attitudes and Practices

In 1789, Benjamin Franklin wrote, "In this world nothing is certain except death and taxes." His comment reflects an awareness and acceptance of death that was common until the era of modern medicine. Prior to the last century, the leading cause of death was infection. Infant and child mortality rates were high; few families escaped the loss of a child. Death was familiar—a common experience that was highly visible to people of all ages. Illness and death were most likely to occur in the home, with family members and friends gathered around. It was the custom for each member of the family to bid the dying person farewell. In return, the dying person gave his or her blessing to favored relatives. The deathbed scene often included advice and charges to the survivors—to develop certain virtues, care for other survivors, gain honor for the family name.

In some cultures and religious traditions, death was (or still is) celebrated as a release from the troubles of this life and a welcome passage to a happy and trouble-free existence in "the hereafter." Mourning was public, as well as private. A widow was expected to wear black for at least a year following the death of her husband. Men wore a black band on the left sleeve as a public display of mourning for the deceased. The survivors did not participate in social events for many months. There were frequent visits to the cemetery. The gravemarker and subsequent care of the grave symbolized respect for the deceased and the devotion of the survivors. In many other ways survivors demonstrated to relatives and the community their love and respect for the deceased. Until recently, both illness and death were a family affair.

Beginning in the early 1900s, infection was brought under control through improved sanitation and immunization. During the late 1930s and 1940s, the sulfa drugs and penicillin were discovered. These changes in the treatment of infection resulted in a dramatic decrease in deaths due to infection, especially among infants and children. As the life span increased, the primary causes of death became heart disease, cancer, respiratory diseases, and accidents. Care of the sick and injured shifted from the home to the hospital. Responsibility for care of the sick was delegated to health care personnel, with family members in the role of bystanders. This trend resulted in isolation of the patient from family members. Children, especially, were excluded from contact with the hospitalized patient. Illness and death ceased to be a family affair.

For Discussion and Reflection

Consider how death was viewed by your family or community of origin. What cultural or religious traditions influenced these views? Has your own view of death changed over time?

Today, many people have never been personally involved with serious illness or the dying process. They have never had the opportunity to learn to accept death as a part of the cycle of life. Death is now perceived by many people as a terrible tragedy that "ought not to happen, especially to me and my family."

These changes of the past 75 years have great significance for emotional and mental health. Due to the invisibility of the dying process and the abandonment of many mourning rituals, there is a growing tendency to deny death. In many American subcultures, it is almost as though there is a conspiracy of silence. One just does not talk, or even think, about death until it strikes within one's circle of relatives or friends.

When death does touch a family, there may be a tendency to deny the grief process. Today, the community generally does not provide for bereaved people the kind of long-term support that can facilitate the grief process. Instead, survivors are expected to "pick up the pieces and get on with their lives" soon after the funeral.

In the work setting, life may go on as usual the day after a colleague's funeral, with no one willing to introduce the subject of death into the informal communication channels. The formal communication channel may acknowledge this loss of a member of the organization with a memorandum or floral offering. Otherwise, the work routine continues with minimal recognition that a member is missing.

Within other subcultures, however, a death can bring family members together. Friends and relatives may travel from significant distances to be with the bereaved family. Family members may share meals and spend time sharing memories about the deceased person. This approach is more conducive to healthy grieving and emotional healing.

Current Attitudes and Practices

Changes in infant and child mortality have had a particular effect on societal attitudes toward death as it relates to age. Although death is acceptable for older people (generally age 65 and above), it is viewed as inappropriate for someone under the age of 30 to die. Yet less than a hundred years ago, parents felt blessed if half of their children survived to age 12. Today, we find it especially tragic—unacceptable and terribly unfair—when a child dies.

Changes in the health care system have contributed to changes in societal attitudes toward death. In fact, a highly significant change in attitudes toward death has occurred *within* the health care system. Instead of accepting death as an inevitable outcome of some diseases, death is perceived as an enemy to be conquered with whatever resources the system can offer: new and better drugs, life-support systems, surgical replacement of body parts, heroic measures to restore vital functions. Some physicians believe they have a responsibility to maintain life in the physical body as long as possible, regardless of the patient's potential for recovery or a meaningful existence. Concern for the *quantity of life* has replaced concern for the *quality of life*. When all measures available prove inadequate to keep a patient alive, some personnel view the death as a personal failure ("If only I had made rounds 30 minutes sooner!") or as a failure of the system ("If we had been able to use such-and-such, we could have saved that patient.").

There is increasing awareness of a need to examine societal attitudes toward death and care of the dying. Some hospitals have modified their policies regarding visitors, some even permitting small children to visit a dying grandparent, parent, or sibling. Hospice and home care of a dying person are increasingly recognized as alternatives to hospitalization. More families now participate in the dying process, thereby permitting the dying person to retain a sense of family membership until the end. These recent trends recognize and respect the *human needs* of the dying person.

The Emergence of Thanatology During the 1950s a new interest and concern about death and dying emerged, largely due to the work of Dr. Elisabeth Kübler-Ross, sociologists, social workers, and pastoral counselors. Many professionals who were working with dying patients recognized that their educational programs had not prepared them for this role. The concern of these professional workers to meet the needs of patients with terminal illness led to the emergence of **thanatology**, the study of death and dying, and to death education for health care professionals and for the public.

Thanatology involves people from a variety of disciplines: sociology, theology, psychology, counseling, social work, nursing, and medicine. Their work has led to increased awareness of the needs of dying persons, the importance of the grief process, techniques for helping patients and their families cope with death and **bereavement**, and the need for death education.

The Meaning of Death

An important aspect of death education is learning to accept one's own mortality. In the past, this important lesson was learned early in life through direct experience with serious illness and death itself, usually in the home. Current practices that isolate dying patients prevent this direct involvement. But death education can help people think through the meaning of death, resolve their fears, reach some level of personal acceptance, and come to terms with their own mortality. In addition, death education can prepare people to accept their feelings as legitimate reactions when they do have to cope with a death crisis. It is especially important that health care professionals who care for dying patients resolve their own fears about dying, because subconscious fears about death influence how one interacts with a person who is dying.

The meaning of death for each person is influenced by cultural background, religious beliefs, and life experiences. Following are examples of beliefs about death:

- Death is the end of existence.
- Death is only the end of physical existence.
- Death is a natural, biological event that concludes life.
- Death is the loss of everything—life itself, the future, loved ones, possessions.
- Death means separation from loved ones.
- Death means a reunion with loved ones who have already died.

and wishes regarding end-of-life care and about any medical interventions that are not wanted. Without such meaningful discussions at intervals, there is risk that one's wishes will be ignored, even if an advance directive has been completed.

It is not necessary to involve a lawyer in preparing a living will. Each state has a specific form. A living will form should be filled out according to the instructions, signed in the presence of witnesses who are not family members or beneficiaries, and then signed by the witnesses. The original should be filed in a safe place; copies should be provided to members of the family. Upon admission to a hospital, a copy should be added to the patient's chart; *a family member should obtain a receipt from a hospital representative, acknowledging that an AMD for that patient is on file.*

The Durable Power of Attorney

The medical DPA is a document that designates a specific person to make medical decisions if the patient is unable to do so. The desires of the individual should be made clear to the decision maker at the time the document is prepared. When illness or accident occurs, the decision maker is responsible for seeing that the patient's wishes are carried out. Some DPA forms include statements pertaining to life support, resuscitation, and artificial feeding, so that specific instructions are included in the legal document. The advance health care directive may refer to a living will, a durable power of attorney, or both.

The Patient Self-Determination Act

Under the PSDA, any hospital, nursing home, hospice, or health maintenance organization (HMO) that receives federal funding (Medicare and Medicaid) must inform patients about their rights, specifically the right to refuse certain types of treatment. This federal law also prohibits health care professionals from discriminating against a patient who elects to forgo life-sustaining procedures. The PSDA specifies that any patient who enters a hospital or nursing home must be informed about:

- The right to make decisions about medical treatments
- The right to refuse a treatment (medical or surgical)
- The right to prepare an AMD if the patient does not already have a living will or medical DPA
- The procedure in that institution for preparing an AMD
- The right to have an AMD made part of his or her medical record

This law resulted from the proliferation of court cases regarding the right to die. A number of families have experienced emotional trauma and incurred tremendous legal expense in the effort to allow their loved one, in a state of irreversible coma, to die. Health care professionals, regardless of their own opinions, must respect the wishes of patients that have been stated in an AMD. Box 17-1 shows some of the requirements of the Patient Self-Determination Act.

As a health care professional, you may encounter situations in which a patient asks your opinion or advice about treatment or end-of-life care, such as whether to accept or refuse a treatment or whether to sign a DNR. Keep in mind that your role is to provide information about the patient's rights and choices, but not to influence the patient's decision or discuss your personal beliefs.

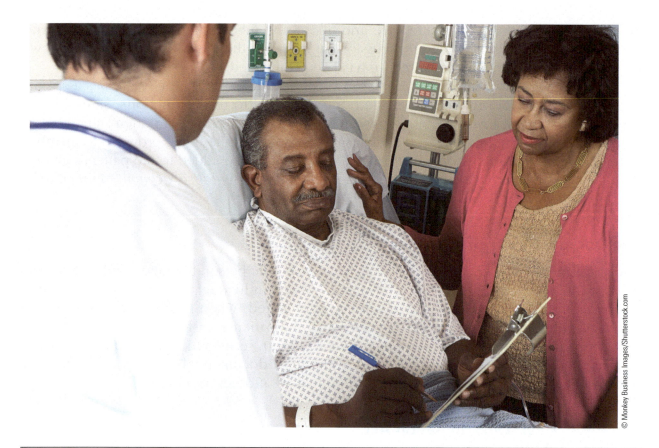

FIGURE 17-2 As a health care professional, your role is to provide information about the patient's rights and choices, not to influence the patient's decision or discuss your personal beliefs.

Involvement of the Courts in Health Care Decisions

Increasingly, the legal system is becoming involved in health care decisions. This is most likely to occur when (1) relatives of a comatose person believe life support should be discontinued, but there is no advance directive, (2) an advance directive is ignored by health care personnel, or (3) the family wants to do "everything possible" for their loved one, even though the physician and hospital believe life support/nutrition should be discontinued.

In the first situation, the courts use one of two standards for determining whether or not life support may be discontinued. The "substituted judgment" standard recognizes that many individuals have not prepared advance directives and that their loved ones can best decide that individual's preference for end-of-life care. The "clear and convincing evidence" standard requires that the patient's preferences have been clearly stated to relatives or friends prior to the patient becoming unable to make medical decisions personally.

The second situation is discussed under the topic "A Challenge for Health Care Professionals." The third situation is less common, in that most families of a comatose patient accept the recommendation of the physician. If a family does demand that treatment continue, even though there is no hope of improvement in the patient's condition, the hospital or physician may request that the court appoint a **conservator**. The responsibility of the conservator would be to evaluate the situation and recommend a course of action based on what the patient probably would choose, if able to express those preferences.

Box 17-1

The Patient Self-Determination Act

Provisions of the PSDA apply to all health care agencies that receive federal funds (Medicare and Medicaid reimbursement).

Each health care institution will:

- Provide written information to each patient regarding:
  a. The right to make decisions concerning medical care, including the right to refuse medical or surgical treatment.
  b. The right to prepare AMDs.
  c. The institution's policies concerning the implementation of such rights.
- Document in the patient's medical record whether or not the individual has completed an advance directive yet.
- Provide care without discrimination against the patient who has completed an advance directive.
- Establish policies and procedures to ensure compliance with state law regarding advance directives.
- Provide educational activities for staff and the public on the matter of advance directives.

The Department of Health and Human Services will:

- Provide a national public education campaign.
- Develop written materials explaining patients' rights, to be distributed by health care facilities.

A Challenge for Health Care Professionals

Sometimes health care personnel choose to ignore an AMD, believing that they are obligated to do everything possible to keep a patient alive. This behavior involves conflict between the health care professional's philosophy of health care and the legal rights of patients. The conflict may extend beyond the staff, involving hospital policy and established procedures.

Liability for Performing Unwanted Treatment

Performing heroic measures to restore breathing or a heartbeat can be enormously satisfying. As shown in many movies, it is an exciting part of being a health care professional. But keeping someone alive who has provided written instructions that prohibit life-support measures not only violates the patient's rights but is also illegal. Ignoring a DNR can result in prolonged suffering, further medical expenses for the patient and family, and possibly litigation against health care professionals and the hospital. Every health care professional should understand the legal aspects of AMDs; knowing which patients have advance directives is the responsibility of each caregiver.

Preparation for Death-and-Dying Situations

You may or may not be preparing for a role in health care that includes the care of dying patients. Regardless of your expected role, you should take the following steps to prepare for participation in a life-or-death situation, either in your career or in your personal life:

- Know the provisions of federal laws and the laws of your state pertaining to the rights of patients and their families.
- Know the policies of your employing health care agency.
- Be aware of your own beliefs about death and dying.

The concept of death with dignity, knowledge about AMDs, and awareness of the provisions of the PSDA should help you accept that patients have a right to participate in decisions about end-of-life care. You should also learn to accept the inevitability of death, the limitations of medical science, and the inappropriateness of heroic measures in some situations. *It is especially important that you develop your own philosophy about death, which includes facing your own fears about death and accepting your own mortality.*

Thoughtful consideration of the following questions will help you clarify your beliefs and develop your own philosophy of death:

- What do I believe about death?
- What do I believe about my own death?
- What fears do I have about dying?
- What would I have to give up if I were dying?
- What work do I want to complete before I die?
- What relationships do I want to mend before I die?
- What do I want to say to my loved ones before I die?
- What do I want to say to a loved one before he or she dies?
- Who should dispose of my possessions following my death? Who is to receive what?

By developing your own personal philosophy of death, you will have clearer beliefs about the care of a dying patient. If the health care professional role you expect to assume does not involve caring for dying patients, you may be tempted to ignore this exercise. But you cannot be sure what the future holds—in your career or in your personal life. So in terms of "What do I believe about the care of a patient who . . ." consider the following:

- Does not want to be resuscitated if a cardiac arrest occurs?
- Refuses intravenous fluids or tube feedings during the final stages of an illness?
- Refuses dialysis, even though the kidneys are not functioning?
- Refuses chemotherapy, even though the oncologist insists there is a 20 percent chance it will help?
- Begs the doctor, "Just let me die?"
- Begs the doctor, "Just put me out of my misery?"

For Discussion and Reflection

1. Consider one or more of the questions listed above. What actions you can take within the next month based on your answers to the questions?
2. Identify a time when a child or teen in your community has died. What were your reactions? Do you react differently to the death of a young person than to the death or an older person?

Inadequate management of pain is the reason some patients wish for death or consider suicide. The expression of a wish for death, then, may mean that the patient needs improved management of pain. However, many dying patients have accepted death and are ready—mentally, emotionally, and spiritually—even before the physical body ceases to function. Be sensitive to the needs of such patients, and especially to a patient's readiness for death.

As a health care professional, you may experience a range of emotions when a patient dies. Although you are expected to remain professional, it is not necessary or advisable to deny all feelings of grief. A brief statement of sincere grief or compassion can be very meaningful to the family of the deceased.

Ethics Committees

The Karen Ann Quinlan court decision included a recommendation that ethics committees, rather than the courts, should handle controversial patient care situations. In 1995, the Joint Commission on Accreditation of Health Care Organizations began requiring that health care facilities set up a code of ethical behavior. As a result, most hospitals have established ethics committees to review patient care conflicts. Some ethics committees involve patients' families in hearings, thereby ensuring that all viewpoints will be heard and increasing the probability that a decision will be acceptable to the hospital, the physician, and the family. In other hospitals, the ethics committees exclude families from the hearing, relying on reports of the medical staff for rendering a decision. The latter approach carries the risk of having the patient's end-of-life choices ignored in favor of aggressive medical treatment.

Ideally, ethics committees would always protect the patient's well-being and respect the expressed wishes of the patient and family for end-of-life care. Ethics committees can and should encourage staff training in the legal and ethical issues most often involved in patient care/institutional conflict.

Numerous issues have been addressed in the medical community, the mass media, and the courts: definition of death, when life support may be discontinued, when artificial feedings for persons in a persistent vegetative state may be discontinued, the right of a patient to choose accelerated death, culpability of a person who assists a patient to commit suicide, and the moral/ethical/legal aspects of euthanasia. Legal issues will likely continue to be addressed as medical technology advances. Everyone involved in end-of-life care must resolve for themselves the ethical and moral issues related to the dying process.

FIGURE 17-3 By developing your own personal philosophy of death, you will have clearer beliefs about the care of a dying patient.

Activities

1. Interview a friend or family member who is older than you. Ask how illness, death, and dying were handled in the community in which they grew up and what changes they have observed over time in attitudes and practices toward death and dying.

2. At the top of a blank sheet of paper, write "What I believe about death." List your present beliefs. Now write "What I believe about the care of a dying patient." List your present beliefs.

3. Participate in a class discussion about the following topics:

   - Withholding artificial feedings from a patient who is in an irreversible coma
   - Withholding artificial feedings from a patient who is conscious but approaching death
   - "Do not resuscitate" orders
   - A patient's right to refuse a treatment the doctor wants to administer
   - Discontinuing life support for a patient in a persistent vegetative state
   - Discontinuing life support for a conscious patient who requests that it be discontinued
   - Discontinuing dialysis for a patient who does not want to live as a quadriplegic

4. Use the Internet to learn about one of the following cases: Terri Schiavo, Mary Beth Cruzan, Karen Ann Quinlan, Brittany Maynard. Share your findings with a classmate.

5. Obtain a copy of the legal document used in your state for AMDs. Read through the document. Is it a living will? Is it a medical DPA? What rights does it give the patient? What rights does it give the family?

6. Describe challenges you may face as a health care provider when caring for a dying person.

References and Suggested Readings

American Medical Association. (n.d.) Physician assisted suicide. https://www.ama-assn.org /delivering-care/ethics/physician-assisted-suicide

Jansen, L., Wall, S., & Miller, F. (2019). Drawing the line on physician-assisted death. *Journal of Medical Ethics, 45,* 190–197.

Mondal S. (2021, July). Truth-telling to terminal stage cancer patients in India: A study of the general denial to disclosure. *OMEGA: Journal of Death and Dying.* doi:10.1177/00302228211032732

World Federation Right to Die Societies. (2020). What is aid in dying? https://wfrtds.org /what-is-aid-in-dying/

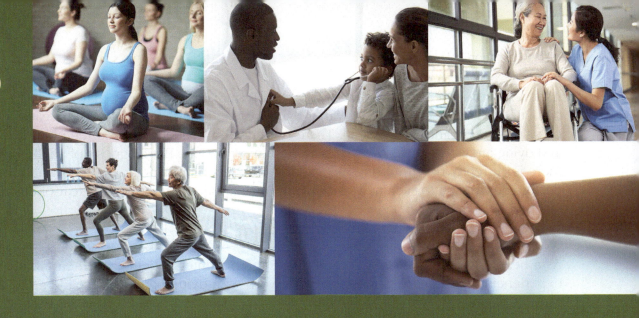

18

Chapter

Caring for the Dying Person

Objectives

After completing this chapter, you should be able to:

- List the five stages of dying, as proposed by Dr. Elisabeth Kübler-Ross, as well as limitations of Kübler-Ross's model.
- Explain how dying can be approached as a time of healing and growth.
- Discuss personal and family decisions related to the care of a dying person.
- Describe medical issues related to care of a dying person.
- Identify the rights of a dying person.
- List guidelines for health care professionals taking care of a dying person.

Key Terms

Hospice

Palliative care

As a result of current practices in the care of terminally ill patients, many people today have had little or no personal contact with a dying person. Their experience with death is limited to occasional attendance at a funeral. There is a universal tendency to fear the unknown, so death and dying are taboo topics of conversation for most people. But diagnosis of an illness for which there is currently no cure brings a patient and family members face to face with the reality of death. The reaction to such news includes fear—fear of the unknown and fear of death.

Reactions to Diagnosis of a Terminal Illness

As a health care professional, you are likely to encounter patients and their families who are experiencing these fears. Counselors who work with dying patients have identified a number of fears expressed by many patients:

- What happens after death? What lies beyond death?
- Will I be forgotten?
- Will my loved ones be cared for adequately without me? If they can get along without me, does that mean I was not important to them?
- What will become of my work, my lifelong efforts to accomplish something? Will my work be continued by someone else? Will someone else take credit for my work?
- What will happen to my property? Will my possessions be cared for? How will they be distributed?
- Will I become dependent on others?
- Will I be a burden? Who will pay my medical bills?
- Will I lose my mind?
- Will I lose control of my life? Who will make important decisions that affect me?
- Will I have more pain than I can bear?
- Will I be left to die alone?

A major responsibility of caregivers is to recognize manifestations of fear and encourage a patient to verbalize them. Expressing fears about death to an understanding listener facilitates the dying process. For example, the following behaviors may indicate that a patient is afraid:

- Being withdrawn or avoiding contact and conversation with others
- Refusing to see family and friends
- Refusing to eat, resisting medication
- Negative comments and behaviors toward health care staff

Stages of Dying

In 1969, Dr. Elisabeth Kübler-Ross published her book *On Death and Dying*, in which she proposed that a dying person goes through five stages, beginning with denial and ending with acceptance that death is approaching. Kubler-Ross's model has been widely used by counselors, therapists, and health care professionals who work with individuals who are dying. Each stage is described below. Understanding these stages can help health care professionals and family members understand a patient's emotions about a terminal illness as well as cope with their own emotions about death.

Denial The first stage of dying involves denial—"No, I am not dying. It just isn't true." This reaction seems to occur regardless of whether or not a person is told directly that he or she has a terminal illness. Denial may be manifested in many ways: changing doctors several times, continuing one's daily routine as though nothing is wrong, refusing to talk about the illness, refusing treatment, or embarking on a search for any and all treatments.

Denial serves a useful purpose. As a defense mechanism, it gives the patient time to deal with the shock of knowing that life is coming to an end. Denial may recur at intervals throughout the dying process. As a health care professional, you should not "push" a patient to talk about death when he or she does not want to, but you can invite patients to talk whenever they feel ready.

Anger The second stage of dying is characterized by anger. As the patient begins to face the reality of terminal illness, the reaction is, "Why me?" During this stage, the patient may direct anger at anyone and everyone. It is a difficult time for health care professionals as well as the family. The caregivers, it seems, cannot do anything right during this period. The patient's behavior is easier to tolerate if one remembers that this patient is in the process of learning to face his or her death.

As a health care professional, you may experience expressions of anger from a patient. It is important to remain professional and not to take angry comments personally. You can validate a patient's feelings with a comment such as "You seem to be angry about having to be here." It is never acceptable for a health care professional to show anger in return. If a patient's angry behavior persists or makes you uncomfortable, you can use I-statements to respond, set limits (discussed in Chapter 14), or consult your supervisor.

Bargaining In the third stage of dying, the patient begins to bargain—with God, fate, the doctor or nurses, or the family. This bargaining may be unknown to the caregivers, or it may be shared. Perhaps the patient prays to stay alive until some particular event—the birth of a grandchild, a wedding, a child's graduation. Perhaps the patient promises to change behavior or lifestyle, if he or she can have a second chance: "If only I can be well again, I'll never take another drink." Bargaining may take the form of being a "good" patient—cheerful and cooperative regardless of annoying treatments or pain.

Depression The fourth stage is marked by depression. With increased symptoms, especially pain or weakness, the patient can no longer maintain denial; bargaining seems pointless; anger gives way to sorrow over impending losses. Dr. Kübler-Ross believes that this period involves two different types of depression: (1) a *reactive depression* to the impending losses faced by the patient and (2) a *preparatory depression* related to the impending separation.

Acceptance The fifth stage is one of acceptance. *Provided the patient has enough time and is helped work through the previous stages*, this stage represents several accomplishments:

- The patient is neither depressed nor angry.
- The patient has grieved for the many losses.
- The patient is tired and/or weak and dozes frequently for short periods.

The stage of acceptance is not a happy stage. It is more likely to be, according to Dr. Kübler-Ross, devoid of feeling. But the patient is at peace.

Kübler-Ross's stages provide a framework for a compassionate understanding of grief and loss. The five stages of grief are still widely used by many counselors and therapists. At the same time, some experts in the field of thanatology have suggested that Kübler-Ross's stages of grief have limitations:

- People who are grieving do not always move smoothly from one stage to another.
- The idea that people need to reach a state of acceptance or closure may be unrealistic. In some instances, people may continue to grieve a loss for many years, and doing so is not necessarily a sign of pathology.
- Though based on Kübler-Ross's clinical experience, the stages have not been empirically validated.
- The Kübler-Ross model does not account for cultural differences in how people experience grief.

Keeping these limitations in mind, you may find that Kübler-Ross's stages provide a helpful way to understand the emotions and behaviors of patients and family members as they come to terms with dying. However, keep in mind that each patient's experience is unique. Kübler-Ross's or any other model should be viewed as a tool for understanding, not a rigid process that every person must follow.

Dying as a Growth Process

When death is viewed in light of the many losses involved, it is difficult to think of dying as an opportunity for growth. Viewed in terms of the emotional changes and the *transformation* that may occur as the dying process is completed, both spiritual and emotional growth become evident.

For Discussion and Reflection

Think about your first experience with death. How old were you? Was the deceased an important person to you? Did you participate in or witness any part of the dying process?

The dying person has a choice: to withdraw in despair, to suppress negative emotions, or to reach out to others. It is through the third option that growth occurs. Growth requires commitment to experiencing self, becoming aware of one's own identity, communicating one's experience to others, and accepting that one's life had purpose and meaning. These changes are facilitated by a support network of loving and caring people, who also have the opportunity for growth as they share in the dying experience.

Many people need the help of a skilled counselor to work through the negative aspects of life experiences. The goal of helping a person work through the dying process is to have the individual achieve emotional adjustment and live life to the fullest during whatever time remains. Arrival at the stage of acceptance with a sense of peace indicates successful resolution of the emotions of the dying process. Once the dying person can deal with the notion of having an illness for which there is no cure, the person can enrich the time remaining through a series of activities:

- Review one's life—various experiences and relationships and the meanings of each.
- Visit places and people that are important.
- Review memories with friends and relatives.
- Make up for missed opportunities.
- Resolve old conflicts.
- Think through and talk over with loved ones such questions as "What will happen to my survivors?" and "How will my place be filled?"

Although these activities may be painful, there will also be joy as these experiences are shared with others who have been a part of one's life experience. The following conditions contribute to successful adjustment of dying patients:

- Supportive relationships with relatives, family, and clergy
- Relatively good adjustment and past patterns of successfully coping with problems
- Willingness to talk about the illness and approaching death
- Control of pain, because pain interferes with adjustment

In addition to striving for emotional adjustment, the patient must face a number of challenges. The illness and impending dependence on others necessitates changes in lifestyle and relationships. For those who have a high level of independence, certain changes in self-concept are difficult, but necessary:

- From "I am an independent person" to "I must let others do some things for me."
- From "I am self-directing, capable, and in control of my life" to "I must let others have control over some aspects of my life."

In addition to these changes in self-concept, there must be a change in planning. Instead of thinking "Some day I will . . .," a dying person must think, "Today I will . . ." It is also important that the dying person continue to feel that life has meaning.

Personal and Family Issues Related to Care of the Dying

When a person is diagnosed with an incurable illness, certain decisions must be made. What treatments should be used? Should drugs or treatments that are known to have serious side effects be used? Should experimental drugs or procedures whose effects are not fully known be used? Should the patient find another physician? Another clinic? Another medical center that may have "a new cure"?

If the patient's condition is deteriorating or the patient is in the terminal phase of illness, questions about care must be decided. Should the patient be in a hospital or nursing home? Should the patient be at home? Who will provide care? Can this responsibility be rotated among family members? Or will one person have to provide around-the-clock care? Is there a home health service that could provide skilled care as needed? Is there a hospice in the community? The most important questions are:

1. Where does the patient want to be during his or her final days?

2. If the patient wants to die at home, is the family willing and able to undertake the care of a dying person at home?

3. If the patient or family members request counseling to assist them in coping with the emotions involved in the dying process, what resources are available in your community? In many communities, grief counseling is available through hospice.

Home Care

In *Coming Home: A Practical and Compassionate Guide to Caring for a Dying Loved One*, Deborah Duda states that dying at home is "the old, natural way which most of the world never questioned." She describes advantages of dying at home as well as conditions under which this decision would not be appropriate. Among the advantages she lists are that the dying person feels wanted, can influence surroundings, has more freedom and control, maintains respect and dignity, can enjoy home-cooked food, has the opportunity to express feelings to various relatives and friends, and the familiar setting is conducive to family support as the patient does the inner preparation for death. Another advantage, not included in Duda's list, is privacy; the patient's last days are family-centered, with minimal intrusion by outsiders. Also, the monetary cost of dying at home can be much less than the costs of intensive care and life-maintenance procedures commonly used in hospitals during the final days of a patient's life.

Dying at home is *not appropriate*, according to Duda, when either the patient or the family actively prefers institutional care. Some families are not able to provide care, either because of their own limitations or because the patient's needs cannot be met in the home setting. If family members cannot handle the emotional drain, the physical demands of caring for someone who is terminally ill, or the overall stress of such a situation, then choosing to die at home would not be appropriate. If the patient has arranged to be an organ donor and the specific terminal illness does not preclude use of the organs, then the patient's death should occur in the hospital setting, with a surgical team on call to harvest any usable organs as soon as the patient is pronounced dead.

Arranging for someone to die at home requires careful planning. The family should contact hospice and home health services to arrange for assistance and consultation services as needed. Roles should be discussed and agreed upon; the primary caregiver should be selected, with others agreeing to assume care at specific times. This may draw family members closer together as they share the common goal of providing loving care for the person they

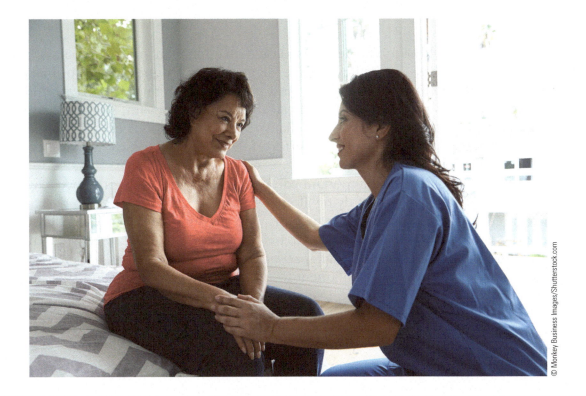

FIGURE 18-1 **For some patients, home health care is a positive alternative to institutional care.**

will soon lose. Or the family may become divided by disagreements and unequal division of responsibilities, with one or two persons carrying most of the burden. Careful advance planning may prevent the latter situation and allow the patient to spend his or her final days in a harmonious family setting.

Hospice Care

Hospice care can be provided at home, in a nursing facility, or in an assisted living facility. According to the National Hospice and Palliative Care Organization, 1.61 million Medicare recipients received hospice care in 2019. Home care with the supportive assistance of hospice personnel is an appropriate choice if the patient does not need or want to be in a facility. Hospice care is provided by a team: the patient's physician; nurses to assess the patient's needs, develop a care plan, and provide skilled nursing care as needed; home health aides to provide personal care and, in some cases, assist with household needs; a social worker to provide emotional support and direct the family to community resources as needed; a chaplain and/or the patient's religious advisor; trained volunteers to provide visitation, companionship, and emotional support. Other benefits of hospice care include providing periods of respite for the primary caregiver and, later, offering bereavement counseling for the survivors. Compared to the hospital setting, hospice provides a more caring and comfortable way for a patient to live out their final days and also provides support and guidance for family members.

Palliative Care

Palliative care is the field of medicine focused on managing pain and symptoms of patients who have a serious illness, regardless of the diagnosis or prognosis. The primary focus of palliative care is *comfort*, both physical and psychological, rather than *cure*. Effective palliative care provides relief from such physical symptoms as pain, shortness of breath, and nausea. For patients who are dying, palliative care also includes emotional support to relieve anxiety, accept the dying process, grieve for impending losses, and to say "good-bye" to loved ones.

Family and close friends are an important part of palliative care. Their presence may relieve a patient's fear of abandonment—of dying alone. Frequent visits by the person designated as "agent" in an advance medical directive may provide reassurance that end-of-life decisions will be honored. Many patients who have prepared an advance medical directive do not want "high-tech" interventions, believing that *such measures prolong dying, rather than living*. Many physicians, with a strong commitment to prolonging life, recommend such measures as additional chemotherapy, mechanical ventilation, artificial feeding, or dialysis, even when the patient is in the final stages of dying. The patient, the family, and the "designated agent" should question the benefit of such recommendations and keep in mind the patient's right to refuse treatment.

Financial Concerns For terminally ill patients and their families, financial concerns can add to the already difficult decisions that must be made. Even for patients who have insurance and/or Medicare, out of pocket costs for long-term care can be significant. Other expenses can include modifying one's home to accommodate a wheelchair, hospital bed, or other medical equipment. Family members who serve as caregivers may lose work income if they are not able to maintain employment while providing care. When appropriate, health care professionals can provide information about community organizations that offer financial counseling or financial assistance.

Medical Issues Related to Care of the Dying

Diagnosis and prescription of therapy are responsibilities of the physician. When the diagnosis of a fatal disease is confirmed, the physician faces several difficult questions:

- Does an adult patient have a right to know the diagnosis?
- Does an adult patient have a right to decide who should be given information about his or her condition?
- Does a physician have a duty to inform a patient that they are dying?
- How much information should the patient be given?
- How and when should the patient be told that he or she is dying?

Past medical practice has been to tell the family that the patient is dying, but "protect" the patient by telling him or her as little as possible. This is a departure from ethical practices related to confidentiality. Does a dying patient have less of a right to confidentiality than one who is not dying? Several studies have revealed that (1) many physicians do not make a practice of telling patients that they are dying and (2) most people believe they would want to be informed.

How the information is given is important. It is possible to convey in a tactful and caring manner that the illness will be fatal. People listen selectively, so patients are likely to deal consciously only with as much of the message as they are able to handle at that moment. There are several reasons why patients should be informed:

- A patient who is not told that she is dying is deprived of opportunities to talk about the illness and dying. This "conspiracy of silence" results in the patient feeling isolated.
- A dying patient needs to get her affairs in order. This pertains to everyone, not just the wage earner or a businessperson. Getting one's affairs in order includes personal as well as business and financial decisions.
- Many dying patients want to deal with spiritual matters in preparation for dying.
- Lack of correct information may lead the patient to seek help from one practitioner after another, until finances have been exhausted. A second opinion often is desirable, but a fruitless search for a nonexistent cure may be avoided by honest communication.

Some patients want to have full information about their disorder, the treatment options available, and the probable course of the illness. In general, defense mechanisms provide some protection against being overwhelmed. The patient focuses on some aspects of the illness and ignores others, according to her capacity for coping. Other patients do not want to be told and are willing to delegate control and all treatment decisions to the physician. It would be destructive to try to force such a patient to "face the truth." On the other hand, such patients are likely to ask questions that indicate a need for reassurance. These patients usually suspect the truth, and their questions indicate a need to talk. Active listening may reveal underlying fears and anxieties for which the patient needs reassurance that they will be cared for and that pain will be alleviated.

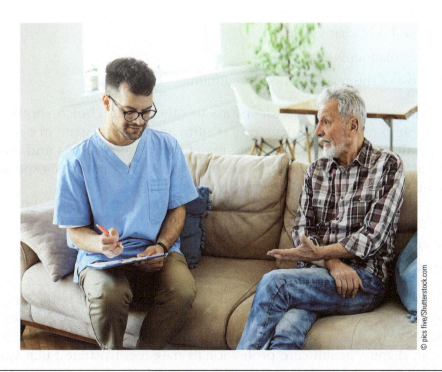

© pics five/Shutterstock.com

FIGURE 18-2 Many patients find comfort in talking about their illness and dying with a sensitive caregiver.

Many physicians provide information to their patients gradually and try to balance bad news with something positive. Later, they give additional information according to the patient's readiness. How much to tell the dying patient must be decided by each physician, based in part on each patient's situation and emotional stability.

Health care professionals involved in care of a dying patient should know what the physician has told the patient so they can respond appropriately to questions from the patient and family. Many patients find comfort in talking about their illness and dying with a sensitive caregiver. Frequent contact with caring people who *listen* results in the patient coming to terms with the illness. When there is good communication with family members, relationships improve. Good communication with health care personnel increases the patient's trust.

Rights of the Dying Person

Some issues discussed in previous chapters pertain to rights of patients. Patients' rights issues are also concerned with truth, informed consent, control, choices, and protection of personal dignity. A patient who signs an agreement to undergo surgery or certain other treatments should do so only after being given full information:

- What is the probability that the surgery or treatment will help?
- What are the possible side effects?
- Will irreversible body changes result?
- Are alternative treatments available?
- What is the cost of the recommended treatment?

Some patients prefer to delegate decisions to others; that choice should be respected. Many patients wish to retain some degree of control and to participate in decisions; this, too, should be respected. Choices regarding life-maintenance procedures and advance medical directives have already been discussed. Some other choices of patients, especially during the final days, include:

- Solitude versus being surrounded by significant others
- Remaining at home versus being in the hospital
- Remaining alert versus being sedated

Choices made by the patient or family members may conflict with what a health care professional considers to be "best" for the patient. This is a conflict of values. If the patient and family have arrived at acceptance of impending death, and if they are concerned about death with dignity, health care professionals may feel frustrated that various available procedures are not being used to prolong life (or prolong the dying process, depending upon one's view). It may help the health care professional to keep in mind that the Patient Self-Determination Act, advance medical directive legislation, and informed consent statutes all resulted from practices that forced unwanted procedures on dying patients.

Each individual's experience with death is unique. While the guidelines in this chapter will help prepare you for assisting a patient who is dying, each patient's needs will be individual. Ultimately, the patient has the right to make decisions based on personal preferences, values, and financial needs.

Roles of Health Care Professionals

Terminal illness by definition results in death. The goals of care for terminally ill patients, therefore, are different from the goals for patients who have the potential to regain physical well-being. It is difficult for many health care professionals to accept any goal other than "getting better." Working with dying patients requires that a health care professional be able to *substitute palliative goals for curative goals*. Palliative goals include keeping the patient comfortable, being available to listen, providing comforting touch as appropriate, accepting the patient's choices, and respecting the patient as a human being, even if comatose and nonresponsive.

The stages of dying proposed by Dr. Kübler-Ross can help health care professionals to understand and accept some of the behaviors manifested by a dying person. For example, anger directed at a caregiver is more easily accepted if it is viewed as one manifestation of a specific stage of the dying process. But attempting to "place" a patient in one stage or another does not serve the patient's needs. Rather, effective care demands the utmost in caring, always keeping in mind that this patient's emotional needs are paramount.

© VGstockstudio/Shutterstock.com

FIGURE 18-3 Effective care requires keeping the patient's emotional needs in mind.

Guidelines for Care of a Dying Person

These guidelines can be useful as you strive to provide *humane* care consistent with the choices and needs of a dying patient:

- Reassure the patient as needed that you will be there and that you will do all possible to provide comfort. Then keep your word.

- Be aware of the patient's emotional state. Respect the patient's unique way of reacting to the illness and dying.

- Allow the patient to talk about dying; do not deny the fact that the patient is dying with statements such as "Oh, you have lots of time left."

- Allow the patient to express feelings. Anger, crying, remorse, and similar feelings help the patient to deal with the impending loss of life.

- Do not make promises that you cannot keep. Such expressions may make you feel better, but deny the reality of the patient's dying process.

- Let the patient know that you care. Use touch as appropriate and be with the patient as much as your other duties permit.

- Listen—a patient provides clues to their specific needs.

- Do not force your feelings or your beliefs on the patient.

- Whenever appropriate, allow the patient to express a preference about their care.

- Respond to a patient's request for prayer, a religious reading, ritual, or service. Call the hospital chaplain or the patient's spiritual advisor as appropriate.

By keeping these guidelines in mind, the health care professional can become the patient's ally in dealing with the process of dying.

Activities

1. Describe the stages of dying as proposed by Dr. Elisabeth Kübler-Ross.

2. Explain how dying can be seen as a time for growth and healing.

3. Locate contact information for a hospice agency in your community, if applicable, and for other agencies that can provide counseling and support for a person who is terminally ill.

4. What factors should medical professionals consider when deciding how much to tell a patient about their illness?

5. In a class discussion, consider the following questions:

   a. How can the rights of a comatose patient be protected?

   b. What are the rights of a dying patient whose organs could be used as transplants for patients in the same hospital?

6. Participate in a class discussion to identify various ways health care professionals could meet the following needs of a dying person:

   a. Relative freedom from pain and discomfort

   b. Maintaining as much independence as possible

   c. Satisfaction of any remaining wishes ("things I wish I had done")

   d. Maintenance of self-esteem when it becomes necessary to yield control to others

   e. Achievement of emotional adjustment, acceptance of impending death, and a state of inner peace

References and Suggested Readings

American Association of Retired Persons. (n.d.) Family caregiving: Grief, loss and end of life. https://www.aarp.org/caregiving/grief-loss-end-of-life/

Duda, Deborah. (2010). *Coming home: A practical and compassionate guide to caring for a dying loved one*. Synergy.

National Hospice and Palliative Care Organization. (2021). *NHCPO facts and figures report, 2021 edition*. Author.

National Hospice and Palliative Care Organization. (2022). Hospice care overview for professionals. https://www.nhpco.org/hospice-care-overview/

Parkes, C. M. (2013). Elisabeth Kübler-Ross, *On Death and Dying*: A reappraisal. *Mortality, 18*(1), 94–97. doi:10.1080/13576275.2012.758629

Trends in Health Care

Health care in the United States is changing rapidly. As a health care professional, you should be informed about current trends and issues, especially those that affect roles and relationships of health care personnel.

Much of the public is now well-informed about health matters; with increasing knowledge, many people want to participate in health care decisions. Lifestyle and stress management are widely recognized as major factors in both treatment and prevention of illness. And more people are using alternative (nonmedical) approaches to health care.

Some patients enter the health care system with a passive attitude: "I'm sick. Fix me. Make me well." These patients are not likely to refuse treatments or seek alternative therapies. Other patients ask questions, expect answers, may refuse an invasive procedure or specific treatment, and may even question whether or not orthodox medicine can help with their health problems. Inadequate answers or a judgmental attitude on the part of a health care professional interferes with establishing rapport or, worse, may alienate the patient. Health care professionals need to understand and accept those patients who wish to assume more responsibility and actively participate in decisions about their health care.

Section VI is designed to help you learn about selected trends in health care as a basis for working with today's patients and for expanding your understanding of holistic health, healing, and the role of stress management in health maintenance.

Chapter 19

Health Care Through the Ages

Objectives

After completing this chapter, you should be able to:

- Describe how healing was viewed in early civilizations.
- List scientific or medical advances during the past 400 years that provided the foundation for current health care practices.
- Define allopathic, alternative, complementary, holistic, integrative, and Eastern medicine.
- Discuss reasons that some innovations in science and medicine are initially rejected.
- Describe potential conflicts among different models of medicine.
- Discuss appropriate attitudes of health care professionals toward new developments in health care.

Key Terms

Allopathic	Empirical	Psychoanalysis
Alternative therapy	Herbalism	Psychopharmaceuticals
Ayurveda	Holism	Scientific method
Complementary therapy	Holistic health care	Synergism
Dolorology	Neurotransmitters	Variables

The history of science and health care includes numerous examples of innovative ideas that were rejected initially by those in power at the time. Many of these innovative approaches were eventually accepted by orthodox medicine. Some innovations were premature—they required changes the culture was not yet ready to accept. Innovations—new ideas—may conflict with existing beliefs and may be perceived as a threat by current practitioners. Many scientists who proposed a new idea or a new method have been subjected to criticism, ridiculed, or even persecuted. Yet some of those innovators who suffered persecution are now recognized as heroes of medicine or a particular field of science. Understanding how health care has evolved throughout history will provide a context to help you understand current innovations and new developments in health care.

Healing in Early Civilizations

For thousands of years the healing practices of each culture were handed down from one generation to the next. The role of healer was highly respected; possession of the secrets of healing conveyed power second only to the power of the ruler. The priests and priestesses performed religious services and were also guardians of healing secrets. The role of *healer* was a *power role*.

Greece and Rome

Although early Greek mythology attributed illness to supernatural causes, it was the Greeks who eventually separated healing from religion and the role of physician from that of priest.

FIGURE 19-1 The Greek physician Hippocrates established a systematic approach to diagnosing illness based upon careful observation and collection of information.

Hippocrates, a Greek physician who lived during the period 460–377 BCE, is known as "the father of modern medicine." Hippocrates insisted upon careful observation and the collection of factual information, thereby establishing a systematic approach to diagnosis of illness. His treatments included diet, fresh air and sunshine, and healthful personal habits and living conditions—what we today refer to as "a healthful lifestyle." Hippocrates demonstrated that illness results from natural causes, rather than from evil spirits or the anger of the gods. This established medicine as the healing profession. Thereafter, religion was the domain of priests and care of the sick was the domain of physicians. Hippocrates also emphasized a code of behavior for physicians—the beginnings of medical ethics. The Hippocratic oath is still used by many medical schools as part of the graduation exercise for medical students.

Early Judeo-Christian Period

Jews and early Christians believed in a divine cause for illness and divine intervention as the basis for healing. The Greeks and Romans, with their many gods, could attribute illness to the wrath of one god and healing to the kindness of another god. Jews and Christians, however, believed in one God. This raised an important question: How could the same being who causes illness also heal the sick? This dilemma was resolved by associating illness with sin. If a person became sick, then certainly that person had sinned and was being punished. These beliefs are still reflected in some religions today, with illness considered a punishment for an individual's "sinful" lifestyle choices.

Evolution of Modern Health Care

The Middle Ages (also known as the Dark Ages) lasted over 1,000 years, from the fall of the Roman Empire to the Renaissance. Throughout this period, epidemics and plagues recurred, especially in crowded cities. But there was no organized health care system as we know it. Many monasteries had gardens in which various therapeutic herbs were cultivated; the monks performed simple healing procedures. In communities far from a monastery, an older man (the village "wise man") or woman (the village "crone" or "wise woman") served as healer for the community. Perhaps these healers possessed natural healing abilities. It is likely that they possessed methods of healing that had been passed down from one generation to the next. Eventually, the influence of the wise healer was perceived as a threat to the power of the local priest. A healer who was especially successful might be condemned as a heretic or witch. Many were tortured and then executed via such methods as hanging or burning at the stake. Persecution of healers who were neither priest nor physician continued up to the 1800s. Once a system of medicine had become established, natural healers were then condemned as "quacks."

The Renaissance (a French term meaning "rebirth") followed the Dark Ages and lasted about 400 years. There was renewed interest in science, art, music, and literature and less emphasis on religion. This was a period of discoveries, of new insights and theories, many of which provided the foundation for the **scientific method** that is an integral part of modern medical research.

Developments in Science

During the 1500s, Andreas Vesalius (1514–1564) studied the human body and made accurate anatomical drawings. Existing beliefs about human anatomy were based on dissection of animals, because it was illegal to dissect a human body. Therefore, in order to obtain cadavers for his anatomical studies, Vesalius removed bodies from the gallows at night. As a result of these secret studies of human anatomy, Vesalius corrected many misconceptions about the structure of the human body. Vesalius was ridiculed by his colleagues for proposing that their beliefs about human anatomy were erroneous, but today he is credited with establishing anatomy as a science. His book of anatomical drawings is a classic.

Just as dissection of human bodies was necessary to identify internal structures, the development of the microscope was a necessary prelude to the discovery of bacteria, the study of cell and tissue structure, and the identification of chromosomes and genes—the basis for modern genetic research. Zacharias Janssen is thought to have invented the compound microscope around 1590. But it would be over 200 years before refinements in lens-making made it possible to magnify objects without distortion. Meanwhile, Anton van Leeuwenhoek (1632–1723) used a simple microscope to study a wide variety of subjects, including various body fluids. As an amateur scientist, van Leeuwenhoek systematically recorded his observations and made detailed drawings. His work provided the foundation for the science of microbiology, even though he was widely criticized when he first published his observations.

The Germ Theory and Antisepsis

It was not until the nineteenth century, around 200 years ago, that handwashing was proposed as a means of preventing infections. A Hungarian physician, Ignaz Philipp Semmelweis (1818–1865), noticed that women who were assisted in childbirth by doctors who had just come from the autopsy room invariably developed "childbed fever." He proposed that doctors should wash their hands after completing an autopsy, to protect their patients. For making this suggestion, Semmelweis was persecuted by his colleagues to such an extent that he eventually suffered a nervous breakdown.

Ironically, in 1865, the year of Semmelweis's death, Joseph Lister (1827–1912) introduced antisepsis to the practice of surgery. The beginning of surgical asepsis was a major event in the history of medicine. Dr. Lister was such a renowned surgeon that his innovation was accepted, and he did not experience rejection and persecution by unconverted colleagues. Lister's use of antisepsis introduced control of infection as an integral part of medical practice. It is noteworthy that Lister's introduction of antisepsis preceded any proof of the existence of microorganisms. Two other scientists, working separately, were to provide proof that microorganisms are present on hands and all objects, thus providing the scientific basis for both handwashing and medical asepsis.

Robert Koch (1843–1910), a German scientist, was responsible for a scientific breakthrough that we now know as the *germ theory*. Through his study of microorganisms, Koch determined the specific cause of several infectious diseases, including tuberculosis. He also established the rules for proving that a specific organism was the cause of a particular infection; this provided the foundation for the field we know today as bacteriology. Development of the germ theory was a major event that established the scientific basis for asepsis, immunization, and modern sanitation.

Many scientists had observed microorganisms under a microscope, but it was Louis Pasteur (1822–1895) who established that those tiny objects were living things that reproduced themselves. He demonstrated that wine could be preserved by destroying the microorganisms present. The process he used is known as "pasteurization" and is still used today to ensure that milk and various other foods are safe.

Later, Pasteur developed a vaccine to prevent rabies in people who had been bitten by a rabid animal, thus sparing them a horrible death. Pasteur's contributions are numerous, yet he, too, was subjected to ridicule by his colleagues, even though he was a highly respected scientist. His contributions were recognized prior to his death, however. The Pasteur Institute, founded in 1888 in his honor by the French government, continues to conduct research on the causes, treatment, and prevention of disease.

Control of Infectious Diseases

The work of Koch and Pasteur led to the development of vaccines to protect people against certain diseases, especially the group of infections known as "childhood diseases." In the past hundred years, the most devastating diseases have been caused by viruses, rather than bacteria: smallpox, poliomyelitis, HIV, influenza (flu), SARS, and COVID-19.

In 1796, an English physician by the name of Edward Jenner (1749–1823) developed a method of protecting people from smallpox, a serious disease with a high mortality rate. Smallpox victims were seriously ill for two to three weeks. Those who survived had numerous small scars, known as pockmarks. Widespread use of the smallpox vaccine eliminated the disease in Europe and North America by 1950, but epidemics killed thousands of victims in other parts of the world. Between 1950 and 1970, intensive worldwide efforts to vaccinate the total population of any country where smallpox occurred resulted in eradication of this disease. Because the disease was considered to have been eradicated, vaccinations were discontinued except for persons traveling to remote areas where exposure was a possibility. Meanwhile, the smallpox virus was kept alive in various laboratories, presumably for the purposes of scientific research. Unfortunately, terrorists now threaten to use these stores of smallpox virus as a weapon of mass destruction. With two generations of unvaccinated populations in Europe and the Americas, the potential for a worldwide epidemic now exists.

Until the outbreak of HIV, the viral threat of the twentieth century was poliomyelitis, also called "infantile paralysis" because children were very susceptible and many were left with permanent paralysis. During the 1940s and 1950s, polio epidemics occurred with increasing frequency, especially during the spring and summer months. The mortality rate was high; many survivors were handicapped by paralysis. In 1953, Dr. Jonas Salk's vaccine became available. The Salk vaccine was widely administered and is now required in some states for admission to the public schools. Polio has not been completely eradicated, but cases are now relatively rare. Jenner and Salk made it possible to protect entire populations against two serious viral infections.

For many viral infections, widespread vaccinations have reduced fatalities. However, some viruses, including influenza and COVID-19, mutate rapidly, creating the need for ongoing research and the development of updated vaccines. To reduce the risk of infection, the public is urged to practice good health habits, especially handwashing, covering the nose and mouth when sneezing or coughing, and wearing a face mask in areas where cases are numerous.

The Discovery of Radiation

Two physicists in France, Pierre (1859–1906) and Marie (1867–1934) Curie, laid the foundation for radiation therapies. Together they studied radioactive substances and identified two previously unknown elements: radium and polonium. After her husband's death, Marie Curie discovered that radium had created an image of a nearby key on a piece of film. This discovery revealed what is now basic knowledge—namely, that radioactive materials give off invisible rays that affect nearby substances.

Marie Curie and her daughter, Irene, then only 17 years old, took a portable X-ray machine to the front lines during World War I to make X-rays available to doctors treating wounded soldiers. After the war, Irene did research on radioactive substances with her husband and her mother for many years. The contributions of the Curies are basic to various diagnostic and therapeutic procedures in current medical use.

Concurrently with the work of the Curies in France, a German physicist by the name of Wilhelm Konrad Roentgen (1845–1923) accidentally discovered X-rays. After conducting some experiments that involved passing an electric current through a special type of glass tubing, Roentgen noticed that some nearby photographic plates had become fogged. His investigation of the cause led to further experiments that resulted in the identification of invisible rays that could pass through soft tissues, but not through bone or metal. This discovery revolutionized diagnostic practices in medicine. Again, the dangers of radiation and X-rays were not known in the beginning. Many radiologists died of leukemia before it was recognized that health care professionals must have adequate protection when they are working around any type of radiation.

© Everett Historial/Shutterstock.com

FIGURE 19-2 Physicist Marie Curie won two Nobel Prizes for her research on radiation and radioactivity.

The Beginnings of Psychiatry and Psychosomatic Medicine

The pioneers just discussed all contributed to medicine as it pertains to physical health. Psychiatry, the medical specialty concerned with mental illness, began with the work of Sigmund Freud, an Austrian physician who first recognized the power of subconscious memories to affect health. Freud developed **psychoanalysis**, a technique for helping patients explore the unconscious part of the mind. Although many of Freud's theories are not accepted by modern practitioners, his writings and those of his students provided the foundation for psychotherapy. He was truly a pioneer, daring to explore territory that had never before been explored by physicians. Freud made the mind and emotions a concern of medicine, which had previously limited its focus to the physical body.

For Discussion and Reflection

1. Discuss one of the historical developments in health care described above. How has this development influenced health care today?
2. Which historical development in health care was most interesting to you? What did you find interesting?

Brain Chemistry The division between physical illness and mental illness has been clouded further by the discovery of a biochemical factor in several mental illnesses, especially unipolar disorder, bipolar disorder, and schizophrenia. Several chemicals, known as **neurotransmitters**, are produced by certain cells within the brain. These chemicals affect mental alertness, memory, ability to concentrate, thought processes, judgment, mood, sleep patterns, sexual behavior, irritability, energy, and other factors that influence the ability to perform one's daily activities. An increase or decrease in certain neurotransmitters may have a profound effect on behavior. The discovery of differences in certain neurotransmitter levels of psychiatric patients versus "normal" individuals has led to the development of a new class of drugs. These **psychopharmaceuticals** influence either the production of a specific neurotransmitter or its transmission from one cell to another. The availability of psychopharmaceutical drugs has had a radical effect on the psychiatric field. Many psychiatrists have abandoned "talk therapy" and now limit their practice to diagnostic evaluations and prescription of one or more psychopharmaceutical drugs to manage a patient's symptoms.

Psychologists, clinical social workers, and counselors now provide most of the psychotherapy, often in conjunction with a psychiatrist who prescribes psychopharmaceutical drugs. Individual therapy is often combined with group therapy sessions, which seem to be especially beneficial for those patients who need the interaction and support that group sessions can provide.

The Genetic Factor The line between "physical" and "mental" illness has also been clouded by sociological studies and gene research that demonstrate a genetic tendency toward certain mental illnesses. These findings give weight to the hereditary aspect. At the individual level, biorhythms, exposure to light, sleep patterns, REM (rapid eye movement) sleep, and dreams have been found to differ from "normal" in psychiatric patients. One relatively common problem, seasonal affective disorder (SAD), occurs during the winter months, when daylight hours are decreased and cloudy days occur frequently. This disorder is a depressive state precipitated by the seasonal decrease in light. Victims of SAD tend to become depressed in the late fall, then improve as winter draws to an end and spring approaches.

These individual patterns and environmental factors further cloud the question of what a "physical" illness is and what a "mental" illness is.

Multiple Causation The previous discussion indicates the fallacy of the "mental illness stigma," still pervasive in American society. That bias is no more justified than a bias against diabetes, a disorder involving faulty sugar metabolism. But diabetes, hypertension, autoimmune disorders, and many other physical illnesses are now considered to have an emotional and/or stress-related component. Even the infectious diseases, once blamed on the causative bacteria or virus, are now viewed in terms of numerous factors that impact an individual's immune system.

Allopathic Medicine and Alternative Approaches

The literal meaning of **allopathic** is "utilizing drugs." Orthodox medical practice in the United States relies primarily on drug therapy and surgery. *Allopathic medicine* is used in current literature on health care to refer to orthodox medicine as practiced in this country. In this text, the terms *conventional* and *orthodox* are used interchangeably, with *allopathic* used to refer to the existing system of medical practice in the United States. The terms **alternative therapy** and **complementary therapy** refer to a wide variety of nonmedical therapies, many of them based on a holistic concept of health and health care. Because "alternative therapy" implies a therapy that is used *instead of* medical care, the more inclusive term *complementary therapy* is preferred by many practitioners, most of whom have clients who are also receiving some type of allopathic care.

A complementary therapy may be provided by someone with a professional level of educational preparation (college degree plus professional training), someone with formal educational training leading to a certificate and/or licensure, or someone who has been trained in a specific therapeutic technique. **Holistic health care** takes into consideration the patient's total being (physical, mental, emotional, spiritual, life context, nutrition, lifestyle) and uses a variety of therapeutic techniques, according to the specific needs of each patient.

Some of these complementary therapies are "innovative" only from the perspective of health care in the United States. The Chinese have been using acupuncture for at least 5,000 years. Homeopathic medicine has been practiced throughout Europe for 200 years. Chiropractic techniques were developed in the early 1900s. Being over 90 years old, chiropractic no longer qualifies as "innovative." It is a form of therapy now widely accepted by the American public and by many physicians.

Holistic and Integrative Medicine

With increasing evidence of multiple causation of disease, the allopathic approach to treatment of symptoms is being replaced by emphasis on removal or treatment of causes. The search for causes leads naturally to a holistic approach to the care of each patient as an individual with a particular lifestyle, stressors related to occupation and family dynamics, and behavior patterns developed over a lifetime. Any of these could be contributing to the current health problem.

A new treatment emphasis is emerging, calling for treatment of *causes* of illness, rather than management of symptoms. Holistic practitioners focus on the total patient. They insist that treatment must include the mental, emotional, and spiritual aspects of the person, as well as the physical aspects. Holistic medicine requires taking time to identify and deal with causes, rather than treating symptoms only. A holistic approach requires taking a detailed history—both family and individual—and conducting a lifestyle inventory to address some or all of the following:

- Genetic clues to the patient's illness may be found in the family history.
- Individual clues may be found in the individual's own history, such as abuse or neglect on the part of the primary caregiver, or the existence during childhood of attention deficit hyperactive disorder.
- A description of the patient's home life and work situation may yield clues about whether or not stress is a contributing factor.
- The patient may experience additional symptoms, such as sleep disturbances.

Holistic treatment of the patient can begin even before a final diagnosis has been established. Holistic health care utilizes the skills of many different therapists; it includes the techniques of allopathic medicine as appropriate, but extends the role of the physician into areas beyond orthodox medical practice. Consider the following examples:

- If stress is obviously a causative factor, the patient can be taught stress management techniques.
- If emotional factors are revealed, appropriate therapy for constructive expression of emotions can be planned.
- Assertiveness training can be recommended to help a patient learn to cope with life problems effectively.
- If faulty dietary habits are revealed, instruction in healthful eating may be given.

Thus, each possible causative factor is dealt with in order to *heal the total patient*.

Eastern Medicine and Ayurveda

Eastern medicine, or traditional Chinese medicine, has been used for centuries in China and has gained popularity in the United States and other Western countries. Ayurveda, the traditional medical practice of India, is another ancient healing system that has gained worldwide popularity. Both of these modalities emphasize treating the whole patient, not isolated symptoms.

Traditional Chinese Medicine

Traditional Chinese medicine (TCM), which is becoming more popular in the United States, differs from Western medicine in many ways. The licensure designation for the U.S. practitioner is doctor of Oriental medicine (OMD). Many practitioners are trained in both Eastern medicine and Western medicine and integrate these two systems into their practice. TCM, the prevalent form of medicine throughout Asia, uses a wide range of remedies, with herbalism being the predominant therapy.

TCM is based on the concepts of **holism** (i.e., wholeness) and balance of *yin* and *yang*. The basis of yin/yang theory is that everything is either yin or yang and is balanced by the polar opposite. Yin embodies feminine characteristics: the moon, night, passivity, coldness, blood, and body fluids. Yang is masculine: the sun, day, activity, heat, energy, growth, and metabolism. Both yin and yang embody some degree of the other; the ideal is perfect balance, but the relationship is flexible. Perfect balance leads to health, wholeness, and harmony.

A problem in one part of the body affects the whole, so treatment must restore the body to a state of wholeness. The perfect balance of yin and yang is disturbed when either yin or yang becomes excessive; each organ is either yin or yang. Excessive yang is indicated by acute pain, spasms, and headaches; excessive yin is indicated by coolness, dull aches and pains, and fatigue. Illness is viewed as evidence that a state of imbalance exists, so treatment is aimed at restoring balance.

Ayurveda

Ayurveda has been practiced in India for several thousand years. *Ayurveda* is a Sanskrit word that means "science of life," and the focus of this approach to health care is on various factors that affect one's life: diet, *prana* (the breath), exercise, spiritual practices, and one's relationship to nature based on body type (*dosha*).

Doshas are three types of vital energy believed to exist throughout nature: *vata*, *pitta*, and *kapha*. Each dosha is a combination of two of the five elements: ether, air, fire, water, and earth. Each human body is primarily one type of dosha, but may also exhibit some characteristics of one or both of the other two doshas. In the human body, doshas are affected by foods, the time of day, seasons, emotional states at any given time, stress, and the elements of that specific dosha. *Prana* refers to life energy that is taken into the body through breathing and food.

Imbalance in the doshas or any blocks to the flow of prana result in a toxic condition and illness. Ayurvedic healing emphasizes detoxification of the body. A cleansing routine is followed by specific therapeutic modalities: a strict dietary regimen that includes a prescribed eating schedule appropriate to the patient's dosha; herbs; and various approaches to improving the flow of prana, such as massage, yoga, meditation, and specific exercises. Therapy is designed to restore balance to the doshas and improve the flow of prana.

As a health care professional, you will very likely work with patients who have received one or more alternative therapies in the past or are currently receiving them alongside conventional treatment. It is outside the scope of your role to either recommend or discourage specific therapies. However, a general familiarity with commonly used therapies can assist you when communicating with patients. You can ask open-ended questions, such as "Tell me more about that" or "How did that treatment work out for you?" in order to better understand the patient's experience. Specific questions about treatments should be referred to the patient's physician.

Innovations in Modern Medicine

Increasingly, the powerful influence of emotions and stress on health is being recognized. The onset of diseases such as cancer is most likely to occur when the immune system is depressed. It is well known that disorders such as ulcers and high blood pressure have an emotional component, but the emotional component may be the result of long-term stress. Several physicians who acknowledged the roles of stress and emotional factors in the onset and course of illness provided the early foundation for holistic medical practice. They believed that strategies for managing stress and resolving emotional factors must be incorporated into the therapeutic protocol. Their contributions led to changes in cancer therapy, pain control, management of hypertension, and the use of medical intuitives in diagnosis.

Cancer Therapy

Dr. O. Carl Simonton is an oncologist who noted that the cancer patients who met with him regularly for group counseling seemed to "hold their own" better than cancer patients who did not participate in the group sessions. Some members of the group actually improved. In 1976 the Institute of Noetic Sciences sponsored a project in which Dr. Simonton and his wife, Stephanie (a counselor), provided psychological counseling to cancer patients who had been labeled "terminal" by their own physicians. Only patients who had received orthodox medical therapies for their cancer were accepted into the project. In addition to participating in counseling sessions, each patient was encouraged to write three sets of objectives, one set for three months in the future, one set for six months, and one set for twelve months. Each set of objectives had three components:

1. Meditate for 20 minutes at least twice a day

2. Exercise for 20 minutes five days each week

3. Have one hour of play per day, seven days per week

Play time could not be accumulated; if a patient played two hours on Saturday, there still must be an hour of play on Sunday. Time spent watching television could not be counted as play time. Patients had to specify their play activities in writing. In regard to exercise, the patient would choose something he or she was capable of doing safely. One patient might be able to walk a mile. Another, confined to bed, might be limited to flexing and extending the fingers and arms periodically. Dr. Simonton helped his patients *program themselves for living*, as opposed to programming themselves (or allowing others to program them) for dying.

Long-term follow-up of these patients indicated that about one-third lived longer than expected, some experienced complete recovery, and those who did not survive experienced a higher quality of life up until the time of death. "Higher quality" means less pain, increased activity, slower decline, and increased participation in family and community life, as opposed to lying in bed helpless and in pain for weeks prior to dying. According to Dr. Simonton, the patients who improved the most were those who were willing to get in touch with any negative aspects of their lives during the counseling sessions.

Publication of the results of this therapeutic approach met with skepticism and criticism from the medical community. Does this rejection of an innovative treatment sound familiar? Some of the historical figures discussed earlier did not live to see their innovations accepted into common practice. The Simontons are more fortunate. Their approach emphasizing psychological factors was premature. Medicine was not yet ready to give up the notion that cancer is a *physical* disease or to accept the powerful influence of mind and emotions on physiological processes. But within 10 years, numerous physicians had accepted the Simontons' approach and were incorporating purposeful, regular counseling into the treatment protocol for cancer patients.

Pain Management

Dr. C. Norman Shealy is a neurosurgeon who practiced the conventional methods of his specialty until he became aware that many of his patients gained only temporary relief of symptoms, even from extensive surgical procedures that were supposed to correct the problem. Dissatisfied with these results, and especially concerned about the number of neurosurgical and orthopedic patients with chronic pain, Dr. Shealy searched for more effective methods. Collaborating with a young electrical engineer, he spent two years

For Discussion and Reflection

In your view, how do thoughts and emotions affect the prognosis or quality of life of an individual with cancer or another life-threatening illness?

designing a low-voltage electrical unit that could short-circuit pain by preventing the pain sensation from traveling up the spinal cord to the brain. This research led to a device now known as the transcutaneous electrical nerve stimulator, or TENS. It is widely used for control of acute temporary pain and also for long-term, chronic pain. When this technique was first developed, it was an example of "alternative medicine."

Because Dr. Shealy was able to demonstrate the effectiveness of TENS to the satisfaction of other neurosurgeons, this example of "alternative medicine" quickly assumed a place within conventional medical practice. Dr. Shealy, the first physician to specialize in management of pain, coined the term **dolorology** for this new medical specialty. (*Dolor* is the Latin word for "pain.")

Management of Hypertension

Dr. Herbert Benson, a professor at the Harvard Medical School, became concerned about increasing evidence that heart attacks, strokes, and hypertension are now occurring in men approximately 13 years earlier than in their fathers. Believing the stress of modern life to exact a high price, both psychologically and physiologically, he studied approaches to stress management outside conventional medicine's use of tranquilizers and/or sedatives. Drugs can control some symptoms related to stress, but do not eliminate *sources* of stress, reverse the physiological effects of prolonged stress, or correct an underlying psychological problem.

Harvard research studies have shown that control of involuntary body processes, such as blood pressure, heart rate, and flow of blood to a specific part of the body, may be learned through the use of biofeedback. After reviewing research related to conscious control of body functions, Dr. Benson raised the question, "Can we influence our own physiological reaction to stress through individually controlled mental practices?"

Dr. Benson began his search for a practical, *easily learned* means of physiological control. He found that people who used Transcendental Meditation experienced certain body changes within a few minutes after achieving the meditative state. These changes were different from the physiological changes that occur during sleep and hypnosis. Eventually, Dr. Benson and his research team demonstrated that hypertensive patients could lower their blood pressure by using a simple meditative technique twice a day. Many patients were able to discontinue their blood pressure medication and maintain a normal blood pressure simply by incorporating meditation into their daily routines.

Three modern medical pioneers—all seeking more effective therapy for their patients—concluded that meditation, practiced at least twice a day for 20 minutes, has therapeutic effects. Dr. Simonton found that this simple practice benefitted cancer patients, even those considered to be terminal by their own physicians. Dr. Shealy found that meditation could be used to manage pain, especially chronic, long-term pain. And Dr. Benson demonstrated that meditation enabled many hypertensive patients to control their blood pressure. Each of these physicians used an alternative practice to enhance the therapeutic benefits of conventional medicine for his patients. Their findings are widely accepted now; in fact, many health care agencies now offer wellness programs that include meditation instruction.

These innovators influenced the practices of some physicians and the breadth of services offered within some health care agencies. The effect on the roles of various health care professionals remains to be seen, however. Ultimately, each health care professional's open-mindedness will determine whether or not he can adapt successfully to the role changes required by a holistic approach to health care.

The Scientific Model

Today, the scientific model is considered by the medical community to be *the method* for proving the effectiveness of a specific technique, drug, or procedure. Complementary procedures are criticized by members of the medical community because they have not been "proven effective" by the scientific method. Yet many current medical practices have never been subjected to rigorous scientific research. At present a double standard exists, in which complementary practices are rejected or viewed with suspicion by members of the scientific community because of a lack of rigorous research, but certain long-standing medical practices that have never been subjected to such research are accepted without question.

The scientific model requires an approach in which the experimental treatment is administered to certain subjects (the experimental group), whereas an ineffective treatment is administered to other subjects (the control group); sometimes, there is a third group that receives no treatment. The experiment is called a "double-blind study" if neither patients nor caregivers know which subjects are in the experimental group and which are in the control group. A blind study prevents patients' and caregivers' expectations from influencing the outcomes of an experiment.

FIGURE 19-3 The scientific method is used to prove the effectiveness of a specific drug, technique, or procedure.

For Discussion and Reflection

How might researchers measure the influence of emotions and attitudes on health and recovery? What are the challenges of measuring emotions and attitudes?

Studies on the effects of drug therapy have shown that the expectations of those conducting an experiment influence the results. For example, the health care professional who knows that a patient is being given the experimental drug expects it to help the patient. This expectation can affect the patient's response to the drug. Factors that influence the outcome of an experiment are known as **variables**.

The scientific model requires that only one or two variables be manipulated, while all other influences are carefully controlled. After treatment, the experimental subjects (those receiving a specific treatment) are compared with subjects in the control group (who did not receive the treatment). A treatment is considered effective only if there are significant differences between the treatment group and the control group. Research findings are considered valid (proven correct) only if other researchers can repeat the experiment and get the same results.

It is relatively easy to measure and record the effects of a precise amount of a drug on blood pressure. It is more difficult to measure an emotion such as fear and prove that minimizing a preoperative patient's anxiety results in faster postoperative recovery. It is impossible to see or measure a patient's "will to live." Yet emotions, belief systems, and factors such as intention (to get well or to escape one's present life situation by dying) are known to be powerful influences on the course of illness. Health care professionals often see two patients who have the same diagnosis and are receiving the same treatment. One recovers, but the other declines and dies. The big question: What made a difference in the outcome of these two patients? The "difficult to measure" variables are ignored by researchers who are committed to the scientific model—that is, precise measurement (quantitative data) of the effects of the specific variable being studied. Some members of the scientific/medical/healing community who are open to alternative approaches are now designing studies that adapt the scientific method to the study of intuitive diagnosis and influences on healing, such as prayer and Healing Touch. No one, however, has devised a method for measuring such powerful factors as the will to live, expectation, or intention.

Empirical Evidence

Empirical refers to experience and observation; *empirical data* are observations collected without the rigorous design of the scientific method. Many alternative therapies involve counseling, meditation, massage, and other procedures that affect the emotional state, tension level, and perhaps even the beliefs of the patient. Practitioners who use various nonmedical therapies have accumulated a large body of empirical data, but their methods are criticized by members of the scientific community who demand numerical data obtained through research procedures that fit the scientific model. In spite of the difficulties, researchers are now making progress in designing such experiments.

Meanwhile, more and more physicians, seeking better results for their patients, are sufficiently impressed by the empirical data to include certain nonmedical techniques in their practice. Yet many physicians continue to practice allopathic medicine without an awareness of or interest in the potential value of complementary therapies. Thus, allopathic medicine and holistic medicine represent *two very different belief systems* that have a profound effect on each practitioner's approach to patient care.

Dilemma of the Health Care Professional

A health care delivery system in the process of significant change presents something of a dilemma for members of the health care team. What is the appropriate response for you, a health care professional, to a patient who is using a complementary therapy in addition to medical treatment? Should you question the legitimacy of the treatment? Should you tell the physician that the patient is not complying with the medical regimen prescribed? Does compliance mean that the patient must follow the medical protocol and forgo any other type of therapy? These questions are less relevant to the average hospitalized patient than to a patient with a chronic health problem, long-term illness, or life-threatening disease. The probability of your caring for such a patient depends on your role, the particular health care setting in which you perform your role, and the extent to which you interact with each patient.

Issues in Health Care

The conflict between orthodox medical practice and complementary therapies is especially evident in several areas: pharmaceuticals versus natural remedies, herbal remedies, nutrition, and nutritional supplements. A full discussion of each of these topics is beyond the scope of this book, so the following paragraphs are intended only to introduce each topic as an area of concern for health care professionals. Many books and journals are available to those who want to become informed about any of these topics. Because of the wealth of information now being published, ongoing study will be necessary to keep up with new developments.

Pharmaceutical Drugs

Pharmaceutical companies constitute a multibillion-dollar industry. The industry justifies the high prices of drugs in the United States on the basis of costs involved in research and obtaining approval from the Food and Drug Administration (FDA). Yet those same drugs sell for much lower prices in other countries. Some cost factors that pharmaceutical companies do not reveal to the public include incentive programs (all-expenses-paid trips, hospitality rooms at professional meetings) to influence doctors' prescription choices, financial support to researchers in university settings, payments to public figures to promote a particular drug, and the costs of advertising. Company representatives visit doctors' offices regularly with gifts for doctors and the office staff, as well as literature and free drug samples.

In addition, drug companies now promote specific drugs to the public, with the FDA's approval. Television commercials and full-page advertisements with beautiful, smiling people tout the benefits of specific drugs for common ailments, such as arthritis and osteoporosis. The risk of side effects is presented with rapid-fire dialogue on television or in the fine print of an advertisement. The purpose of advertising is to sell drugs—by priming patients to pressure their doctors for a specific drug prescription.

Many drugs available today save lives, control symptoms, and prolong life. But the long-term effects of many new drugs are unknown; most drugs receive FDA approval on the basis of short-term research. Thousands of deaths per year are due to prescription drugs: unexpected side effects, incorrect dosage, drug interactions, allergic reactions, or damage to vital organs, especially the heart, liver, or kidneys. For example, the diabetes drug Rezulin was approved by the FDA in 1997; it was withdrawn from the market in 2000 after being linked to numerous fatalities due to liver damage. With increasing public awareness of these problems, many people are using herbs, natural remedies, homeopathic remedies, nutritional healing, and other alternatives to pharmaceutical drugs.

Herbalism

Herbalism, the medicinal use of plants, is perhaps the oldest form of healing. Healers throughout the ages have used the roots, stems, leaves, flowers, nuts, and fruits of plants to treat illnesses and injuries. This knowledge was passed down from generation to generation by word of mouth, although certain ancient cultures recorded their healing practices on papyrus or clay tablets.

Plants contain many different components that work together. Even when the active ingredient has been identified, it is probable that other components of the plant support and facilitate the effects of the primary active ingredient. The enhancement of an effect by a combination of ingredients is known as **synergism**, which is considered by herbalists to be a major advantage of herbs over prescription drugs.

Nutrition and Health

Traditionally, nutrition education has focused on the components of a balanced diet—proteins, fats, and carbohydrates—and the major food groups from which they are derived. As the health movement developed over recent decades, with its emphasis on exercise and healthful eating, greater attention has been directed to other components of the diet—vitamins, minerals, trace minerals, amino acids, and fiber:

- Vitamins are organic nutrients that serve numerous functions in the body; a severe deficiency results in a medically recognized condition, such as scurvy or rickets, but symptoms of a mild or moderate deficiency may not be recognized and correctly diagnosed.

- Minerals are inorganic substances that the body needs in relatively large amounts (e.g., calcium); trace minerals are those the body needs in tiny amounts (e.g., copper).

- Amino acids are the building blocks of the body; there are 20 amino acids, of which 8 are essential and 12 are nonessential. An essential amino acid must be obtained from foods, whereas a nonessential amino acid is one the body can synthesize from other nutrients.

The body must have an adequate supply of these various components in order to build and repair tissues—an ongoing process throughout life—and to carry out various body processes.

Nutrition has become a national concern. Obesity and diabetes are epidemic, indicating that large numbers of people do not eat healthful meals. Instead of a home-cooked dinner, prepared from homegrown vegetables, many people eat at fast-food restaurants or serve a dinner of convenience foods. Corporate farming provides stores with fruits and vegetables of questionable nutritive value and, possibly, contamination with chemical herbicides and pesticides. The food industry is using chemical additives whose effects on health are unknown. Many meats contain antibiotics and hormones. These and numerous other factors contribute to growing concern about practices within the food industry that alter or modify a food from its natural state.

Anyone who wishes to have a healthful diet must find a source of organically grown foods or grow their own. Free range chickens and eggs and organic meats are available, although more expensive. The grocery shopper must read labels to avoid foods that contain chemical additives, usually as preservatives, artificial ingredients, unhealthful forms of fat, or dyes. These choices are not convenient or affordable for everyone. Nor are most people concerned enough to focus on healthful eating. So the adverse effects of unhealthful eating have significance for health care professionals. Holistic practitioners consider diet to be an important factor in health, and possibly a contributing cause of any chronic illness. But healthful eating may require more than wholesome food.

Healthful eating is a primary requirement for maintaining health and for treating illness, but diet alone may not be enough to protect one's health against stress and the many pollutants to which we are all exposed. Full protection and a therapeutic plan for healing requires supplementation.

Nutritional Supplements

Although obstetricians and pediatricians have recommended vitamins to their patients for many years, most allopathic practitioners do not. Naturopathic schools and chiropractic schools emphasize nutrition in accordance with their holistic philosophy. Nutritionists who are associated with holistic health centers are more likely to counsel patients about all aspects of nutrition, including the use of supplements, than dietitians in an allopathic agency. Anyone seeking guidance about nutrition should find a qualified counselor and/or embark on a self-education program. If *nutrition therapy* is needed, then professional consultation is essential.

Vitamin, mineral, and amino acid supplements are all available as tablets, capsules, and powders. Natural products sold in health food stores and holistic centers are preferable to the synthetic products marketed through chain stores. A multivitamin is preferable to taking several vitamins separately, which can lead to an imbalance. The B vitamins should be taken in the form of B complex, again because the ratio of the different vitamins should be balanced.

As a health care professional, you will find it beneficial to become knowledgeable about nutrition, healthful eating habits, and supplements. This will help you maintain a high level of wellness and enable you to protect yourself against health risks to which you may be exposed in your work. It will not be within your role to prescribe, but it will be appropriate to suggest sources of information if a patient asks you about nutrition or supplements. You may occasionally have an opportunity to suggest a change in eating habits that could enhance a patient's nutritional status.

Staying Informed

Many issues now confront society and the health care system:

- Reproductive rights
- The threat of viral infection from COVID-19 and other viruses
- Genetically modified foods
- Organ transplants
- Prolonged use of life-support systems
- Patients' rights (including the right to refuse treatment), a patient's right to die, and advance medical directives
- Malpractice litigation

Some of these are moral and ethical issues; some have direct implications for certain roles, and therefore are of special concern to health care professionals. Many of these issues are highly emotional; the proponents of one side or the other may base their arguments on catch phrases that arouse strong emotional reactions in the listener.

For Discussion and Reflection

Which if the topics listed above is of most interest to you? What personal experience or prior knowledge do you have about this topic? Where on the Internet might you find reliable, unbiased information about this issue?

A full discussion of these issues is beyond the scope of this book; they are mentioned here because every health care professional should be informed about them. Being informed makes it possible to avoid emotionalism and examine an issue thoughtfully. Read, attend meetings, consider various viewpoints, and use every opportunity to become informed; then decide what *you* believe instead of blindly adopting the opinion of someone else. Strive to keep an open mind, combined with a healthy dose of skepticism.

For a large segment of the population, the major issues in health care are *accessibility* and *cost*. For professionals of health services, the major issue relates to the patient-physician relationship and *who should make decisions about health care options*. For third-party payers (insurance companies), the major issue is maintaining greater income (through insurance premiums) than is paid out for health care services—*making a profit*. The Affordable Care Act, passed in 2010, was designed to improve access to health care. While many individuals have benefitted from the opportunity to purchase low-cost health insurance, other individuals have seen the cost of insurance rise as a result of the act. Health care costs and access continues to be a hotly debated political topic, one that raises the following questions:

- Who is entitled to health care?
- What is *essential* health care and what is *nonessential*?
- Who should decide whether a specific service for a specific patient is essential or nonessential?
- What is a reasonable cost for each type of service?

- What is a reasonable income for each health care professional?
- Who will pay for essential services?
- Who will pay for services that are deemed nonessential, but are desired (or demanded) by a patient?

The issues of accessibility and cost are of personal concern to you and your family, even though you, as a health care professional, will probably have ready access to health care. These issues are of great concern to many of your patients, however. As you interact with a patient who is dissatisfied with his health care plan, you may be the object of that patient's displaced anger. Do not take it personally. Be a good listener, and be aware that the complaints you are hearing may be all too true. Meanwhile, we can all hope that eventually everyone will have access to affordable health care.

> **For Discussion and Reflection**
>
> Describe your experience with health insurance. Have you been successful in finding affordable coverage for yourself and your family? What challenges have you or your family personally experienced regarding the costs of health care?

The Health Care System Today and Tomorrow

You are preparing to assume an important role in today's health care system. But that system exists because of the many significant contributions of scientists, physicians, and others throughout history. Some of those contributions were initially rejected and their proponents ridiculed. Today, health care innovations and new theories, or new viewpoints regarding accepted theories, are appearing frequently. Some are rejected by orthodox medicine as quackery or, at best, "not scientifically proven." Some are tried by the more open-minded members of the orthodox medical establishment and, upon proving to be clinically effective, are incorporated into an established medical practice.

What is the appropriate attitude toward such innovations for you in your role as a health care professional? What is an appropriate attitude toward an innovative therapy that is provided by someone whose practice is not under the immediate direction of a medical doctor? Eventually you will need to deal with these questions and decide what will be your attitude toward innovative therapies.

Technological Advances

Today's health care system is a dynamic (i.e., ever-changing) system. Many current innovations are technological—new, sophisticated equipment for laboratory tests, new techniques for identifying and mapping physical changes in the patient's body, modifications in therapeutic devices, complex machines for maintaining vital functions. These technological innovations tend to be readily accepted into the existing system, though the high cost of some equipment may limit its use to large facilities. Some technological innovations require additional training for health care professionals. The expanded role or time-saving feature of some innovations results in ready acceptance. This is especially true of equipment and techniques that contribute to diagnosis.

Emerging Therapies and Roles

Other innovations—primarily therapeutic approaches—are less readily accepted. Rejection by medical personnel often is based on the fact that a particular technique is performed by someone who is not under the direction of a physician. Techniques such as acupressure, Shiatsu, Structural Integration, therapeutic massage, and craniosacral therapy require highly specialized training. Others, such as acupuncture and chiropractic techniques, require completion of a lengthy formal educational program. In addition, professional counselors such as psychologists, social workers, and counselors are assuming a greater role in patient care. Many of these have completed a doctoral program (i.e., PhD, EdD, DC) as lengthy as medical education. Some of these nonmedical practitioners are required to be licensed by the state. But education or training, certification, or licensure do not guarantee acceptance by all allopathic physicians.

Because public acceptance of these complementary therapies is increasing, you are encouraged to keep an open mind, listen to patients, and withhold judgment until you have enough information to make a rational evaluation.

Activities

1. How was healing viewed in early civilizations? How are these views similar to or different from views today?

2. Select one of the scientific advances described in this chapter. How did this advance impact modern medical care?

3. What has your personal experience been with allopathic, alternative, complementary, holistic, integrative, or Eastern medicine?

4. Explain why innovations in science and health care are often rejected at first.

5. What are the potential benefits and challenges for patients who wish to combine alternative treatment modalities with conventional treatments?

6. As a health care professional, how would you respond to a patient who asks your opinion about an experimental treatment or an alternative therapy?

References and Suggested Readings

Department of Health and Human Services. (2022). On 12-year anniversary of the Affordable Care Act, new HHS report shows ways the Biden-Harris administration's American Rescue Plan Investments are lowering health care costs and expanding coverage. https://www.hhs.gov/about/news/2022/03/23/12-year-anniversary-affordable-care-act-new-hhs-report-shows-ways-biden-harris-administrations-american-rescue-plan-investments-lowering-health-care-costs-expanding-coverage.html

Johns Hopkins Medicine. (2022). Ayurveda. https://www.hopkinsmedicine.org/health/wellness-and-prevention/ayurveda

Johns Hopkins Medicine. (2022) Chinese medicine. https://www.hopkinsmedicine.org/health/wellness-and-prevention/chinese-medicine

LaMattina, J. (2022). *Pharma and profits: Balancing innovation, medicine, and drug prices.* Wiley.

What Is Healing? Who Is the Healer?

Objectives

After completing this chapter, you should be able to:

- Describe the role of the immune system and mind/body connection in healing.
- Explain how the therapeutic environment and the patient's intention influence patient outcomes.
- Discuss characteristics of holistic health care.
- List strategies for evaluating whether a particular therapy is legitimate.
- Explain the role of health care professionals in helping patients make informed decisions about therapies.

Key Terms

External locus of control
Integrative medicine
Intention

Internal locus of control
Nocebo effect
Placebo

Placebo effect
Psychosocial

Every health care professional has wondered at times why one patient recovers from a serious illness, while another patient with the same disease and therapy slowly declines and eventually dies. What triggers the healing process in some patients, even when the prognosis is grim? What is the relationship between a patient's attitude and beliefs and the outcome?

Factors That Affect Healing

Also puzzling is the fact that in an epidemic, some people get sick and others, even members of a victim's family, do not contract the infection. This raises questions about the immune system. Why does it protect sometimes, but not always? How do both attitudes and genetics influence health outcomes?

The Immune System

It is now known that all of us have cancer cells in our bodies, but certain components of the immune system destroy those abnormal cells with great efficiency until . . . what? Why does the immune system stop destroying those abnormal cells? What change permits those cancer cells to reproduce and form a tumor? Can internal factors such as emotions and stress or external factors in the environment trigger this process?

These questions have led to a number of discoveries about what affects the immune system. Physicians in ancient cultures observed that a grieving person was likely to develop cancer within a year or two following a significant loss. But at that time, the existence of the immune system was completely unknown. Modern clinicians and researchers have established the validity of that ancient observation. Certain emotional states, especially grief, depress the immune system and render it less capable of destroying abnormal cells present in the body. The result is a favorable climate for the growth of cancer cells.

This particular body–mind–emotions relationship is now widely accepted. Yet much research on cancer still involves searching for an external intervention. This type of thinking denies the powerful mind/body relationship, clinging instead to the "old" way of attributing both the cause and the cure of disease to external influences. Even though today's research techniques enable scientists to study the immune system more effectively, there are still many unanswered questions.

The Placebo Effect

Another puzzle is the **placebo effect**—improvement or recovery when the "drug" administered to a patient is actually a **placebo**, an inert substance such as a sugar pill. This phenomenon is also called *placebo response*. Researchers use placebos in studies of new treatments to determine whether the treatment produces better outcomes than the inert substance. However, research shows that patients may improve even when given a placebo because of expectation and conditioning—they expect to feel better following treatment, and they have been conditioned to experience an improvement in symptoms following the administration of treatment or consultation with a doctor.

For Discussion and Reflection

In your opinion, does a person's state of mind influence their physical health? For example, do emotions, attitudes, and stress levels contribute to health or illness?

Why does the patient improve, even though the "treatment" administered is not medically acknowledged as having therapeutic value? Studies of placebo effect have led to recognition that expectation may influence the outcome of treatment. Expectation applies to both patients and health care professionals; if either or both believe that a treatment or drug is going to cure the patient's illness, improvement is more likely to occur. Placebo effect is a problem for researchers who are trying to test the effectiveness of a new treatment, because it is difficult to control. This is why double-blind studies are used to test the effectiveness of a new drug.

The placebo effect can be seen as a puzzling variable in medical research, but it can also be viewed as further evidence of the role of emotions, intention, and expectation on the healing process—in other words, the mind/body connection.

The Mind–Body Healing System

Mind–body medicine is an approach to health that acknowledges the interconnection between mind, body, and spirit. Emotions and beliefs, including unconscious beliefs, influence a person's physical health. This approach incorporates findings from disciplines including neurobiology, developmental psychology, behavioral medicine, and spiritual healing.

Mind–body medicine includes a number of different therapies and treatment modalities. These various modalities all emphasize the mind–body connection, but the treatment itself might primarily focus on the physical (acupuncture), the mental (hypnosis), or both (yoga). Mind–body techniques have shown promise in treatments of the following illnesses, to name a few:

- Hypertension
- Coronary artery disease
- Headaches
- Gastrointestinal disorders
- Chronic pain
- Anxiety
- Cancer

One of the benefits of most mind–body techniques is that they can be used alone or in conjunction with conventional medical treatments. The practice of combining mind–body or alternative treatments with conventional treatments in order to achieve the best outcome for patients is known as **integrative medicine**.

Who Gets Sick? Who Gets Well?

Some clinical practitioners and researchers are proposing new ways of looking at the causes of disease. One theory is that there are *several* contributing causes in any illness, rather than a single cause. Some of the causative factors lie *within* the individual:

- Immune system function (specifically resistance and susceptibility)
- Emotional states, which we now know to have powerful effects on the immune system

For Discussion and Reflection

Consider the healthy lifestyle changes recommended above. Which healthy habits have you already incorporated into your life? What changes could you make in the future to reduce your risk of illness?

- Physiological changes due to chronic stress
- Subtle factors—beliefs, attitudes, will to live, and, possibly, an unconscious desire to escape one's life situation
- Lifestyle factors, including diet, exercise, and substance use

According to the Centers for Disease Control and Prevention (CDC, 2019), lifestyle changes could significantly reduce death rates from the top five causes of deaths in the United States:

- Heart disease
- Cancer
- Unintentional injuries
- Chronic lower respiratory disease
- Stroke

In 2017, these five causes accounted for 61 percent of deaths in the United States. The CDC recommends the following lifestyle changes to reduce an individual's risk:

- Avoid tobacco
- Increase physical activity to 150 minutes per week of moderate activity or 75 minutes per week of vigorous activity
- Eat a healthy diet by increasing fruits, vegetables, and whole grains and reducing consumption of red meat and processed meats
- Limit exposure to sun and UV rays
- Limit alcohol consumption

All of the above contributors to illness or injury involve *choices*, and the choice each individual makes is based on a combination of beliefs, values, and attitudes that influence behavior. From a holistic perspective, persons who choose unhealthful practices are also choosing to increase their risk of sickness or injury in the future.

The Therapeutic Environment

As a health care professional, you need to provide a therapeutic environment that will facilitate the healing process. You have already learned that a therapeutic climate includes physical comfort and correct technique in performing procedures, but is something else required for a truly therapeutic climate?

Perhaps you have noticed that the patients of some physicians and some therapists seem to recover more readily than the patients of other physicians and therapists. Perhaps the same surgery was performed, the same drugs prescribed, the same therapeutic techniques used. What makes the difference in results? Does the difference lie within the patient, or can it be attributed to some characteristics of the health care professionals?

FIGURE 20-1 When the therapeutic environment instills a sense of trust and being cared for, the patient is more likely to develop a positive attitude toward treatment.

All medical treatments occur in a **psychosocial** context. Many factors can influence the patient's treatment experience and likelihood of recovery. Some of the factors that contribute to the psychosocial context around the patient and the therapy include the following:

- Personal beliefs and expectations of the patient
- Interaction with other patients
- Memories about previous therapies
- Words of doctors and medical personnel
- Sight of health professionals, hospitals, and medical instruments
- Color, shape, smell, and taste of medications
- Being touched by needles and other devices

When the therapeutic environment helps to instill a sense of trust and being cared for, the patient is more likely to develop a positive expectation regarding treatment. On the other hand, when a patient has a negative experience with health professionals, whether in the past or the present, the patient's expectation can be negative. When a patient experiences stress, side effects, or increased pain as a result of negative expectations or perceptions, this is known as the **nocebo effect**.

Intention

Current thinking, then, emphasizes both the role of the patient and the role of positive, supportive relationships in determining the outcome of illness. This presents a *new dimension* to the role of health care professional. Patient care that consists of carrying out the physician's orders or performing assigned procedures is a limited role. The challenge to health care professionals is to perform patient care with the *conscious **intention*** of helping the patient to heal. This does not require additional time or effort. It does require concentration—*giving full attention to the patient* and *focusing on caring, positive thoughts throughout a procedure* for the purpose of providing a healing climate.

Would this make a difference? There is evidence that *intention does make a difference.* Each health care professional must make a personal decision about whether or not to strive for creating a truly healing climate in each contact with a patient. Be aware also that healing occurs only if the patient has the *intention* to get well. Intention, in turn, is affected by such factors as belief systems, faith, and will to live. A newly recognized challenge for health care professionals is acceptance—*nonjudgmental acceptance*—of a patient who does not intend to get well.

Who Survives?

"When you are hit by adversity or have your life disrupted, how do you respond? Some people feel victimized. . . . Some shut down. They feel helpless and overwhelmed. . . . A few, however, reach within themselves and find ways to cope with the adversity" (Siebert, 2010, p. 1). With these words, Dr. Al Siebert, a psychologist, introduces his book *The Survivor Personality.* Dr. Siebert believes that survivors differ from other people only in their ability to "*reach within* themselves and *find ways to cope.*" For many years, he has studied people who survived various types of life crises, including the diagnosis of an incurable disease. Dr. Siebert discusses the reluctance of the medical profession to acknowledge that some patients survive despite medical predictions of imminent death. As noted earlier, when such patients improve and no longer exhibit symptoms of their "fatal" illness, most doctors label the improvement as "spontaneous remission" and make no effort to determine the factors that may have contributed to the patient's improvement.

Dr. Siebert's research led to the identification of several common factors in the stories of people who survived medical diagnosis of a terminal illness; such patients:

- Develop their own strategy for survival after finding that they cannot get guidelines for survival from their physicians
- Recognize that they must search and experiment to find the survival strategy that is unique to their own situation
- Perceive their health crisis as a wake-up call—something in their lifestyle is contributing to the illness, and survival requires change
- Accept that survival may require modifying their belief system
- Decide to make changes in ways of living, relationships, thought patterns, beliefs, and/or expression of feelings in order to improve the quality of life

A factor that Dr. Siebert believes differentiates survivors is a psychological concept known as locus of control. People with an **external locus of control** believe that their lives are

FIGURE 20-2 People with an internal locus of control are more likely to seek ways of dealing with adversity.

controlled by factors external to themselves: illness is caused by some outside force (germs, an accident, punishment for one's sins), and any cure will also be an external force (e.g., the physician, a drug, a special treatment). This type of person looks to the doctor to make her well or, if that is not possible, to manage her illness. She does not want advice about what she can do for herself.

People with an **internal locus of control** feel responsible for what happens to them; consequently, they are likely to seek ways of dealing with any adversity, including a serious illness. This type of person seeks information and wants to know what worked for others. People characterized by a strong internal locus of control want to participate in treatment decisions and may seek complementary types of therapies, learn to meditate, and make extensive changes in lifestyle. Also, they are likely to view the adverse situation as a learning experience or "wake-up call." Some survivors refer to a past adversity as "the best thing that ever happened to me," meaning that the experience led them to examine their life situation and make significant changes in their lives.

For Discussion and Reflection

Have you, or has someone you know well, survived a serious illness or injury? If so, consider what factors supported recovery.

The Holistic Approach to Health Care

You have learned about many of the factors that influence a person's health, including individual choices. The belief that illness is the result of outside influences (e.g., germs, accidents that "just happen") affects the choices people make. Thinking, "Other people get sick or have accidents, but I don't," may result in carelessness. How people feel about themselves influences their choices and self-care. Behaviors that indicate lack of self-care and unhealthy choices include:

- Being a workaholic
- Not allowing oneself time to play (not using leisure time for recreating oneself)
- Eating "on the run" or eating mostly convenience meals
- Ignoring bodily sensations that may be early warning signs of illness
- Ignoring the effects of stress on the body, mind, and emotions
- Ignoring safety precautions in the workplace
- Driving fast or recklessly
- Not wearing a seat belt

Life choices are increasingly recognized as contributing causes of illness or accident. Modern living exposes us to many stressors not known by earlier societies. Each day we encounter air pollution, food additives, building materials and home furnishings that give off toxic fumes—the list is almost endless. But the greatest stressors for many people are time pressures and interpersonal relationships.

For Discussion and Reflection

List the responsibilities you currently have—for example, parenting, taking classes, and working part time. How do you balance these responsibilities with self-care?

Job responsibilities plus home responsibilities plus commuting time plus errand-running leave little leisure time for many people. Time pressures interfere with the development of satisfying and mutually supportive relationships, even within a family setting. Relationship problems may continue for years because "there just isn't time to work on it." People are risking their health when they fail to make time to cope with stress and improve relationships.

Characteristics of Holistic Health Care

The holistic philosophy recognizes that each individual is unique. Health, sickness, and healing are related to a balance or imbalance among body, mind, emotions, and spirit. The holistic philosophy also emphasizes that disease is the result of multiple factors, not just one. When a patient's treatment is based on a single cause and other contributing factors are ignored, the patient is likely to experience a sequence of illnesses.

Diagnosis and Therapy from a Holistic Perspective

Preventive medicine recognizes *unmanaged stress as a major contributor to illness*. It also recognizes that *healing* in modern society requires the learning of stress management techniques. Chapter 21 discusses stress management in greater detail. From the holistic perspective, several approaches emerge as essential to healing:

1. Concern for the patient's total being: emotional, mental, and spiritual, as well as physical aspects
2. Having the patient participate in a planned program of health care, including lifestyle changes

3. Teaching the patient stress management techniques

4. Helping the patient face and resolve emotional issues

5. Helping the patient assume responsibility for their illness, health, and well-being

It may take weeks or months to make all the changes needed, to deal with emotional issues that may underlie the illness, or to experience the full benefits of therapy. Many patients are not willing to take responsibility for their own health, and therein lies the problem: Even those who are willing to take some responsibility may find it hard to change their lifestyle, deal with painful issues, or even to persist in a long-term plan until the benefits become apparent.

There is also a problem from the standpoint of health care delivery. The holistic approach is time consuming. It requires going beyond the physical examination and related diagnostic studies to study the "whole patient" and the life context within which that patient lives and works. It involves *teaching people*, rather than providing a quick cure. It requires patience and persistence to help people identify underlying causes of illness and make significant lifestyle changes.

Regardless of the delivery system, it is desirable that health care encompass the holistic concepts that (1) each patient is an individual who lives and works within specific settings that impact that person's health and (2) therapy must address all dimensions of that individual's being: emotional, mental, and spiritual as well as physical. In addition, the information provided in this unit makes it apparent that stress management must become an integral

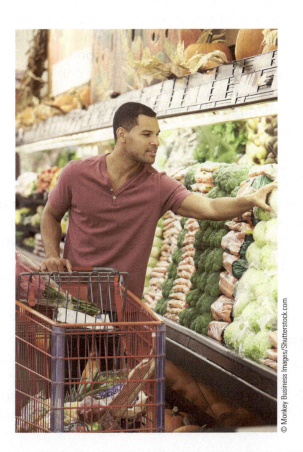

FIGURE 20-3 The holistic approach to health care emphasizes making healthy life choices.

part of health care for prevention and health maintenance, as therapy for chronic conditions, and as a significant part of the treatment protocol for persons recovering from serious illness or injuries. Because of growing recognition of the importance of stress management within the medical community, Chapter 21 is designed to help you, as a future health care professional, learn several techniques for managing stress. *Only as a practitioner of stress management will you be prepared to help others learn about the importance of managing their own stress.*

There will always be patients who prefer orthodox medical care to holistic care, and there will be health care professionals who find greater job satisfaction in one system than in the other. As a health care professional, you may eventually have the opportunity to pursue your career in either type of health care setting. Your own beliefs about health and healing should be considered when you are faced with such a choice.

Increasing numbers of people are using alternative and complementary therapies to assist in stress reduction or to alleviate a specific health problem. An *alternative therapy* refers to treatment used instead of orthodox treatment. For example, a patient may choose to use herbal medicine or a homeopathic remedy rather than taking a prescribed pharmaceutical drug. A *complementary therapy* is treatment used in conjunction with orthodox treatment. For example, a patient might take prescribed medication to treat hypertension while also practicing meditation to reduce stress. Integrative medicine is a patient-centered, holistic approach in which orthodox and alternative treatments are used together in an effort to treat the whole patient.

In the past, alternative and complementary therapies were viewed with great skepticism by most allopathic physicians, although both alternative and complementary therapies have long been used effectively by many cultures outside the United States. In recent years, with the rise of integrative medicine, both the medical community and American society as a whole have become more open to the idea of using complementary therapies alongside orthodox treatments. As a health care professional, you should keep an open mind when learning about alternative therapies, but you should also carefully evaluate the evidence for the therapy's effectiveness.

What Is Legitimate Therapy?

A legitimate health care professional does not make false promises. A legitimate health care professional employs appropriate therapies and encourages each patient, even in the presence of serious illness, to maintain hope and a positive attitude. On the other hand, one should be suspicious if practitioners:

1. *Promise* a "cure"
2. Claim to have a *secret method* not available to other practitioners
3. Demand a large payment "up front"
4. Become defensive or evasive about their qualifications

Recognizing unrealistic claims of curative power is the first line of defense in protecting oneself from a fake healer. The second line of defense is determining the qualifications of the practitioner.

Education and Credentials

Many roles in health care services require formal education. Qualified *professional* practitioners display in their offices at least two college or university degrees and a license from the state or a certificate from a recognized professional organization. Qualified practitioners of a complementary therapy also have documentation. Educational programs that prepare a specific type of practitioner issue a certificate or diploma to those who successfully complete the program of study. In some states, certain complementary practitioners must be licensed by the state.

If such documentation is not displayed, ask to see written evidence of a practitioner's qualifications. A potential client has the right to know the qualifications of a practitioner, especially when a fee is involved. If questions regarding licensure, certification, or educational preparation make the practitioner defensive, evasive, or even uncomfortable, seek help elsewhere.

Implications for Health Care Professionals

As a health care professional, you may be asked for a recommendation or opinion about an alternative therapy or a particular practitioner. Exercise caution in responding to such a request. Your best and safest approach is to help that person obtain the information needed for (1) evaluating the proposed therapy or practitioner, and then (2) making their own decision. Do not make such a decision for someone else. Instead, point out the educational, licensure, or certification requirements for the therapy being considered. You should also know what constitutes a legitimate title. Anyone may call themselves "counselor," "therapist," or "healer." But the terms *licensed* and *certified* can be used legally only if the practitioner has been granted that title by the state, an educational program, or a professional association.

Each person who considers the services of a nonmedical therapist has a responsibility to evaluate the qualifications of the practitioner, then make a *conscious decision* based on information about that specific therapy and that particular practitioner. After a reasonable trial period, another *conscious decision*—to continue or not continue—should be based on whether or not the therapy is beneficial. The need for careful evaluation of a therapy and professional is less critical if the therapy is offered through a holistic health center headed by a physician or other health-related *professional* practitioner. The employing agency has a responsibility to check credentials and determine if the practitioner is competent.

As a health care professional, your role is to provide information, not opinions, if a patient asks about an alternative or complementary therapy. Opinions are subjective based on your own ideas and experiences. However, by providing facts and information, you can empower patients to make their own informed decisions about a particular course of treatment.

For Discussion and Reflection

If you were considering a complementary therapy, what information would you get before receiving treatment?

The Self-Help Trend

Public interest in holistic health evolved out of the self-help movement that focused on freeing oneself from psychological and mental blocks. That movement resulted in a flood of "pop psychology" self-help books on such topics as assertiveness, self-esteem, communication, interpersonal relationships, and sexuality. The result was a marked change in attitudes toward responsibility for increasing one's effectiveness in coping with life situations and improving relationships. Various health organizations began to emphasize exercise and a healthful diet, further encouraging individual responsibility for health and well-being.

The current interest in complementary therapies seems to be a natural outgrowth of these earlier movements. Most people recognize that modern life involves high levels of stress. One can seek escape from stress and life problems through medication or alcohol. Or one can utilize stress reduction techniques and modify lifestyle to eliminate some sources of stress. If a chronic health problem exists for which allopathic medicine offers only symptomatic relief, one can choose that approach or seek an appropriate complementary therapy.

The person who is seeking techniques for self-help probably has already assumed some degree of responsibility for health management. That does not mean that the individual fully understands all that is involved in achieving optimal health. If you have the opportunity to help such a person, encourage the individual to learn about wellness rather than to seek help for a single problem. That means considering lifestyle, stressors in the life situation, stress management techniques, nutrition, exercise, and any mental/emotional factors that may be affecting physical health. By now you surely recognize that this is the holistic approach. High-level wellness (and, in the case of chronic diseases, recovery) cannot be achieved without a holistic approach. The goal for every patient should be true healing, so that optimal health, whatever that might be *for that individual,* can be achieved.

Some self-help techniques can be learned from books and articles. Others, such as identifying emotional factors that need to be resolved, may be accomplished more readily with professional help. The person who begins a self-help program alone may experience improvement, then become aware of the need for help. Whatever the approach, most of the following will contribute to improvement in one's overall health:

- Awareness of choices that affect health
- A *conscious* choice to modify lifestyle
- Daily use of a stress management technique
- Self-study, workshops, and/or counseling to release feelings related to old traumas, unmet needs, and/or unresolved conflicts
- One or more techniques for directing the flow of body energies and releasing blockages

For Discussion and Reflection

1. In your opinion, what are the advantages and disadvantages of the self-help trend described above?
2. With health information readily available online, do you think many patients have researched symptoms and treatments before they visit a health care professional? What are the advantages and disadvantages of using the Internet to research health information?

Integrative Medicine

Currently, there is an increasing move toward integrative medicine, in which conventional treatment and therapies which were once considered complementary or alternative are used together. For example, a cancer patient might undergo chemotherapy, a conventional treatment, but also participate in a support group and use visualization or meditation to relieve pain and aid healing.

The following are examples of therapies that may be included in an integrative approach:

- Botanical medicine
- Integrative approach to nutrition
- Chiropractic and osteopathic care
- Acupuncture and East Asian medicine
- Ayurvedic medicine
- Movement and body-centered therapies
- Homeopathy
- Physical activity and exercise
- Spirituality and health

By selecting the treatments most suited to a patient's needs, integrative medicine offers a more holistic, patient-centered model of medical care than orthodox medicine alone has traditionally offered.

© AYA images/Shutterstock.com

FIGURE 20-4 Integrative medicine combines conventional and complementary medical practices.

Role of the Health Care Professional

Increasingly, medical doctors are open to holistic health care and some complementary therapies. Numerous medical doctors have written books about their expanded approach to therapy, some providing anecdotal reports of their patients' healing experiences. Some patients are writing about how they took responsibility for their own healing and recovered from a supposedly irreversible disease.

As a health care professional, you have a responsibility to encourage patients to believe in their doctors and in their prescribed therapies. Inevitably, however, you will encounter a patient, relative, or friend who asks your advice about a complementary therapy. It would be appropriate for you to help such a person obtain information, but that person should make the decision to use or not use a specific therapy. Use your best judgment in each situation without exerting influence in either direction. An open mind combined with healthy skepticism is a good combination. Do not deny someone the potential benefit of a complementary therapy simply because you are unfamiliar with it or because it is not offered in your particular health care agency at this time.

Activities

1. Participate in a class discussion of one or more of the following statements:
   - Love, including self-love, is essential to health and well-being.
   - Harmony among body, mind, emotions, and spirit is essential to health and well-being.
   - Life choices can increase the probability of illness.
   - Life choices can increase the probability of an accident.
   - Life choices can promote health and well-being.

2. Drawing on your personal experience (relatives, friends, acquaintances) and your clinical experience, list examples of people who:
   a. Recovered from a life-threatening illness, contrary to the expectation of their physicians.
   b. Recovered from a serious illness through medical intervention, such as surgery, only to develop symptoms of another serious illness within a year.

   Refer to one of the examples you listed above and consider what factors may have contributed to recovery. What traits characterize that person?

3. Use the Internet to research the mirror box, which is used to reduce phantom pain following an amputation. Describe how the use of the mirror box illustrates the mind–body connection.

4. Explain what to look for when researching a therapy you are unfamiliar with to decide whether it is legitimate.

5. Participate in a class discussion about how a health care professional should respond to a request for advice about using a specific complementary therapy for a chronic problem.

References and Suggested Readings

Centers for Disease Control and Prevention (CDC). (2019, November 8). Potentially excess deaths from the five leading causes of death in metropolitan and nonmetropolitan counties: United States, 2010–2017. *Surveillance Summaries, 68*(10), 1–11.

Kreitzer, M., & Koithan, M. (2018). *Integrative nursing* (2nd ed.). Oxford University Press.

Siebert, Al. (2010). *The survivor personality.* Perigee.

Managing Stress

Objectives

After completing this chapter, you should be able to:

- Identify causes of stress and describe the physiological changes that occur as a result of stress.
- Discuss strategies for managing stress.
- Describe the physiological changes that occur as a result of relaxation, exercise, and mindfulness.

Key Terms

Mental chatter   Relaxation response
Mindfulness   Stress management

Perhaps you are wondering how the topic of stress management relates to the information discussed in previous chapters. The truth is, stress impacts your well-being and that of your patients significantly. It has been estimated that 75 percent or more of doctor visits to general practitioners are for stress-related conditions. A few examples include heart disease, high blood pressure, irritable bowel syndrome, tension headaches, obesity, sleep dysfunction, and neck and shoulder pain. While stress is not always the direct cause or the only cause of these conditions, chronic stress has been shown to increase the likelihood of developing health problems.

Not only does chronic stress contribute to illness, dealing with illness can create additional stress for patients and their families as they deal with disruptions in their routines, physical discomfort, the financial burden of treatment, and making decisions about medical care. Learning to deal effectively with your own stress is one of the best investments you can make in your own personal care, as well as in your preparation to be an effective health care professional. You have a responsibility to yourself and your family to maintain the best possible state of health. That includes learning about stress management and including stress management in your daily routine.

It is not within the role of nonphysician health care professionals to prescribe **stress management** for a patient, because diagnosis and prescription of a therapeutic plan are the domain of medicine. In some circumstances, however, it is appropriate for any health care professional to talk with a patient about the importance of stress management. Your participation in helping a patient learn about stress management is more likely if you are working with a holistically oriented medical practitioner.

Understanding Stress

As you have learned, stress is a physiological and emotional response to thoughts or events that an individual perceives as threatening or overwhelming. For most people, just thinking about a threatening event, whether real or imagined, produces a reaction much like they would experience if the threatening event actually occurred. When the brain perceives a threat, it activates the sympathetic nervous system, triggering the "fight or flight" response to prepare the individual to respond to danger—even if the danger is only imagined. The following physiological changes occur:

- Heart rate and respiratory rate increase.
- Muscles tighten.
- Adrenaline and cortisol are released.
- The mind may begin to "race" with fearful or distressing thoughts.

When these changes occur, it is much more difficult for an individual to think clearly, make a rational decision, and process information.

In an actual emergency, these physiological changes enable us to run faster, fight harder, or react more quickly to danger. However, when this heightened state becomes a frequent part of our lives, over time we are likely to experience one or more of the following adverse effects:

- Chronic headaches or stomachaches
- Digestive problems, including heartburn, diarrhea, or constipation
- Difficulty sleeping
- Cardiovascular problems
- Weight gain, due to high levels of the stress hormone cortisol
- Reduced immune system functioning

Sexual and reproductive functioning are also impacted by high levels of stress over time:

- In men, chronic stress affects testosterone levels and sperm production, and it may contribute to erectile dysfunction and impotence (APA 2018).

- In women, chronic stress may contribute to irregular menstrual cycles, increased symptoms of premenstrual syndrome (PMS), and lowered sexual desire (APA 2018).

A distinction can be made between stress and anxiety, though the two are closely related emotional responses. Stress is the result of an external threat or perceived threat. *Perceived threat* refers to an individual's thoughts and feelings of being threatened, whether or not an actual threat exists. For example, for some people, giving a speech in front of a group is "no big deal," while for others, giving a speech feels extremely threatening and creates stress.

Anxiety, on the other hand, is an emotional response to thoughts and feelings that are not caused by an immediate external event. For example, remembering past situations that were upsetting or imagining what might happen are examples of thoughts that produce anxiety. For many people, "wondering and worrying" create feelings of anxiety. Both anxiety and stress can be managed using similar strategies; the difference is that to successfully manage anxiety, individuals need to work on their thoughts and mindset in addition to practicing strategies to reduce the physiological effects of stress.

Everyone feels stress and anxiety at times. Having a daily stress management practice and managing our thoughts and self-talk can prevent stress from becoming overwhelming. However, anyone who finds that stress and anxiety have increased to the point of interfering with enjoyment of life and the ability to perform daily activities is encouraged to seek the help of a counselor or other mental health professional.

> **For Discussion and Reflection**
>
> Would you rate your current level of stress as low, medium, or high? If you selected medium or high, what are the main causes of stress in your life right now? How many of these are in your control?

Managing Stress

Our goal is not to avoid stress entirely. A certain amount of stress is inevitable in life, and in small doses, stress is beneficial, providing a burst of energy that can help us handle a specific situation more effectively. In moderate doses, short-term stress can stimulate memory and brain function. However, when stress becomes chronic, or ongoing over a period of time, we increase the risk of facing the adverse effects described earlier.

Various external factors can cause chronic stress. Examples include the following:

- Jobs that involve dangerous or challenging situations on a regular basis

- Relationships that involve frequent disrespect, conflict, or abuse

- Systemic discrimination based on race, nationality, religion, gender identity, sexual preference, or other factors

- Local or national events such as pandemics, natural disasters, military conflict, or economic problems

Internal factors such as emotional and behavioral patterns contribute to anxiety. Some examples include the following:

- Recalling painful events from the past over and over
- Worrying about the future or about "what might happen"
- Expecting events to go a certain way, and becoming frustrated when they do not
- "Finding fault" with others because they do not behave as we would like
- Repeatedly blaming, criticizing, or negatively labeling ourselves

The first step to managing stress and anxiety is to reflect and identify the external and internal situations which cause our stress. For most people, there may be several causes. Once the causes of stress have been identified, consider whether the *situation* needs to be changed, whether *your reaction to the situation* needs to change, or perhaps both. For example, if your job has become increasingly challenging, you may decide to look for other employment. On the other hand, you may decide that by changing your attitude and taking more time for self-care, you can handle the challenges of your job without as much stress.

Stress management refers to various techniques you can use to counter the physiological effects of stress. These techniques help promote the **relaxation response** of the parasympathetic nervous system, which is the opposite of the stress response. When you relax, your heart rate and breathing slow down, your blood vessels dilate, and you can think more clearly.

There are many ways of coping with stress. Some people have a daily exercise program that significantly reduces their stress level. Others participate in a sport at least once a week. Sports may or may not reduce stress, depending upon one's level of competitiveness. If winning is important, then losing a game may increase stress, rather than reduce it.

Certain activities that people think of as "relaxing" do *not* have stress management value. For example, watching a show, partying, going to the beach, a weekend skiing trip, and other such recreational activities are diversions—escapes from the daily pressures of the job and home responsibilities. Though pleasant and possibly self-renewing, recreational activities do not bring about the physical and psychological changes that are essential to managing stress effectively.

Three approaches that have proven useful for managing stress are relaxation, exercise, and mindfulness. For each of these approaches, a variety of practices and techniques can be used.

Reducing Physiological Effects of Stress

Relaxation

Relaxation techniques are designed to consciously evoke the body's relaxation response, which includes slower breathing, a slower heart rate, relaxed muscles, and a sense of peace, calm, and well-being. The National Center for Complementary and Integrative Health (2020) describes the following evidence-based relaxation techniques:

- *Biofeedback-assisted relaxation* uses electronic devices to measure heart rate, muscle tension, or other body functions and provide feedback so you can learn to control these functions.
- *Progressive relaxation* involves tightening and then relaxing one muscle group at a time throughout the body.

Many professional counselors teach relaxation techniques, and many books and websites also provide instructions for relaxation. Although relaxation techniques should not be used as a substitute for medical care when you have a medical condition, the techniques are considered safe for almost everyone and can often complement other types of treatment.

Exercise

When you exercise, your body releases *endorphins,* chemicals which block pain and promote a sense of well-being. Endorphins are responsible for the well-known "runner's high." Unless you are a serious athlete, however, low- to moderate-intensity exercise, rather than high-intensity exercise, is recommended for stress management.

Non-competitive activities such as walking, swimming, yoga, and tai chi are generally more effective for stress reduction than competitive activities in which players are focused on winning. Notice that exercising for stress management is different than "working out" to increase your fitness level. A 10-minute walk in the park may not help you reach your target heart rate for cardio training, yet it can release tension and provide a sense of calm and well-being.

> **For Discussion and Reflection**
>
> Do you exercise regularly? What type of exercise do you enjoy? Have you noticed a difference in your level of stress after exercising?

Mindfulness

Mindfulness refers to the practice of giving our full attention to what is happening at the present moment. Most people pay only partial attention to the present as they go throughout the day. Their attention is divided between what they are doing, such as driving, cooking dinner, or attending class, and listening to an ongoing stream of **mental chatter** that runs in the background of their thoughts.

© shurkin_son/Shutterstock.com

FIGURE 21-1 For stress reduction, noncompetitive activities such as walking, swimming, yoga, and tai chi are generally more effective than competitive activities.

Stored memories provide the content for mental chatter; it may be factual or psychological, useful or destructive. When mental chatter arouses negative feelings associated with a past experience, we relive a bad experience that cannot be changed. Thus, mental chatter may be the source of ongoing anxiety. Mental chatter can be so engrossing that a person is out of touch with what is happening at the moment. By taking conscious control, however, an individual can learn to avoid feelings associated with past experiences and anxiety related to some anticipated future event.

Mindfulness can be practiced both in everyday activities and through *meditation*. As you move through your day, practice focusing your full attention on what you are doing at the moment. If you are driving, notice the vehicles around you. Notice the color of the sky, the flowers growing beside the highway, and so on. If you are talking to someone, look directly at the person and focus on what they are saying. While there are times when we all need to "multitask," look for opportunities throughout your day to put away distractions, turn off the mental chatter, and give your full attention to the task at hand. When you give your attention to the present situation, you are more effective in your daily activities and less likely to be drawn into a cycle of worry by your mental chatter.

Meditation is a practice which combines breathing and mindfulness, allowing you to clear your mind of thoughts and focus your attention on your breath, a lit candle, a specific word or phrase, or some other calming focal point. Although many ancient spiritual traditions include meditation, you do not have to practice a specific religion, or any religion at all, to meditate. According to the National Center for Complementary and Integrative Health (2020), mindfulness-based meditation is considered safe and has been shown to be effective for many people. There are many ways to practice meditation, but they have four common elements:

- A quiet location free from distractions
- A comfortable body position such as sitting or lying down
- A focal point for the attention
- A nonjudgmental attitude, letting thoughts come and go without judging or holding on to them

Many people learn meditation from a counselor, therapist, or other practitioner, but others teach themselves using books, recordings, or online videos. When practiced over

© Zdenka Darula/Shutterstock.com

FIGURE 21-2 Meditation combines breathing and mindfulness, allowing you to clear your mind of thoughts and focus your attention on your breath or other calming focal point.

time, meditation has been shown to produce positive changes in the body and brain. Like relaxation, meditation should not be used as a substitute for medical care, but research has shown that it often complements medical treatments.

In addition to its physical benefits, meditation has profound psychological benefits when practiced over time. People who meditate regularly often report the following experiences:

- Changes in perception of self, others, and life events
- Reevaluation of values and beliefs
- A freeing of emotions, especially suppressed emotions
- Greater compassion
- Increased capacity for self-love and love for others
- Greater readiness to accept love
- Improved ability to cope with life situations
- Increased awareness of "self"

Using Positive Self-Talk

To combat the effects of mental chatter described above, many people use *affirmations*, or positive statements that provide an alternative to negative self-talk. An affirmation should be short, positive, and related to feelings or beliefs. It should be stated in the present tense: "I am . . ." rather than "I will be . . ." The affirmation can be repeated silently during relaxation or in a quiet moment at the beginning or completion of a meditation. The affirmation can also be written on a card that you carry with you, tape to your mirror, or place in any location where you will see it frequently. Repeat your affirmation mentally at intervals throughout the day to maintain a positive state of mind and reinforce the positive feeling or belief. Examples of affirmations include the following:

- I am happy, healthy, and joyful.
- I am strong, courageous, and confident.
- Today I let go of old habits and choose to create new ones.

You have now learned several methods for managing stress and anxiety. As students in a health care educational program, you experience the stress of assignments and tests. As you carry out clinical assignments, you experience the stress of the health care setting, which may be somewhat overwhelming to you at first. In addition, you experience the stress associated with your other life roles. Recognize that you are subject to many stressors and be good to yourself. Eat right, sleep right, take time to play, and use a stress management technique at least once each day!

Activities

1. Describe what causes stress and how stress affects the body.
2. For one week, list the stressors you experience in class, in the clinical area, at home, and in your various relationships. For each stressor you listed, note whether the stressor is within your control, partly within your control, or outside your control.

3. To become aware of your mental chatter, complete the following exercise:

A. Settle into a comfortable position, note the time, close your eyes.

- For three minutes, be aware of any thoughts that occur to you.
- Notice how one thought leads to another, in endless procession.
- Begin to label each thought as it occurs: a memory, an expectation about a future event, a judgment about an event or someone, or something you like or dislike.
- Become aware of any feelings that arise as certain thoughts occur: fears, anxieties, anger, guilt, pleasure.
- For the next two minutes, count the thoughts that occur. Open your eyes and note the position of the second hand and the minute hand. Now, give your full attention to your breathing, excluding all thoughts of any type. As soon as a thought occurs, note the positions of the second hand and minute hand. How long were you able to focus on your breathing without any thought occurring? You probably maintained the focus on your breathing for only a few seconds, certainly for less than a minute. This illustrates the power of mental chatter.

B. To learn how mindfulness can control mental chatter:

- Observe your breathing—the movement of air in and out of your nostrils, the movement of the chest wall, or the expansion and contraction of the abdomen during inspiration and expiration.
- When a thought occurs, be aware that your attention has shifted from focusing on the breath to focusing on mental chatter. Without trying to control it, just quietly observe your mental chatter. *Note that as you observe without getting involved*, your body becomes more relaxed.
- Gently return to focusing on the breath. Each time a thought occurs, repeat these two steps. The length of time you can maintain your focus on the breath will increase with practice. Now, you should also be more aware of how mental chatter automatically controls your attention, *unless you take conscious control.*

References and Suggested Readings

American Psychological Association (APA). (2018). Stress effects on the body. https://www.apa.org/topics/stress/body

American Psychological Association (APA). (2019). Healthy ways to handle life's stressors. https://www.apa.org/topics/stress/tips

Lupien, S., Juster, R., Raymond, C., & Marin, M. (2018). The effects of chronic stress on the human brain: From neurotoxicity, to vulnerability, to opportunity. *Frontiers in Neuroendocrinology, 49,* 91–105. https://doi.org/10.1016/j.yfrne.2018.02.001

Lupien, S., Leclaire, A., Majeur, D., Raymond, C., Jean Baptiste, F., & Giguère, C. (2022). "Doctor, I am so stressed out!" A descriptive study of biological, psychological, and socioemotional markers of stress in individuals who self-identify as being "very stressed out" or "zen." *Neurobiology of Stress, 18,* 100454. https://doi.org/10.1016/j.ynstr.2022.100454

National Center for Complementary and Integrative Health. (2020). Mind and body approaches for stress and anxiety: What the science says. https://www.nccih.nih.gov/health/providers/digest/mind-and-body-approaches-for-stress-science.

Glossary

abstinence: voluntary avoidance of a specific substance or behavior.

abuse: improper treatment; may be verbal or physical, resulting in injury to the victim; also, may be sexual, involving a child or unwilling adult.

ADD: acronym for *attention deficit disorder*.

addiction: physiological dependence on a substance; cessation results in withdrawal symptoms.

ADHD: acronym for *attention deficit hyperactivity disorder*.

adjustment: the degree to which one is dealing successfully with life situations.

adrenaline: the hormone produced by the adrenal glands during emotion-arousing situations; increases muscular strength and endurance; prepares the individual for "fight or flight."

advance medical directive (AMD): a legal document which specifies an individual's wishes in regards to end-of-life care.

alcoholism: physiological dependence on alcohol.

alcohol use disorder: a medical condition characterized by an impaired ability to stop or control alcohol use.

allopathic: pertaining to therapy that relies primarily on drugs; as currently used, refers to medical practice in which drug therapy and surgery are the most common forms of treatment.

alternative therapy: a nonallopathic therapy; term preferred by most practitioners is *complementary therapy*.

alternatives: two available choices.

altruism: concern about the well-being of others; may lead one to perform charitable acts.

ambiguity: vagueness or lack of clarity.

AMD: acronym for *advance medical directive*.

analgesic: substance that relieves pain without causing loss of consciousness; less potent than a narcotic.

anticipatory grief: grieving experienced during a terminal illness, or before the death of a loved one.

aptitudes: natural tendencies, talents, or capabilities. Those who have an aptitude for a specific area (e.g., mathematics) learn material related to that area more easily than someone who does not have that aptitude.

aspiration: goal, desire for achievement.

assisted suicide: ending one's own life with assistance from another person, who provides medication, information, or other means of ending life.

assumption: acceptance of something as fact without evidence or proof.

attention deficit disorder (ADD): a chronic condition characterized by inattention, or difficulty focusing on and completing tasks.

attention deficit hyperactivity disorder (ADHD): a chronic condition characterized by inattention and hyperactive or impulsive behavior.

attitude: disposition toward something specific; includes feelings, beliefs, and behavior.

autism spectrum disorder: one of several related developmental disorders, which include the disorders previously referred to as classic autism, Asperger's syndrome, and pervasive development disorder—not otherwise specified (PDD-NOS).

autonomy: the state of functioning independently, without outside control or direction.

ayurveda: a traditional system of natural medicine developed in India.

behavioral genetics: a field of study which investigates how behavioral traits and disorders are influenced by heredity and environment.

bereavement: separation from or loss of someone who is very significant in one's life.

bias: prejudice in favor of or against a person or group.

burnout: a state of physical and mental exhaustion due to cumulative stress.

chromosomes: rod-shaped bodies that carry the genes containing hereditary characteristics; each cell (except the germ cells) has 46 chromosomes in the nucleus.

clarification: explanation or qualification of something.

client-centered care: treating clients with respect while honoring their values and personal wishes.

codependency: relationship in which the dysfunctional behavior (usually alcoholism or drug addiction) of one person meets certain needs of the other (e.g., a wife receives satisfaction from "rescuing" her alcoholic husband).

compassion: concern for the suffering or misfortune of another.

compensation: (1) a defense mechanism in which a substitution of some type provides temporary relief from the discomfort of an unmet need, but does not actually satisfy the need; (2) some form of payment or reward.

complementary therapy: a nonallopathic therapy.

condolences: expressions of sympathy.

conformity: tendency to be like others, to observe the conventions of a group.

congenital: a condition present at the time of birth.

consequence: the result of an action or behavior.

conservator: one who has been legally designated to protect the interests of a person who is unable to manage his or her affairs.

coping skills: the skills needed for dealing effectively with various life experiences.

covert: hidden, not observable; opposite of *overt*.

cultural competence: knowledge and skills which enable one to work effectively with individuals from various cultural backgrounds.

cultural awareness: recognizing that individuals have different beliefs, values, and customs based on their background.

cynicism: distrustful of human nature or motives.

debilitating: weakening; impairing one's strength.

dehydration: condition in which the body lacks adequate water to maintain body functions; if severe, can lead to a life-threatening imbalance of body chemistry.

dependency: reliance on someone or something for support.

desertion reaction: a form of withdrawal that may occur when a very young child or an elderly person is left in the care of someone other than a family member.

developmental disorders: physical or mental disorders which affect a child's development, often causing the individual to learn or to meet developmental milestones at a slower than typical rate.

digital: using the fingers or toes.

discrimination: different treatment of a person because of some specific characteristic, such as age, gender, race, religion, national origin, or economic status.

disguised behavior: behavior used by a person to cover up true feelings.

displacement: a defense mechanism in which strong feelings (usually anger) about one person are transferred or directed to someone else who did not initially arouse the feelings.

DNA: acronym for *deoxyribonucleic acid*, the substance that contains the hereditary makeup of each cell.

DNR: acronym for *do not resuscitate*.

do not resuscitate (DNR) order: a legal document that states that an individual should not be resuscitated in the event of cardiac or respiratory arrest.

dolorology: a medical specialty concerned with pain management.

DPA: acronym for *durable power of attorney*.

durable power of attorney (DPA): a legal document designating an agent to act on one's behalf in the event one becomes incapacitated.

dysfunctional: faulty or disturbed function.

dyslexia: a developmental disorder that affects reading.

egocentric: concerned primarily with self.

empathy: ability to identify with another person's situation and understand the feelings and reactions of that person.

empirical: based on observation and experience, rather than on experimental data.

empowerment: becoming stronger and more confident.

enabler: one who facilitates another's addictive behavior by helping the addict gain access to the addictive substance.

enunciation: the uttering of sounds; may be clear or unclear to the listener.

equity: offering support to remove barriers such as transportation, language, or finances so that all individuals have an opportunity to receive services.

ethics: standards of conduct, a code of behavior for a specific group; medical ethics are the standards of conduct to be observed by health care providers.

euthanasia: administration of a lethal substance to a person who is dying and in great pain; also called *mercy killing*.

expectation: something one thinks will occur.

external locus of control: the belief that various factors outside oneself control the events of one's life.

family dynamics: the interactions between and among members of a family.

fetal alcohol syndrome (FAS): a pattern of growth, mental, and physical problems that a child develops as a result of the mother's consumption of alcohol during pregnancy.

fixed mindset: the belief that one's abilities, such as intelligence or talent, are fixed and unchangeable.

frustration: any blocking of progress toward a desired goal.

gene: unit that carries a hereditary trait.

genetic: carried by the genes; pertaining to heredity.

genotype: the specific hereditary makeup of a person.

grief work: the process of working through the emotional reaction to loss; generally considered to last at least one year.

growth mindset: the belief that one's abilities can be improved and developed through practice and hard work.

habituation: psychological dependence, need, strong desire.

hallucinogenic: causing a person to hallucinate, to perceive sights and sounds that are not actually present.

hassle: an annoyance.

herbalism: the use of herbs for a variety of purposes, including medicinal uses.

hereditary: traits inherited from the parents.

heredity: the transmission of characteristics from parents to offspring.

hierarchy: arrangement in a specific order or rank from lowest to highest; vertical relationships.

holism: the belief system that encompasses holistic ideas.

holistic health care: perceiving the whole and all of its parts; the philosophy that healing occurs most readily when all aspects of the patient are considered.

hospice: a facility for the care of terminally ill patients, based on a death-with-dignity philosophy.

hostility: anger, either specific or general; may be the basis for aggressive tendencies.

Human Genome Project: a scientific research project between 1990 and 2003 that identified all the genes in human DNA.

hypnosis: trancelike condition usually induced by another person, in which the subject is receptive to suggestions.

incapacitated: incapable of functioning.

incest: sexual intercourse between persons whose blood relationship makes it illegal for them to marry; usually involves parent/child, brother/sister, or uncle/niece; may be an aspect of child abuse.

incompatible: unable to exist together harmoniously.

inconsistency: differing from one occurrence to another.

integrative medicine: a health care approach that emphasizes wellness and treating the whole person using a combination of allopathic, complementary, and alternative therapies.

intention: a specific purpose (a conscious thought) for a particular action.

internal locus of control: the belief that one can utilize inner resources to influence events.

I-statement: a communication technique used to express feelings or needs by stating them in the first person.

lethargy: abnormal drowsiness, sluggishness.

living will: a document stating a person's wishes for medical care in the event that the person is incapacitated and unable to express those wishes directly.

manipulative: using various strategies to influence others in order to obtain something.

martyr complex: psychological condition in which a person derives satisfaction from being taken advantage of by another person.

mental chatter: the stream of thoughts and memories that runs through the mind when it is not focused on a mental task or on an experience that requires attention; may interfere with going to sleep; if uncontrolled, can be a source of stress.

mindfulness: a practice which involves being aware, attentive, and intentional in the present moment.

mindset: mental readiness to react in a specific way.

mortality: subject to dying.

narcotic: addictive type of drug used medically to relieve pain.

necrosis: death of tissues in a limited area.

neglect: failure to pay appropriate attention or, in the case of a child, provide essential needs.

neurotransmitter: chemical substances that transmit impulses in the brain and nerves.

nocebo effect: an inert substance or treatment which causes an adverse effect on the recipient; opposite of *placebo effect*.

noradrenaline: hormone produced by the adrenal medulla during emotion-arousing situations.

overt: obvious, observable; opposite of *covert*.

palliative care: relieving or controlling symptoms without healing the underlying disease process.

paraphrase: restate; express a meaning in different words.

paraverbal: the tone, volume, and rate of speech, all of which can alter the meaning of a statement even when the same words are used.

passive aggression: indirect resistance, sometimes while giving the appearance of cooperation; may be due to covert hostility.

Patient Self-Determination Act (PSDA): a law passed by Congress in 1990 requiring health care facilities to inform patients about advance health care directives upon admission to the facility.

pedophilia: sexual activity between a child under the age of 13 and someone 5 to 10 years older than the child; a type of child abuse.

perception: use of the senses to become aware of something.

perfectionism: excessive concern about order and what is right; holding *perfect* as the standard of what is acceptable.

perpetrator: one who commits, or has committed, some type of offense or crime.

phenotype: an organism's physical type; a set of characteristics that establish physical appearance.

physiological: dealing with the functions and vital processes of living organisms; the physical aspect of being, rather than the mental, emotional, or spiritual aspects.

placebo: an inactive substance administered instead of a specific therapy.

placebo effect (placebo response): the beneficial effect of a placebo, usually reflecting the expectations of the patient, health care provider, or both.

procrastinate: to put off doing something until a later time.

proficient: skillful.

prognosis: predicted course or outcome of a disease or injury.

projection: a defense mechanism which involves blaming one's own shortcomings on someone else or on circumstances.

prosthesis: an artificial replacement for a missing body part.

proxy: one who has been designated to act on behalf of another person.

PSDA: acronym for *Patient Self-Determination Act*.

psychoanalysis: method of treating mental/emotional disorders by discovering and analyzing repressed memories, emotional conflicts, and past traumas.

psychopharmaceutical: a class of drug that has specific effects on the mind, emotions, or mood, usually by altering brain chemistry.

psychosocial: related to both psychological and social factors.

psychotherapy: the treatment of mental and emotional illness through one or more psychological techniques.

rapport: a relationship in which there is mutual acceptance, understanding, and respect.

rationalization: a defense mechanism which involves offering a socially acceptable explanation for behavior when the true reason would be too painful to admit.

regression: exhibiting behaviors that are appropriate to an earlier stage of development.

relaxation response: in stress management, a physical response which includes lowered blood pressure and stress hormones, relaxed muscles, and a feeling of well-being.

repressed: unconscious.

REM sleep: the phase of sleep during which dreaming occurs.

repression: a defense mechanism which involves forcing an unpleasant memory into the subconscious mind.

resentment: chronic anger that is not consciously expressed, but may be an unconscious influence on behavior.

resilience: the ability to bounce back after a bad experience.

role: the duties and behaviors expected of a person in a specific situation.

scientific method: a systematic procedure for conducting measurements, observations, and experiments and forming and testing hypotheses.

selective observing: a tendency to notice certain details of a situation while ignoring or overlooking other details.

self-awareness: recognizing one's own characteristics, feelings, and beliefs.

self-concept: self-image, beliefs about oneself.

self-confidence: believing in oneself as a competent person.

self-deception: seeing oneself incorrectly; lack of self-awareness.

self-reliant: able to depend upon oneself; confident in one's own judgment, decisions, abilities, and coping skills.

separation anxiety: extreme anxiety that a child may develop when a caregiver is absent or about to leave.

sexually transmitted disease (STD): an infectious disease which is transferred from one individual to another through sexual contact.

socioeconomic: relating to a combination of social and economic factors.

stance: a mode of standing or positioning of the body and feet.

standard of performance: a level of quality against which one's work can be measured.

stress: a physiological response (internal and adaptive) to extreme or chronic emotional states.

stress management: techniques which counteract the effects of stress by encouraging relaxation, lowered heart rate and blood pressure, lowered stress hormones, and a sense of well-being.

stressors: outside influences that arouse some type of emotional response.

suffocation: death from lack of oxygen due to the face (nose and mouth) being covered.

suppression: not expressing, holding in or down.

survivor guilt: the tendency of a survivor of a trauma or accident to feel guilty for being alive, especially when someone else did not survive the same experience.

sympathy: concern for another person, especially one who is experiencing illness, trauma, or crisis.

synergism: increased effectiveness or potency of a substance when combined with another substance.

thanatology: the study of death and dying.

transference: unconsciously directing one's feelings about one person toward another person.

trauma-informed care: an approach that recognizes and responds to the effects of trauma on individuals.

variables: factors that has an influence or ability to bring about change.

verbalize: express in words; often used to indicate oral expression, rather than written.

vicious cycle: recurring behaviors or events that maintain an unsatisfactory situation; will continue unless a change is made to interrupt the cycle.

withdrawal (drug-related): withholding a substance to which someone is addicted; the group of symptoms that occur as the body reacts to absence of the addictive substance.

Index